Nursing Research

Critical Appraisal and Utilization

Nursing Research

Critical Appraisal and Utilization

Geri LoBiondo-Wood, Ph.D., R.N.

Associate Professor and
Interim Assistant Dean,
University of Nebraska
College of Nursing,
Omaha, Nebraska

Judith Haber, Ph.D., R.N.

Associate Professor and
Coordinator of Academic Affairs,
College of Mount St. Vincent
Division of Nursing,
Riverdale, New York

ILLUSTRATED

THE C. V. MOSBY COMPANY

ST. LOUIS • TORONTO • PRINCETON   1986

MOSBY

A TRADITION OF PUBLISHING EXCELLENCE

Editor: David P. Carroll
Assistant editor: Megan Thomas
Supervising manuscript editor: Elaine Steinborn
Design: Suzanne Oberholtzer
Production and manuscript editor: Mary Stueck

Printed in the United States of America

The C.V. Mosby Company
11830 Westline Industrial Drive, St. Louis, Missouri 63146

Library of Congress Cataloging-in-Publication Data
Main entry under title:

Nursing research.

   Includes index.
   1. Nursing—Research. I. LoBiondo-Wood, Geri.
II. Haber, Judith. [DNLM: 1. Nursing. 2. Research.
WY 20.5 N9744]
RT81.5.N873 1986   610.73'072   85-28395

GW/VH/VH 9 8 7 6 5 4 3   01/C/020

Contributors

Ann Bello, M.A., R.N.
Associate Professor of Nursing,
Norwalk Community College,
Norwalk, Connecticut;
Doctoral Candidate, New York University,
New York, New York

Harriet R. Feldman, Ph.D., R.N.
Assistant Dean,
Adelphi University,
Marion A. Buckley School of Nursing,
Garden City, New York

Margaret Grey, Dr. P.H., R.N.
Assistant Professor,
University of Pennsylvania
School of Nursing,
Philadelphia, Pennsylvania

Judith Haber, Ph.D., R.N.
Associate Professor and
Coordinator of Academic Affairs,
College of Mount St. Vincent
Division of Nursing,
Riverdale, New York

Carol Noll Hoskins, Ph.D., R.N.
Associate Professor and Chairperson,
Doctoral Program in Nursing,
New York University Division of Nursing,
New York, New York

Bettie S. Jackson, Ed.D., R.N., F.A.A.N., E.T.
Assistant Director of Nursing-Research,
Moses Division/Montefiore Medical Center,
Bronx, New York

Christine Tassone Kovner, Ph.D., R.N.
Assistant Professor
New York University Division of Nursing,
New York, New York

Rona F. Levin, Ph.D., R.N.
Director, Master's Program,
Adelphi University,
Marion A. Buckley School of Nursing,
Garden City, New York

Geri LoBiondo-Wood, Ph.D., R.N.
Associate Professor and
Interim Assistant Dean,
University of Nebraska
College of Nursing,
Omaha, Nebraska

To our families
Pat and Lenny, Laurie, and Andrew

Preface

The foundation of this textbook is the belief that nursing research is integral to all levels of nursing practice. All too often research is perceived as a complex process carried out in an "ivory tower" by expert nurse-scientists and having little or no relevance to the everyday practice of nursing. This dichotomous view of nursing research is not valid. Instead, research is essential to the development of a unique scientific body of knowledge, a hallmark of any profession, and should be utilized to provide the foundation for shaping and guiding theory-based nursing practice.

Therefore, all nurses need to understand, evaluate, and apply research. However, the kind of knowledge appropriate to different levels of education varies. There is a general consensus that the research role of the baccalaureate graduate calls for the skills of critical appraisal; that is, the role of the nurse as a knowledgeable research consumer. Preparing students for this role involves developing their understanding of the research process, their appreciation of the role of the critiquer, and their ability to apply the critical appraisal process to research reports. An undergraduate course in nursing research should teach students how to understand, appraise, and apply research. Thus students need to comprehend the steps of research reports. The development of a basic level of competency in this area is essential to fully integrate research into clinical practice. This is in contrast to the focus of a graduate level research course where the emphasis is on how to understand as well as carry out research.

Nursing Research: Critical Appraisal and Utilization prepares nursing students and practicing nurses to become knowledgeable nursing research consumers by emphasizing the following areas:

- Addressing the role of the nurse as a research consumer with the goal of increasing the appreciation of this role.
- Teaching the fundamentals of the research process as well as the critical appraisal process in a logical, systematic progression. This attitude toward research promotes a spirit of inquiry and encourages systematic thinking and judgment that will enable students and nurses to expand their current knowledge base. This will be reflected in their increased use of the research literature as it applies to their clinical practice.

- Elevating the critiquing process to a position of importance comparable to that of producing research. This enables students and nurses to make judgments regarding the relative utility and merit of a research project. Both consumers and producers of research need to be sophisticated appraisers of the state of the art. Moreover, before becoming a producer of research, the student needs to be a knowledgeable consumer. The goal is the stimulation of thoughtful practice that is both creative and innovative through the use of nursing research.
- Demystifying the notion that research is a complex process restricted to use by learned academicians. Research generated by academicians should be utilized by all practitioners of nursing, but if the process remains mysterious, the majority or practitioners may feel incapable of understanding and utilizing research findings.

The text is organized into two parts. Part I focuses on roles, approaches, and issues in nursing research. This part of the text provides an overview of the nurse's role as a research consumer. It introduces the sources of human knowledge and the characteristics of the scientific approach. Legal and ethical issues related to the conduct of research are introduced.

Part II focuses on the integration of both the research and the critiquing processes. Chapters 4 through 18 delineate each step of the research process, and clinical research studies are used to illustrate each step. The interrelatedness of the steps is examined in relation to the total research process. Critical thinking is stimulated by presenting the potential strengths and weaknesses inherent in each step of the process. These chapters include a section describing the critiquing process for each step, as well as lists of related Critiquing Criteria, designed to stimulate a systematic and evaluative approach to research literature. Chapter 19 summarizes the research and critiquing process by presenting and evaluating a complete research study. Chapter 20 illustrates how the research process is utilized in and integrated with nursing practice.

The accompanying Study Guide, Instructor's Manual, and Questbank complement the textbook and enhance the learning process.

The development of a scientific foundation for clinical nursing practice is the essential priority for nursing research in the future. *Nursing Research: Critical Appraisal and Utilization* will help students to develop a basic level of competency in understanding the steps of the research process that will enable them to critically analyze research studies and apply the findings in their clinical practice. To the extent that this goal is accomplished, nursing will have a cadre of practitioners who derive their practice from theory and research specific to nursing.

Acknowledgments

The completion of any major undertaking is never accomplished alone. There are those who contribute directly and those who contribute indirectly to the success of a project. We acknowledge here with our warmest thanks the following people who have helped and supported us throughout this endeavor:

- Our students, particularly the nursing students at Columbia University, School of Nursing, whose interest and lively curiosity sparked the idea for this textbook.
- Our contributors, whose expertise, cooperation, and punctuality made them a joy to have as colleagues.
- Our editors, David Carroll and Megan Thomas, whose confident and forthright style provided us with support whenever we needed it.
- Our supervising manuscript editor, Elaine Steinborn, and production and manuscript editor, Mary Stueck, for their help with manuscript production and last minute details.
- Our typists, Sharon Moore and Betty Vinci, whose painstaking care with our sometimes disorderly manuscripts made the editorial process much smoother.
- Our families, Pat Wood and Lenny, Laurie, and Andrew Haber, for their unending love, faith, understanding, and support throughout what is inevitably a consuming but exciting experience.

Geri LoBiondo-Wood
Judith Haber

Contents

ONE

NURSING RESEARCH
Roles, Approaches, and Issues

1

The Role of Research in Nursing

Geri LoBiondo-Wood
Judith Haber

LEARNING OBJECTIVES

After reading this chapter, the student should be able to do the following:

- State the significance of research to the practice of nursing.
- Identify the consumer of nursing research.
- Discuss the differences of trends within nursing research before and after 1950.
- Describe how research, education, and practice relate to each other.
- Evaluate the nurse's role in the research process as it relates to the nurse's level of educational preparation.
- Identify the future trends in nursing research.
- Formulate the priorities for nursing research for the remainder of the twentieth century.

KEY TERMS

applied research   consumer
basic research   critique
clinical research   research

As you begin to read the first chapter of this book you may be wondering, why on earth is a research course part of my nursing curriculum? You may be asking yourself, will this course help me pass the state boards when I graduate? You may also wonder, how will learning about research help me practice nursing in a better way? In answer to such questions, the research course you are taking will not specifically help you to pass your state boards. However, it may sharpen your critical thinking skills so that your ability to analyze the exam questions and potential answers is improved. More important, though, is the belief shared by many nurses that a knowledge of nursing research can have a significant effect on the depth and breadth of the professional practice of every nurse.

The purpose of this chapter is to introduce you to the significance and the historical evolution of nursing research and to highlight the multiple roles of the nurse in the research process. We will discuss the current status of research in nursing and then speculate on future directions for nursing research. We hope to engage you in a mutual learning process that begins with this chapter, a process that will clarify the role of the nurse in the research experience.

• Significance of Research in Nursing

The nursing profession has devoted great effort to developing the unique specialized body of knowledge used in the delivery of health care to clients. Indeed, having a specialized body of knowledge that is scientifically based is one of the hallmarks of a profession and is essential for fostering a sense of commitment and accountability to clients.

The current body of scientific knowledge can best be expanded through further research endeavors. But this expansion of knowledge has little meaning for the profession as a whole if it remains only in research journals or in the minds of the researchers. It must be part of the active repertoire of knowledge of those directly engaged in practice.

Today more than ever before nurses are required to be accountable for the quality of client care they deliver. In an era of consumerism and rising health care costs, clients are asking health professionals to document the effectiveness of their services. Essentially, they are asking nursing, "How do nursing services make a difference in my case?" Other groups, including insurance companies and governmental reimbursement agencies such as Medicare, Medicaid, and diagnostic related groups (DRGs) are also requiring accountability for services provided.

Scientific investigations that are practice oriented can contribute significantly to validating the effectiveness of particular nursing measures and to improving the quality of client care. The findings of such studies provide a theory base for decision making about the delivery of nursing care. The nursing profession will be increasingly responsible for preparing its practitioners to be sophisticated producers of research and consumers of scientific literature, so that the new knowledge being generated can be evaluated and applied to nursing practice in a meaningful way.

The Commission on Nursing Research of the American Nurses' Association (1981) has recognized the need for research skills at all levels of professional nursing. Scientific investigation promotes accountability, one of the hallmarks of a profession and a fundamental concept of the American Nurses' Association Code of Conduct. There is a general consensus that the research role of the baccalaureate graduate calls for the skill of critical appraisal; that is, the nurse must be a knowledgeable consumer of research. The remainder of this text is devoted to helping you develop that expertise.

• Research: the Link Between Theory, Education, and Practice

Research is the link between theory, education, and practice. Mercer (1984) states that research is the process through which the knowledge base for nursing practice grows. Theory conceptualizes the abstract nature of the relationship among phenomena. Research, however, is the systematic, logical, and empirical inquiry into the possible relationships among particular phenomena. Educational settings provide a milieu where students can learn about the research process. In this setting they can also explore different theories and begin to evaluate them in light of research findings. Theoretical formulations supported by research findings may potentially become the foundation of theory-based practice in nursing.

At this point you might logically ask how the theory and research content of your course will relate to your nursing practice. The answer is twofold; it may help you to become a beginning producer of research, however, it must help you to become an intelligent *consumer* of research. A consumer uses, applies, and practices in an active manner. To be a knowledgeable consumer, a nurse must have a knowledge base about the relevant subject matter, the ability to discriminate and abstract information logically, and the ability to apply the knowledge that has been gained.

For example, nurses become knowledgeable consumers through educational processes and practical experience. The link between knowledgeably applying the nursing process and being a knowledgeable consumer is research. However, it is not necessary for nurses to conduct research studies to be able to appreciate and utilize research findings in practice. Rather, to be intelligent consumers, nurses must understand the research process and attain the critical evaluation skills needed to judge the merit and relevance of research findings before applying them in clinical practice and in caring for clients.

• Historical Perspective

MID- AND LATE NINETEENTH CENTURY

In the mid-nineteenth century, nursing as a formal discipline began to take root with the ideas and practices of Florence Nightingale. Her concepts have contributed to and are congruent with present values of nursing research. The promotion of health, prevention of disease, and care of the sick were central ideas of her system. Nightingale believed that the systematic collection and exploration of data were necessary for nursing. Her collection and analysis of data on the health status of British soldiers during the Crimean War led to a variety of reforms in health care (Palmer, 1977). Nightingale also noted the need for measuring outcomes of nursing and medical care (Nightingale, 1863). Other than Nightingale's work, there seems to have been little research during the early years of nursing's development. This may be in part because schools of nursing had just begun to be established in the United States, schools were unequal in educational ability, and nursing leadership had just begun to develop.

TWENTIETH CENTURY—BEFORE 1950

Nursing research in the first half of the twentieth century focused mainly on nursing education, but some client- and technique-oriented research was evident. The early efforts in nursing education research were done by such leaders as Lavinia Dock (1900), Anne Goodrich (1932), Adelaide Nutting (1907, 1912, 1926), Isabel Hampton Robb (1906), and Lillian Wald (1915). Nutting's (1907) *The Education and Professional Position of Nurses* and Nutting and Dock's (1907) *History of Nursing* were the earliest studies of nursing and nursing education. These pioneering works consist of documentation gathered for the purpose of reforming nursing education and establishing it as a viable profession.

The continued need for reform in nursing education was met by the Nursing and Nursing Education in the United States Landmark Study, known as the Goldmark Report (1923). Sponsored by the Rockefeller Foundation, the Committee for the Study of Nursing Education was funded to survey on a national level the educational preparation of the faculty and the clinical experiences of the administrators, private duty nurses, public health nurses, and nursing students. The report identified multiple deficiencies and disparate educational backgrounds at all levels of nursing. This study, and others in the first half of the century, recommended reorganization of nursing education and, most importantly, its movement into the university setting.

Clinically oriented research slowly emerged in the early half of the century and mainly centered on the morbidity and mortality associated with such problems as pneumonia and contaminated milk (Carnegie, 1976). A few of these projects were instrumental in the development of client care protocols and the employment of nurses in community settings. An experimental project by Wald and Dock (1902) led to the employment of school nurses in the New York City school system and subsequently in other cities (Roberts, 1954). Though she did not perform formal research, Linda Richards, the first American trained nurse at Bellevue Hospital, was the first nurse to keep written documentation of client care. This documentation was used by the medical profession for their investigations (Carnegie, 1976).

In 1913 the Committee on Public Health Nursing of the National League of Nursing Education (NLNE) studied such concerns as infant mortality, blindness, and midwifery. The committee called for nursing to distinguish its role in the prevention of disease and the promotion of health through the knowledge and use of the scientific approach.

The 1920s saw the development and teaching of the earliest nursing research course because of the influence of Isabel M. Stewart (Henderson, 1977). A course titled "Comparative nursing practice," first taught by Smith and later by Henderson, introduced students to the scientific method of investigation. Students were encouraged to question all aspects of nursing care and to do laboratory experiments on such topics as measuring the oxygen content in an oxygen tent during a client's bed bath to assess whether it dropped below a therapeutic level. Also during this period, case studies appeared in the *American Journal of Nursing (AJN)*. These were used as a teaching tool for students and as a record of client progress (Gortner and Nahm, 1977). Scientific criteria were applied to assess the appropriateness of the methodology used (Gortner and Hahm, 1977).

Other practice-related research focused on improving nursing techniques (Clayton, 1927), handwashing procedures (Broadhurst et al., 1927) and thermometer disinfecting techniques (Ryan and Miller, 1932), among others. Clinical investigations similar to these and subsequent studies of nurses and nursing education were done through the first part of the century.

Social change and World War II affected all aspects of nursing including research. There was an urgent need for more nurses; increased hospital admissions and military needs created a shortage of personnel. In 1943 the U.S. Cadet Nurses Corps was created after the Nurse Practice Act of 1943 was passed. The Corps provided assistance for nurses and after the war offered information that assisted in planning for nursing education. During the war, investigations focused on hospital environments, nursing status, nursing education, and nursing shortages.

After the war, nursing, like the rest of the world, began to reassess itself and its goals. In 1948 *Nursing for the Future* by Esther Lucille Brown was published. This was the culmination of a 3-year study funded by the Carnegie Foundation. This report reemphasized the inconsistencies in educational preparation and the need to move into the university setting and included an updated description of nursing practices. An outgrowth of Brown's report was a number of studies on nursing roles and needs. Also during the immediate postwar period many states carried out studies on nursing needs and resources (Simmons and Henderson, 1964).

TWENTIETH CENTURY—AFTER 1950

The 1950s saw the infancy stages of nursing research begin to develop and bloom. The developments of the 1950s laid the groundwork for nursing's current level of research skill. Nursing schools at the undergraduate and graduate level were growing in number, and graduate programs were including courses related to research. The worth and benefit of research was appreciated by nursing leadership and was beginning to filter to the various levels of nursing. This period saw the inception of the *Journal of Nursing Research* dedicated to the promotion of research in nursing. In 1955 the American Nurses' Foundation was chartered as a center for research; the audience for its publications consisted of receivers and administrators of research monies. Also at the national level of the American Nurses' Association a standing Committee on Research and Studies was formed in 1954. This committee was charged with planning, promoting, and guiding research and studies relating to the functions of the Association (See, 1977). A secondary function of the committee was to collect and unify nursing information that could be used to advise the Board regarding periodic inventories of nurses. Concurrently in 1955 the Commonwealth Fund endowed the National League of Nursing (NLN) with monies for the support of research education and training. Throughout the 1950s these organizations and others, such as the U.S. Public Health Service, put forth funds and personnel to study the characteristics of nursing members and students; the supply, organization, and distribution of nursing services; and job satisfaction.

The first nursing unit for practice-oriented research was set up at the Walter Reed Army Institute of Research. This unit was geared toward chemical research. Even though research during this period was focused on nurses and their characteristics, the fields of psychiatric nursing and maternal-child health care received monies from federal grants to develop nursing content and educational programs at the master's and doctoral levels. Grants were also conferred on individuals who studied the social context of psychiatric facilities and its influence on relations between staff and clients (Greenblatt et al., 1955; Stanton and Schwartz, 1954) and the role of the nurse with single mothers (Donnell and Glick, 1954).

In the late 1950s nursing studies began to address clinical problems. In a guest editorial featured in *Nursing Research* (1956), Virginia Henderson commented that studies about nurses outnumber clinical studies 10 to 1. She stated that "the responsibility for designing its methods is often cited as an essential characteristic of a profession" (p. 99).

Thus in the 1960s there began a reordering of research priorities and a targeting of practice-oriented research. These priorities were supported by the American Nurses' Foundation and other major nursing organizations. However, even with this support, research did not flourish. This may be partly attributed to the lack of educational preparation of nurses in research. Where research education did exist, nurses had not yet developed sufficient expertise in research design and methodology to teach their own research courses. So nurses were, until very recently, dependent on others from related disciplines such as psychology, education, and sociology, who had this expertise to teach these courses. Today this is not usually the case.

Consistent with this need for guidance, many of the studies during the 1950s and 1960s were coinvestigated by individuals from the social sciences and medicine. Another reason for the paucity of research was the small number of nurses with baccalaureate and higher degrees. Although enrollment in these programs had increased by 1960, less than 2% of the employed registered nurses held master's degrees and less than 7% held baccalaureate degrees (ANA, 1960).

During the 1960s, studies on nurses and nursing continued but at the same time the pioneers in the development of nursing theories and concepts, such as Ida Jean Orlando (1960), Hildegarde Peplau (1952),and Ernestine Wiedenbach (1964), called for the development of nursing practice based on theory. Though their theories and those of others have only begun to be tested, the early development of those theories has spurred nurses into a more critical level of thinking regarding nursing practice.

Collaborative efforts in the 1960s on practice-oriented research led to follow-up research by Dier and Leonard (1966) and Dumas and Leonard (1962). These studies done at Yale University explored the effects of nurse-patient teaching and communication on such events as hospitalization, surgery, and the labor experience. Another classic study, the culmination of 8 years of work by Glaser and Strauss (1965), explored various aspects of thanatology among dying patients and their caretakers.

A review of the nursing research studies published during the 1960s reveals that clinical studies were beginning to predominate. These studies investigated a wide gamut of nursing care issues such as infection control, alcoholism, and sensory deprivation. Lydia Hall (1963) published the results of a 5-year study that looked at alternatives to hospitalization for a select group of elderly clients. This study gave rise to a totally nurse-run care facility, the Loeb Center in New York City, that is still in operation and run by nurses today.

The rich history of nursing was also recognized during the 1960s. Nursing archives at Boston University's Mugar Library were established through a federally funded grant with the goal of promoting nursing research. In 1967 the First Nursing Research Conference of the ANA was held. A group of nurses and nursing faculty gathered to report on research and critique the findings presented.

The opening of the 1970s saw the publication of the National Commission for the Study of Nursing and Nursing Education Report or the Lysaught Report (1970). This report, conducted with the support of the ANA, NLN, and other private foundations, surveyed nursing practice and education. It offered the conclusion that more practice-oriented and education-oriented research was necessary and these data must be applied to the improvement of educational organizations and curricula. The call for clinically oriented study was becoming a reality. Carnegie (1976) noted that the majority of research published in the nursing journals was clinically oriented.

The 1970s also saw new growth in the number of master's and doctoral programs for nursing. These programs, along with the ANA, NLN, Sigma Theta Tau, and the Western Interstate Council for Higher Education in Nursing, clearly supported nurses learning the research process as well as producing research that could be used to enhance care quality. In the 1970s newer journals such as *Advances in Nursing Sciences, Research in Nursing and Health,* and *The Western Journal of Nursing Research* were established that promoted the generation of nursing theory and research.

While some may say that not enough has been done, or nursing has not been expedient enough in acknowledging the need for research, a careful review of the history of nursing research shows that it has steadily grown along with the many social and political changes that have influenced the practice of nursing. The 1980s have seen extended growth among upper level programs in nursing, especially at the doctoral level. These nurses, with the knowledge of nursing practice and research processes and methods, are now beginning to take the place of social scientists in the classroom and are teaching research methods as well as practice concepts. Hospitals and service institutions are developing nursing research offices and are funding beginning research. The support and acknowledgment of service and education for research have brought new challenges for nurses, including research production and, more currently, the utilization of research findings in practice.

• The Roles of the Nurse in the Research Process

There are many roles for nurses in research. One of the marks of success in nursing research is the delineation of research activities geared for nurses prepared in different types of educational programs (Fawcett, 1984).

Graduates of associate degree nursing programs should demonstrate an awareness of the value or relevance of research in nursing. They may assist in identifying problem areas in nursing practice within an established structured format, and they may assist in data collection activities (ANA, 1981).

Nurses with a baccalaureate education must be intelligent consumers of research. That is, they must understand each step of the research process and its relationship to every other step. Such understanding must be linked with a clear idea about the standards of satisfactory research. This comprehension is necessary when critically reading and understanding research reports and thereby determining the validity and merit of reported studies. Through critical appraisal skills that use specific criteria to judge all aspects of the research, a professional nurse interprets, evaluates, and determines the credibility of research findings. The nurse discriminates between an idea that is interesting but requires further investigation before implementation in practice, and findings that have sufficient support to be considered for utilization (Batey, 1982).

In this context, understanding the research process and acquiring critical appraisal skills open a broad realm of information that can contribute to the professional nurse's body of knowledge and that can be applied judiciously to practice in the interest of providing scientifically based client care (Batey, 1982). Thus the role of the baccalaureate graduate in the research process is primarily that of a knowledgeable consumer, a role that promotes the integration of research and clinical practice.

Lest anyone think that this is an unimportant role, let us assure you that it is not. Fawcett (1984) states that we are all aware of those who assert that research is the baliwick of "ivory tower" investigators. She goes on to state, however, that it is the average clinical practitioner who is ultimately responsible for utilization of the findings of nursing and other health-related research in clinical practice. To appropriately use such research findings, nurses must understand and critically appraise them. Thus if nursing as a profession is ever to have a genuine theory-based practice, it will be in large part up to nurses in their role as consumers of research to accomplish this task.

Baccalaureate graduates also have a responsibility to identify nursing problems that need to be investigated and to participate in the implementation of scientific studies (ANA, 1981). It is often clinicians who generate research ideas or questions from hunches, gut-level feelings, intuition, or observations of clients or nursing care. These ideas are often the seeds of further research investigations. For example, a nurse working on a psychiatric unit observed that a certain percentage of discharged clients were readmitted to the unit within 2 months of discharge. She noted that there were differences in the discharge procedure and wanted to find out if the type of aftercare treatment made a difference in the readmission rate. Of particular interest was the variation related to whether the client was connected to the aftercare therapist or facility before discharge and how this influenced the readmission rate. The presence and support of an expert nurse-researcher in the clinical setting can often provide leadership and direction for staff nurses in the systematic investigation of such an idea in an on-site clinical research project. Systematic collection of data about a clinical problem contributes to the refinement and extension of nursing practice.

Baccalaureate graduates may also participate in research projects as a member of an interdisciplinary or intradisciplinary research team. The nurse may participate in one or more phases of such a project. For example, a staff nurse may work on a clinical research unit where a particular type of nursing care is part of an established research protocol. In such a situation the nurse administers the care according to the format described in the protocol. The nurse may also be involved in the collection and recording of data relevant to the administration of and client response to the nursing care.

As members of a profession, it is also incumbent on baccalaureate graduates to share research findings with colleagues. This may involve collaborative dissemination of the findings of a study that you have participated in for an article or for a research or clinical conference. Or it may involve sharing with colleagues the findings of a research report that you have critiqued and have found to have merit and potential applicability in your practice.

Nurses who are educationally prepared at the master's and doctoral levels must also be sophisticated consumers of research. However, they are also being prepared to conduct research as either a coinvestigator or primary investigator.

At the master's level, nurses can analyze and reformulate nursing problems so that scientific knowledge and methods can be used to find solutions. They enhance the quality and relevance of nursing research by providing clinical expertise about problems and by providing knowledge about the way that clinical services are delivered. They facilitate the investigation of clinical problems by providing a climate conducive to conducting research. This includes collaborating with others in investigations and enhancing nursing's access to clients and data. At the master's level, nurses conduct research investigations for the purpose of monitoring the quality of the practice of nursing in a clinical setting. They assist others in applying scientific knowledge in nursing practice (ANA, 1984).

Doctorally prepared nurses have the greatest amount of expertise in appraising, designing, and conducting research. They develop theoretical explanations of phenomena relevant to nursing. They develop methods of scientific inquiry and use analytical and empirical methods to discover ways to modify or extend existing knowledge so that it is relevant to nursing. Three types of research are conducted by

• *Table 1-1*   **Types of Nursing Research**

Type of research	Definition	Example
Basic research	Theoretical or pure research that generates, tests, and expands theories that describe, explain, or predict the phenomenon of interest to the discipline without regard to its later use	Fitzpatrick's (1983) study of time perception is part of a larger program of basic research designed to develop the life perspective rhythm theory
Applied research	"Answers questions related to the applicability of basic theories in practical situations," (Donaldson and Crowley, 1978). It tests the practical limits of descriptive theories, but does not examine the efficacy of actions taken by practitioners	Kishi's (1983) study of the relationship between communication patterns used by health care professionals and client recall of information tested the limits and applicability of Flanders Interaction Analysis System, an educational theory, in well-baby clinics
Clinical research	Examines the effects of nursing processes on health status and examines the effects of actual implementation of knowledge in clinical practice settings (Fawcett, ANS, 1984)	Ziemer's (1983) study of the differential effects of information about procedures, sensations, and coping strategies associated with abdominal surgery on postoperative complications

doctorally prepared nurses: basic, applied, and clinical. Table 1-1 provides a definition and example of each type of research. In addition to their role as producers of research, doctorally prepared nurses also act as role models and mentors who guide, stimulate, and encourage other nurses who are developing their research skills. They also collaborate with and serve as consultants to educational or health care institutions or agencies in their research endeavors.

The most important implication of the delineation of research activities according to educational preparation is the necessity of having a collaborative research relationship within the nursing profession. Not all nurses must or should conduct research. However, all nurses can play some part in the research process. Nurses at all educational levels, whether they are consumers of producers of research or both, need to view the research process as something of *integral value* to the growing professionalism in nursing.

Professionals need to take the time to read research studies and to evaluate them using the standards congruent with scientific research. The critiquing process is used to identify the strengths and weaknesses of each study. Nurses should keep in mind that no study is perfect; while the limitations should be recognized, nurses may extrapolate from the study whatever is sound and relevant to be considered for potential use in clinical practice.

FUTURE DIRECTIONS IN NURSING RESEARCH

In a complex health-oriented society such as ours that is increasingly responsive to consumer concerns related to the cost, quality, availability, and accessibility of health care, it is of paramount importance to define the future direction of nursing research (Snyder Hill, 1984).

There is unanimous agreement among nursing leaders that the essential priority for nursing research in the future will continue to be the extension of the scientific knowledge base for nursing practice (Polit and Hungler, 1983; Mercer, 1984, Lindemann, 1984; Fawcett, 1984). This priority will definitely have implications for nursing education and nursing administration.

An increasing number of nurses who have significant expertise in appraising, designing, and conducting research will continue to emerge within the profession. They will be at the forefront of the ongoing refinement of our scientific knowledge base for nursing practice.

Nursing researchers will have increasing methodological expertise. They will be more knowledgeable about computer technology as it applies to the research process. There will be a greater emphasis on measurement issues such as the development of tools that accurately measure clinical phenomena. The increasing focus on the need to utilize multiple measures to accurately assess clinical phenomena will also be apparent. Related to the need to accurately measure clinical phenomena will be the development of noninvasive methods of measuring physiological parameters of interest in high technology settings. This may well be another aspect of utilizing multiple measures to assess particular clinical phenomena.

Nurses who are prepared to direct the conduct of research will head an expanding number of nursing research departments in clinical settings. They, in turn, will involve the nursing staff in generating and conducting research projects as well as critically evaluating existing research investigations. An expanded number of centers for nursing research will be established in university settings as faculty members become qualified to run them.

The collaborative relationship between educational and practice settings will need to intensify. Faculty members from universities will increasingly be invited to work collaboratively with nursing research departments or directly with nursing staff members in hospitals or agencies.

Staff members from clinical settings such as hospitals and other health care agencies will collaborate with students and/or faculty in the university setting to share clinical ideas, observations, and research endeavors. Joint appointments between educational and clinical settings will increase to maximize the sharing of expertise in all areas of the research process in the interest of improving the quality of care for the object of our mutual concern, the client. The net result will be expanded intradisciplinary collaboration. Nurses will also be in a stronger position to engage in interdisciplinary research with members of other professions.

Another trend will be the proliferation of cluster studies, multiple site investigations of clinical problems. Gortner (1975) states that the accumulation of evidence supporting or negating an existing theory will help define the base of nursing practice.

Clinical consortia will help delineate the common and unique aspects of client care for the various health professions.

Replication of research studies will become a valuable component of building the theory base for nursing practice. Mercer (1984) states that the adoption of research findings in practice with their potential risks and benefits, including the cost of implementation, should be based on a series of replicated studies.

The emphasis of research studies will be related to clinical issues and problems. The Commission on Nursing Research of the American Nurses' Association (1981) has stated that the preeminent goal of scientific inquiry by nurses is the ongoing development of knowledge for use in the practice of nursing. Consequently, priority should be given to nursing research that would generate knowledge to guide practice in the following areas:

- Promoting health
- Preventing health problems
- Decreasing the negative impact of health problems on coping abilities, productivity, and life satisfaction
- Ensuring that the care needs of vulnerable groups such as the aged are met through appropriate strategies
- Designing and developing health care systems that are cost-effective in meeting the nursing needs of the population
- Promoting health, well-being, and competency for personal health in all age groups

Nurses with graduate research preparation will be conducting research studies to accomplish these goals. Baccalaureate graduates will be critically appraising the research literature to examine the findings of clinical studies for potential incorporation into theory-based nursing practice. Examples of research consistent with the priorities given earlier include the following:

- Identifying determinants of wellness and health functioning in individuals and families, and identifying factors predictive of successful coping with chronic illness
- Identifying phenomena that negatively influence the course of recovery and that may be alleviated by nursing practice, such as anorexia, pain, sleep deprivation, and nutritional deficiencies
- Developing and testing strategies that facilitate the individual's health enhancing behaviors such as altering nutrition; reducing stressful responses associated with medical management of surgical patients; providing more effective management of high-risk populations such as families with an impaired child; and enhancing the care of clients culturally different from the majority, clients with special problems such as teenagers and underserved client groups such as the poor
- Designing and assessing, in terms of cost and effectiveness, models for delivering nursing care strategies found to be effective in clinical studies

By the year 2000 the population will include an increased proportion of children and elderly who are chronically ill or disabled. People who have sustained life-threatening illnesses will live with new life-sustaining technology that will create new demands for self-care and family support. Cancer, heart disease, arthritis, chronic pulmonary disease, diabetes, and Alzheimer's disease are prevalent during middle and later life and will command large proportions of the available health resources. Mental health problems will result from rapid technological and social change. Alcohol and drug abuse will be responsible for significant health care expenses. Increasingly, the settings where client care is provided for individuals and families will be homes, schools, workplaces, and ambulatory care centers.

In light of the priority given to clinical research issues, the funding of investigations will be increasingly in the area of clinical research projects. This is not to say that other types of research investigations such as those utilizing historical, philosophical, or evaluative designs are not important. In fact, as nurses define their practice, become eligible for third-party reimbursement, and are generally held more accountable for their practice, they will have to engage in more evaluative outcome studies.

It is apparent from the previous discussion that the future directions of nursing research will focus on the scientific validation of nursing practice. Both consumers and producers of research will engage in a unified effort to accomplish this priority.

• Summary

Nursing research provides the basis for expanding the unique body of scientific knowledge that forms the foundation of nursing practice. Research is the link between education theory, and practice. Nurses become knowledgeable consumers of research through educational processes and practical experience. As consumers of research, nurses must have a basic understanding of the research process as well as critical appraisal skills that provide a standard for evaluating the strengths and weaknesses of research studies before applying them in clinical practice.

A historical perspective of nursing research traces its origins to Florence Nightingale. Moving forward to the first half of the twentieth century, nursing research mainly focused on studies related to nursing education. However, some clinical studies related to nursing care were evident. Nursing research blossomed in the second half of the twentieth century; graduate programs in nursing expanded, research journals began to emerge, the ANA formed a research committee, and funding for graduate education and nursing research increased dramatically. Basic, applied, and clinical research studies were carried out by an increasing number of nurse researchers.

Nurses at all levels of educational preparation have a responsibility to participate in the research process. The role of the baccalaureate graduate has been delineated as one of knowledgeable consumer of research. Nurses prepared at the master's and doctoral levels must be sophisticated consumers, but will also be producers of research studies. A collaborative research relationship within the nursing profession will extend and refine the scientific body of knowledge that provides the grounding for theory-based practice.

The future of nursing research will continue to be the extension of the scientific knowledge base for nursing expertise in appraising, designing, and conducting research, will provide leadership in both academic and clinical settings. Collaborative research relationships between education and service will multiply. Cluster research studies and replication of studies will have increased value.

The emphasis of research studies will be related to clinical issues and problems. Priority will be given to research studies focusing on health promotion, the diminution of the negative impact of health problems, the ensuring of care for the health needs of vulnerable groups such as the aged, and the development of cost-effective health care systems. The recipients of health care will increasingly be children and elderly people with chronic health problems. Alcohol and drug-related problems will also increase. The settings where clients will receive care will be homes, workplaces, schools, and ambulatory care centers.

Both consumers and producers of research will engage in a collaborative effort to further the growth of nursing research and accomplish the research priorities of the profession.

• References

American Nurses' Association. (1960). *Facts about nursing,* New York, pp. 109-116.

American Nurses' Association. (1976). Commission on Nursing Research: Preparation of nurses for participation in research, Kansas City, Mo.

American Nurses' Association. (1981). Guidelines for the investigative function of nurses, Kansas City, Mo., pp. 2-3.

Batey, M.V.: Research: A component of undergraduate education, in *Evaluating research preparation in baccalaureate nursing education: national conference for nurse educators,* University of Iowa College of Nursing, 1982.

Broadhurst, J., and others. (1927). Hand brush suggestions for visiting nurses, *Public Health Nursing,* 19:487-489.

Brown, E.L. (1948). Nursing for the future, New York, Russell Sage Foundation.

Carnegie, E. (1976). *Historical perspectives of nursing research,* Nursing Archive, Special Collections, Boston, Boston University.

Clayton, S.L. (1927). Standardizing nursing techniques, its advantages and disadvantages, *American Journal of Nursing,* 27:939-943.

Committee on Nursing and Nursing Education in the United States, Josephine Goldmark, sec., (1923). New York, Macmillan Inc.

Diers, D., and Leonard, R.C. (1966). Interaction analysis in nursing research, *Nursing Research,* 15:225-228.

Dock, L.L. (1900). What we may expect from the law, *American Journal of Nursing,* 1:8-12.

Donaldson, S.K., and Crowley, D.M. (1978). The discipline of nursing, *Nursing Outlook,* 26:113-120.

Donnell, H., and Glick, S.J. (1954). The nurse and the unwed mother, *Nursing Outlook,* 2:249-251.

Dumas, R.G., and Leonard, R.C. (1963). The effect of nursing on the incidence of postoperative vomiting, *Nursing Research,* 12:12-15.

Fawcett, J. (1984). Another look at utilization of nursing research, *Image,* Spring, 16:59-61.

Fawcett, J. (1984). Hallmarks of success in nursing research, *Advances in Nursing Science,* 1:1-11.

Fitzpatrick, J.J. (1983). A life perspective rhythm model. In Fitzpatrick, J.J., and Whall, A.L. *Conceptual models of nursing: analysis and application,* Bowie, Md., Robert J. Brady Co., pp. 295-302.

Glaser, B.G., and Strauss, A.L. (1965). *Awareness of dying* (Observations series), Chicago, Aldine Publishing Co.

Goodrich, A. (1932). *The social and ethical significance of nursing: a series of addresses,* New York, The Macmillan Co.

Gortner, S.R. (1975). Research for a practice profession, *Nursing Research,* 24:193-197.

Gortner, S.R., and Nahm, H. (1977). An overview of nursing research in the United States, *Nursing Research,* 26:10-33.

Greenblatt, M., and others. (1955). *From custodial to therapeutic patient care in mental hospitals,* New York, Russell Sage Foundation.

Hall, L.E. (1963). A center for nursing, *Nursing Outlook,* 11:805-806.

Henderson, V. (1956). Research in nursing practice—when, (editorial), *Nursing Research,* **4**:99.

Henderson, V. (1977). We've "come a long way," but what of the direction? (guest editorial), *Nursing Research,* **26**:163-164.

Kishi, K.I. (1983). Communication patterns of health teaching and information recall, *Nursing Research,* **32**:230-235.

Larson, E. (1981). Nursing research outside academia: a panel presentation, *Image,* October, **13**:75-77.

Lindemann, C. (1984). Dissemination of nursing research, *Image,* Spring, 57-58.

Mercer, R.T. (1984). Nursing research: the bridge to excellence in practice, *Image,* Spring, **16**:47-50.

National Commission For the Study of Nursing and Nursing Education (1970). *An abstract for action,* New York, McGraw-Hill Book Co.

Nightingale, F. (1963). *Notes on hospitals,* London, Longman Group.

Nutting, M.A., and Dock, L.L. (1907-1912). *A history of nursing,* 4 vols., New York, G.P. Putnam's Sons.

Nutting, M.A. (1912). Educational status of nursing, U.S. Bureau of Education, Bull. no. 7, Washington, D.C., U.S. Government Printing Office.

Nutting, M.A. (1926). *A second economic basis for schools of nursing and other addresses,* New York, G.P. Putnam's Sons.

Orlando, I.J. (1961). *The dynamic nurse-patient relationship,* New York, G.P. Putnam's Sons.

Palmer, I. (1977). Florence Nightingale: reforms, reactionary, researcher, *Nursing Research,* **26**: 84-89.

Peplau, H.E. (1952). *Interpersonal relations in nursing: a conceptual frame of reference for psychodynamic nursing,* New York, G.P. Putnam's Sons.

Robb, I.H. (1906). *Nursing: its principles and practice for hospitals and private use,* 3rd ed., Cleveland, E.C. Koeckert.

Roberts, M.M. (1954). *American nursing: history and interpretation,* New York, Macmillan Inc.

Ryan, V., and Miller, V.B. (1932). Disinfection of clinical thermometers: bacteriological study and estimated costs, *American Journal of Nursing,* **32**:197-206.

Simmons, L.W., and Henderson, V. (1964). *Nursing research: a survey and assessment,* New York, Appleton-Century-Crofts.

Snyder Hill, B.A. (1984). Adelphi application health care, practice, education and education administration, *Image,* Winter, **16**:6-8.

Stanton, A.H., and Schwartz, M.A. (1954). *The mental hospital: a study of institutional participation in psychiatric illness and treatment,* New York, Basic Books, Inc.

Wald, L.D. (1915). *House on Henry Street,* New York, Henry Holt & Co.

Wiedenbach, E. (1964). *Clinical nursing: a helping art,* New York, Springer Publishing Co., Inc.

Ziemer, M.M. (1983). Effects of information on post-surgical coping. *Nursing Research,* **32**:282-287.

2

The Scientific Approach to the Research Process

Harriet R. Feldman

·

LEARNING OBJECTIVES

After reading this chapter, the student should be able to do the following:
- Describe the relationship between philosophy and science.
- Identify the major sources of human knowledge.
- Contrast the strengths and weaknesses of the major sources of human knowledge.
- Compare the inductive and deductive methods of logical reasoning.
- Identify the characteristics of the scientific approach as they relate to the research process.
- Define theory.
- Describe the points of critical appraisal used to examine the relationship between theory and method.

KEY TERMS

assumption	inductive reasoning
deductive reasoning	research
generalization	scientific approach
hypothesis	theory

• The Philosophy of Science

Philosophers and scientists pursue a common goal of working toward the expansion of knowledge. Their approaches to understanding reality, however, are different. For example, the philosopher uses intuition, reasoning, contemplation, and introspection to examine "the purpose of human life, the nature of being and reality, and the theory and limits of knowledge" (Silva, 1977, p.60). On the other hand, the scientist observes, verifies, constructs operational definitions, tests hypotheses, and conducts experiments to derive scientific laws and interpret reality. Another contrast is in the kinds of questions philosophers and scientists ask. Philosophy deals with *metaphysical* questions: What is knowledge? Are people inherently good or bad? Science deals with *empirical* questions: How are X and Y related? Does treatment A result in the resolution of problem B?

The development of *nursing knowledge* depends on both philosophy and science. For example, an individual's philosophy of human behavior, health, and client care will guide the intent and direction of a research effort. In addition, through logic and reasoning, the researcher/scientist can organize, formulate, and verify ideas and relationships. For example, Martinson (1979) states:

> Before making observations, the investigator must decide what she is going to observe and where she will make these observations. She must have already articulated in her own mind why she is selecting certain factors for observation and rejecting others. Prior to making such decisions, she must formulate some ideas regarding her study. These ideas, whether in the form of vague hunches or clearly formulated propositions, will serve as a guide in determining what questions are to be addressed by the research and which procedures and tools are to be used in searching for the answers (p.155).

The research consumer can also employ these processes to critically appraise the content, methods, and utility of research projects in light of moral and ethical standards. For example, you might ask the following questions: Does the theoretical rationale reflect a philosophical view of reality as a cause and effect relationship or as an interactional relationship? On what basis are sample delimitations made? Why were identified study variables selected? What are the propositions and how were they derived? Do subject selection and data collection procedures adhere to accepted moral and ethical guidelines?

Science can be viewed from at least two perspectives: it can be viewed as a body of theoretical knowledge (Andreoli and Thompson, 1977; Johnson, 1974) or as a method or process of inquiry (Beckwith and Miller, 1976; Newman, 1979). The body of knowledge perspective is very specifically concerned with interrelated *facts, principles, laws,* and *theories* and not with random or unrelated data. The method or process of inquiry is the medium for *systematically* collecting, quantifying, and evaluating data. It is useful to include both perspectives when defining science.

This chapter will examine the sources or origins of human knowledge fundamental to developing a body of knowledge and the components of the scientific approach that guide the process of inquiry. In addition, the relationship between theory and method will be discussed.

• Sources of Human Knowledge

There are many ways that ideas are generated. Some sources of knowledge are highly structured and are generally bound by defined rules of process or method. Examples include scientific inquiry, critical thinking, and logical reasoning. Other sources are less structured and have few defined rules; they include empathy, intuition, trial and error experience, and meditation. As a research consumer it is important for you to know how information is approached in a research or scientific context. Therefore several of these sources of knowledge will be discussed.

INTUITION

Webster's defines intuition as "the power of knowing, or knowledge obtained, without recourse to inference or reasoning; innate . . . knowledge." Intuition is a frequently used method of problem solving. It can operate in one of two ways, for example, as a form of inference where intuition closely resembles sensory perception or as an extrasensory experience independent of sensory input. Vaughan (1979) says, "Whatever the explanation or belief about it, intuition is widely acknowledged as being essential to problem solving and creativity in many different forms" (p.150).

Intuitive leaps in science and the arts, made by such people as Einstein and Beethoven have led to great contributions to humanity. The following situation illustrates an intuitive leap or an *ah ha*. Each time I teach a course in change theories and strategies, I list the stages of the change process. A few years ago a student enthusiastically blurted out, "That's the same as the nursing process," another student said, "It's also like the research process." Each of these students expressed an insight, and consequently, that insight helped them to have a clearer understanding of the change process. How many times have *you* unsuccessfully sought a solution to a problem, only to awaken in the middle of the night with a creative answer? Some of you may even keep writing materials near your bed to catch the insights while they are fresh!

In the case of research pursuits, intuition also plays a role. While intuition is not a sufficient means to approach information in a research context, it can serve as a guiding and creative adjunct. For example, it is an initial "hunch" or inference that leads many investigators to the examination of anticipated relationships. Furthermore, the logical process of inquiry is often complemented by intuitive insights that bring depth and breadth to the total research experience.

When reviewing research reports, the use of intuition in beginning and throughout the research process may or may not be apparent. Sometimes the introductory section of a research report identifies how the investigators first became aware of the problem they studied. Authors do not always include this information in the introduction, nor do they necessarily document insights that arose along the way.

TRIAL AND ERROR EXPERIENCE

An early approach to problem solving uses the process of elimination. When a problem is identified a solution is attempted. Depending on whether or not the solution works, you either adopt the trial solution or try another one. When the second solution fails, you keep trying, eliminating one solution after another until the problem is actually solved. This can be a very inefficient method of problem solving in terms of both time and energy, because it may take a very long time to find the successful solution. In addition, that solution may have already been determined by someone else. You may wonder how to find out if a solution has been found and how the trial and error method can be short circuited. There are alternatives; for example, you can review the literature pertinent to that problem to see what solutions exist, or you can ask a consultant about possible solutions.

In your role as consumer, you will be evaluating research methodology to see if the approach to solving the problem, as compared to testing the hypothesis, is appropriate to the study. You would ask if the hypothesis directly answers the research problem, if other possibilities were considered, and if the data collection instruments are valid and reliable. Given that the rationale for and the method of hypothesis testing are theoretically sound, it is logical to conclude that trial and error is not the approach used.

TRADITION AND AUTHORITY

Often we are tricked into believing that something is right or acceptable because it is backed by tradition and authority. While it is important to look at tradition and listen to what those in authority are saying, both of these sources of human knowledge must be critically evaluated in light of other available data, for example, related literature and experts in the field. As a research consumer, you have a responsibility to examine the validity and utility of knowledge derived from these sources. This is accomplished by questioning, identifying, and synthesizing all available data sources and noting the ones that clearly and logically support valid solutions.

When trial and error experiences lead to problem resolution, a ready source of known solutions becomes available. That resource pool forms the basis for tradition or precedent. As we become more invested in those traditional solutions, they take on an air of authority. The temperature-taking ritual is an example in nursing of this problem-solving evolution from trial and error to authority. In many instances nurses have come to accept, over time, that individuals require q4h temperature readings simply because they are admitted to an acute care facility. The initial rationale for this procedure has been long forgotten and more current investigations have refuted this practice. In fact, some hospitals have discontinued the q4h temperature-taking routine, based on their own research.

Another example of how tradition and authority have guided practice relates to tracheotomy care. Traditionally the use of sterile technique in tracheotomy care has been advocated and in many cases mandated. The rationale for this approach certainly seems sound and authoritative. However, Harris (1981) reported no statistically significant differences between sterile and clean techniques in her study of tracheotomy patients. In fact, the trend toward infection was greater in the sterile versus clean procedure.

As a research consumer, you must question tradition and authority. The more you challenge the kind of practice that evolved solely by precedent, the sooner nursing will advance toward the development of a scientific basis for practice.

LOGICAL REASONING

The two major methods of logical reasoning are inductive and deductive. As you tackle daily problems, you often utilize these approaches without realizing it. For example, *inductive reasoning* involves the observation of a particular set of instances that belong to and can be identified as part of a larger set. This reasoning moves from the particular to the general. On the other hand, *deductive reasoning* uses two or more variables or related statements that, when combined, form the basis for a concluding assertion of a relationship between the variables or relational statements. This reasoning moves from the general to the particular.

Both approaches to reasoning are useful in arriving at an understanding of phenomena. Knowing how they are used in a scientific or research context will help you to follow the reasoning applied by research investigators in the development of specific theoretical relationships.

Inductive Reasoning

As stated earlier, inductive reasoning moves from the particular to the general. Generalizations are developed from specific observations. For example, Freud gathered a great deal of information by listening to his clients report their dreams before making generalizations about the symbolism identified. As a nurse, you may observe that many of the children you care for behave in a particular way and conclude that the unfamiliar setting of the hospital is very stressful. Unfortunately, as one individual and with a limited number of patients to observe, your conclusion cannot be generalized to the claim that the hospital setting is stressful for *all* children. This pitfall is one you as a research consumer should look for when you critique research, for example, did the investigator overgeneralize? The following questions elaborate on this point: If the study was on an animal population, was the generalization extended to include a human population? If the study involved hysterectomy patients, was the generalization extended to include surgical patients as a group?

In summary, the inductive approach begins with an observation or some other way of obtaining information and leads to a conclusion or hypothesis. In cases where conclusions are arrived at using very specific or limited data, generalization of results can be erroneous. "The only valid conclusion which can be drawn is that a particular relationship existed in a particular situation at a particular point in time, and that further studies are required to test or control for rival hypotheses that may have been instrumental in determining the results" (Downs and Newman, 1977, p.11).

Deductive Reasoning

Deductive reasoning moves from the general to the particular. A specific hypothesis can be deduced from a theory that serves as a more general statement or network of interrelated phenomena. As a result of deduction, observations and predictions can be made. Rather than a source of new information, deductive reasoning can serve as an approach to unveiling existing relationships. For example, if we know that theory R is true, we could anticipate what outcomes and behaviors are logically expected. Here are two examples of how a nurse can use deductive reasoning.

1. Since you know certain physiological changes take place in bedridden clients as a result of continuous or uneven pressure to bony prominences, you could deduce that pressure-relieving methods would decrease the incidence and intensity of decubitus ulcer development.

2. The gate control theory of pain identifies the interaction of motivational, affective, and sensory processing that modulates the perception of and response to pain. Therefore such factors as anxiety, attention, age, culture, meaning of the present event, and pathophysiological findings are associated with the pain experience. Since anxiety and the pain sensation tend to reinforce each other, thereby increasing the intensity of the pain experience, you could deduce that anxiety-reducing measures, for example, empathic interaction, a back rub, an explanation to the client, and promptness in the administration of pain medication would result in decreased pain.

As with inductive reasoning, there may be inherent problems when using the deductive approach. First, not all deductions can be verified, particularly in a case where the measurement methods are poor or undeveloped. Second, a deduction that is based on a tentative premise may result in a conclusion that is logically valid, yet unsound. Finally, an unsound conclusion may be assumed sound, especially if it seems reasonable. If a systematic scientific approach is used to test a hypothesis deduced from a theory, the conclusion is more likely to have soundness and utility.

SCIENTIFIC APPROACH

The scientific approach is the most advanced method of acquiring knowledge. It offers a logical, orderly, and objective means of idea generation. By combining several components, for example, logic and reasoning, order and control, and empiricism and generalization, a rather sophisticated system of inquiry has been developed. This system has limitations, such as moral and ethical problems, measurement and control problems associated with nursing and social science research, and the general difficulty related to studying human beings, but it has been found to be more useful and predictive than other sources of human knowledge such as intuition, trial and error, or tradition and authority.

As a research consumer, you will be evaluating reported studies in terms of the investigators' adherence to the scientific approach. You will ask such questions as: What controls were in effect for this study, that is, what were the delimitations? What research method was used, for example descriptive, experimental, or quasi-experimental? How was the sample selected, and was it representative of the defined population? What steps were taken to control extraneous variables?

A more in-depth discussion of the characteristics of the scientific approach will help clarify these components. Table 2-1 compares the scientific method used for the natural sciences with the research process of th social sciences. Both attest to the logical and systematic process involved in knowledge acquisition.

Components of the Scientific Approach

Kerlinger (1973) defines scientific research as the "systematic, controlled, empirical, and critical investigation of hypothetical propositions about the presumed relations among natural phenomena" (p.11). This definition reflects a complex process. For the scientific approach to yield results that are minimally biased in all aspects, that is, sample selection, theoretical rationale, methodology, tools of analysis, and conclusions, the investigator must pursue an orderly and precise method of inquiry. The following is an examination of the major components of this approach.

ORDER AND CONTROL   As a systematic method of problem solving, the scientific approach requires order, or the use of clearly delineated, ordered steps. For example, you would not develop a hypothesis until a thorough search of the literature had been conducted. Similarly, you would not draw conclusions before you statistically analyze the collected data. This predetermined system or process guides the research so that you have greater confidence in your predictions and outcomes. When reviewing a research report, you should look for the investigator's approach to the problem,

• *Table 2-1* Systematic Ways of Acquiring Knowledge

Scientific method	Research process
State the problem	Formulate and delimit the problem
Gather the facts (collect and organize data)	Review the related literature
Devise experiments to also gather facts	Develop a theoretical framework
Test the hypotheses	Identify the variables
Make the generalizations or deductions	Formulate the hypotheses
Check the truth of the generalization or deduction against reality by means of more experiments and fact gathering	Select a research design
	Collect the data
	Analyze the data
	Interpret the results
	Communicate the findings

study methods, data analysis, and conclusions. Ask if the steps are ordered appropriately and if there is continuity in terms of the focus of the content. Is the conclusion based on actual findings? Is the hypothesis developed from the theoretical rationale?

Control, while almost impossible to achieve totally, is an important facet of the scientific approach (see Chapter 8). To isolate and study specific variables, it is necessary to control as much as possible extraneous influencing factors. To control events and conditions, it is essential to know what these extraneous factors are. For example, it is known that pain perception is influenced by age, sex, culture, and other factors. In examining the relationship between self-esteem and pain perception, the investigator must specify which age group, sex, and culture will be delimited, that is, included and excluded. An alternate approach would be to select a large sample reflecting a variety of ages, sexes, and cultures (see Chapter 14). Then the data would be analyzed for both the total sample and each of the influencing factors. This would yield information about the strength of each factor in terms of study outcomes. In your role as research consumer, you should determine if the sample is representative of the defined population or if there was a bias in the selection process. You should ask how and why the subjects were chosen, whether or not there is support of sample delimitations, and what steps were taken in the procedure for data collection to control the extraneous variables.

EMPIRICISM   Empiricism is the *objectivity* component of the scientific approach, that is, the reality foundation for investigations. Observations are made and verified on the basis of actual information, instead of the personal beliefs or biases of the researcher. In addition, other investigators are able to evaluate and replicate or repeat the empirical inquiry process. Documented evidence of empiricism in research will include objective, appropriate, and stable instruments for data collection, unbiased selection of subjects, and data collection methods and settings that are valid representations of reality. You should evaluate the investigator's use of valid and reliable instruments and unbiased sampling procedures, as well as the controls and setting used in the process of data collection (see Chapters 12, 13, and 14).

GENERALIZATION   One goal of science is to understand relationships among phenomena to predict future outcomes and relationships. Focusing on isolated events would not make it possible to "explain a wide variety of phenomena in a manner that consistently holds and therefore is not tentative" (Chinn and Jacobs, 1983, p.61). The following example will clarify the intent of generalization.

If a nurse-scientist were studying maternal attachment behaviors, there would be more interest in understanding what general factors influence these behaviors, for example, early skin-to-skin contact (Curry, 1982), than in Jane Doe's specific experience. While understanding individuals is important, a more substantive contribution to science can be made based on a broad range of empirical data that have been subjected to repeated investigation.

Questions that elicit information about generalization include the following: When and to whom do the conclusions apply? What are the limits and scope of the findings, for example, in terms of extraneous factors and sample delimitations? Does the investigator generalize beyond the population on which the study was based?

THEORY   As cited in Polit and Hungler (1983), theories "offer an opportunity for bringing together observed events and relationships, for explaining how and why phenomena are associated with one another, and for predicting the occurrence of future events and relationships" (p.22). A theory can be defined as a process of organizing reality into systematically identified relationships among variables to explain and predict phenomena. Through empirical observations and research, theories are developed and tested, and generalizations evolve. As a component of the scientific approach, the theory provides a framework for testing hypotheses. It also guides decision making with regard to defining variables and subsequent interpretation of results. A more detailed discussion of the theoretical framework will be provided in Chapter 6.

Some of the questions to ask as a consumer are the following: Is the theoretical rationale explicitly stated? Are the hypotheses explicitly substantiated, that is, do they clearly emanate from the theory? Are the definitions of variables clear and do they adequately reflect the theory? Are the results interpreted in relation to the theory?

ASSUMPTIONS ABOUT REALITY AND CAUSALITY (DETERMINISM)   Assumptions are basic principles assumed to be true, without need for scientific proof. For example, it has been assumed that people will have pain during their lives, people are mortal, "infants are born with unique, individual characteristics that affect the development of maternal attachment" (Curry, 1982, p.74), and "both nurse-practitioners and physicians identify and manage health problems of their patients" (Chen, Barkauskas, Ohlson, and Chen, 1982, p.164). The first two assumptions are broad and apply to humans in general; the last two are part of the foundations of specific theories. As a final example, Rogers (1970) espouses a particular view of human beings as more than and different from the sum of their parts. This underlying assumption is one of several that form the basis for testing relationships using Rogers' conceptual framework.

Assumptions that guide the scientific approach are that there is an objective reality independent of an individual's perceptions, the world is real, and nature has order, regularity, and consistency. Another assumption relates to determinism, which has to do with causality of phenomena. Events and situations are assumed to have causes. For example, cancer may be the result of several phenomena, such as smoking and certain chemicals and pollutants, and the inflammatory response occurs as a result of certain conditions. This traditional assumption of cause and effect relationships, which has guided much of the activities of scientists, has been challenged in favor of assumptions about mutual and simultaneous interactions among phenomena (Rogers, 1970), from which changed phenomena evolve.

Assumptions are not always stated in an obvious way. They may be implicit rather than explicit, and this is a question you should ask. You should also identify what the assumptions are, if they reflect a specific value orientation, and whether or not there are inconsistencies between assumptions.

• The Relationship Between Theory and Method

As stated earlier, relationships are examined by testing hypotheses that are based on a theoretical framework. That examination takes place under the aegis of order and control, empiricism, assumptions, theory, and generalization. To validate relational statements, an overall design or method must be implemented. That method must also operate in a systematic, controlled way to ensure that "the reality indicators for the conceptual relationship specified by the theory are valid" (Chinn and Jacobs, 1983, p.100). A variety of designs can be used to address the problem under study; however, there must be consistency between the hypothesis or relational statement and the type of design used.

Chapter 8 will focus on the meaning, purpose, and issues related to the research design. Suffice it to say at this point, that as a consumer you should evaluate the overall design and procedure of hypothesis testing, including the setting, instrumentation, conformity to established criteria for implementing the specific design, data collection procedure, and control of extraneous factors, to make sure that there is a relationship between the theory and the method.

• Summary

This chapter serves as an introduction to the sources of human knowledge and characteristics of the scientific approach as they relate to the research process. The relationship between philosophy and science underlies the nursing research effort, a focus of which is the development of nursing knowledge. The philosophical view of the researcher guides the intent and direction of a research project.

There are many sources of human knowledge. Some sources are relatively unstructured, for example, intuition and trial and error approaches; other sources are highly structured, for example, the scientific approach, including inductive and deductive methods of logical reasoning. Both sources play a role in the research process, although the scientific approach is the most advanced and objective method of inquiry.

The scientific approach is a complex process that is systematic and controlled. As an empirical approach, it yields results that are minimally biased in all aspects. Additionally, since a goal of science is to understand relationships among phenomena, a more formal process of inquiry makes it possible to explain a wide variety of phenomena and, at the same time, to make predictions or generalize about future outcomes and relationships.

Theories help organize reality by systematically identifying relations among variables. Through empirical observations and research, theories are developed and tested. Theories also provide a framework for testing hypotheses, that is, statements about relationships, and form the basis for determining the overall design or method of a study. Fundamental to the testing of relationships are the underlying assumptions or the basic principles that are assumed to be true, without need for scientific proof. These assumptions guide the research effort in much the same way as the researcher's philosophical views of human behavior and health.

As research consumers, nurses are called on to judge the soundness of the research approached used, including why and how ideas were generated and related, how hypotheses were derived, what method or design was used, and what assumptions and generalizations were made.

• References

Andreoli, K., and Thompson, C. (1977). The nature of science in nursing, *Image,* **9**:32-37.

Beckwith, J., and Miller, L. (1976). Behind the mask of objective science, *The Sciences,* **16**: 16-19.

Chinn, P., and Jacobs, M. (1983). *Theory and nursing: A systematic approach,* St. Louis, The C.V. Mosby Co.

Chen, S., Barkauskas, V., and Chen, E. (1982). Health problems encountered by nurse practitioners and physicians, *Nursing Research,* 31:163-169.

Curry, M. (1982). Maternal attachment behavior and the mother's self-concept: The effect of early skin-to-skin contact, *Nursing Research,* **31**: 73-78.

Harris, R.B. (1981-82). Clean versus sterile suctioning and inner cannula tracheotomy cleaning technique in relation to level of infection in first week post-operative head and neck surgical patients, *PRN: The Adelphi Report.*

Johnson, D. (1974). Development of theory: A requisite for nursing as a primary health profession. *Nursing Research,* **23**:372-377.

Martinson, I. (1978). Why research in nursing? In N.L. Chaska, ed.: *The nursing profession: views through the mist,* New York, McGraw-Hill Book Co.

Newman, M. (1979). *Theory development in nursing,* Philadelphia, F.A. Davis Co.

Polit, D., and Hungler, B. (1983). *Nursing research: Principles and methods,* 2nd ed., Philadelphia, J.B. Lippincott Co.

Rogers, M. (1970). *An introduction to the theoretical basis of nursing,* Philadelphia, F.A. Davis Co.

Silva, M. (1977). Philosophy, science, theory: Interrelationships and implications for nursing research, *Image,* 9:59-63.

Vaughan, F. (1979). *Awakening intuition,* Garden City, N.Y., Anchor Books.

• Additional readings

Benoliel, J. (1977). The interaction between theory and research, *Nursing Outlook,* **25**:108-113.

Greene, J. (1979). Science, nursing and nursing science: A conceptual analysis, *Advances in Nursing Science,* 2:57-64.

Reynolds, P. (1971). *A primer in theory construction,* Indianapolis, Bobbs-Merrill/Educational Publishing.

Ruchlis, H. (1963). *Discovering scientific method,* New York, Harper & Row, Publishers.

3

Legal and Ethical Issues

Bettie S. Jackson

LEARNING OBJECTIVES

After reading this chapter, the student should be able to do the following:
- Describe the historical background that led to the development of ethical guidelines for the use of human subjects in research.
- Identify the essential elements of an informed consent form.
- Evaluate the adequacy of an informed consent form.
- Discuss the nurse's role in assuring that FDA guidelines for testing of medical devices are followed.
- Describe the Institutional Review Board's role in the research review process.
- Describe the nurse's role as patient advocate in research situations.
- Identify research situations, specifically populations of subjects, that require special consideration when research involving them is considered.

KEY TERMS

anonymity	informed consent
confidentiality	Institutional Review Board
ethics	

Listen, Martin. I am aware that the technique of experimenting on humans without their consent is against any traditional concept of medical ethics. But I believe the results justify the methods. Seventeen young women have unknowingly sacrificed their lives. That is true. But it has been for the betterment of society and the future guarantee of the defense superiority of the United States. From the point of view of each subject, it is a great sacrifice. From the point of view of two hundred million Americans, it is a very small one. Think of how many young women willfully take their lives each year, or how many people kill themselves on the highways, and to what end? Here these seventeen women have added something to society, and they have been treated with compassion. (From Robin Cook, *Brain*, 1981, p.292.)

"When people rely on rules to protect them from harm, they are not interested in pieces of paper but in the conduct of the people who are supposed to be governed by the rules" (Implementing Human Research Regulations, 1983, p.1). Rules and regulations dealing with the involvement of human subjects in research do not necessarily assure that research will be conducted legally and ethically. Researchers themselves and the caregivers that provide for the clients who also happen to be research subjects must be fully committed to the tenets of informed consent and clients' rights. The principle of "the ends justifying the means" must never be tolerated.

This chapter deals with the legal and ethical considerations that must be taken before, during, and after conducting research. Researchers and the caregivers of research subjects should take every precaution to protect the people being studied from physical or mental harm or discomfort (Polit and Hungler, 1983, p.29). It is not always clear what constitutes harm or discomfort. This chapter will trace the historical development of the concept of informed consent. It will discuss the systems that have been established to oversee the rights of people who are potential and actual research subjects. Research on special groups of potential subjects, such as the elderly or the incompetent, will be discussed. The nurse as a client advocate, whether she functions in her role as a researcher or caregiver, will also be discussed.

• Ethical and Legal Considerations in Research

Developments in the field of biostatistics over the last 80 years have enabled scientists to combine their new knowledge with the analytical means to evaluate the effects of their interventions. For example, advanced statistics and computers have made it possible to analyze the outcomes of therapies between control and experimental groups to determine if any differences are statistically significant. These powerful analytic abilities have enabled researchers to experiment with subjects in ways that were not previously possible.

Ethical and legal considerations in regard to research first received attention with the post-World War II Nuremburg Military Tribunal. This Tribunal's prosecution of Karl Brandt and others represented the first major effort of the law to cope with the problems of modern biomedical research. Before the Tribunal could measure the activities of the defendants, a set of basic principles of ethical, moral, and legal concepts for the conduct of acceptable experiments had to be written as the standard (Creighton, 1977, p.337). Among the 10 rules included in the Nuremburg Code still in use today are the following:

1. Voluntary consent of the human subject is essential.
2. Experiments should be so designed and based on the results of animal experimentation* and knowledge of the natural history of the disease or other problems that the anticipated results will justify the experiment.
3. The degree of risk to be taken by the subject should never exceed the potential humanitarian importance of the problem to be solved.
4. Through all stages of the experiment the highest degree of skill and care should be required of those who conduct or engage in it, and the experiment should be conducted only by scientifically qualified persons.†
5. At any time during the course of the experiment, the human subject should be at liberty to end his participation in the experiment.
6. The scientist in charge must be prepared to terminate the experiment at any stage if there is probable cause to believe that continuation of the experiment is likely to result in injury, disability, or the death of the experimental subject.‡

INFORMED CONSENT

Informed consent is simply defined by Polit and Hungler (p.615) as "an ethical principle that requires researchers to obtain the voluntary participation of subjects after informing them of possible risks and benefits." However, informed consent goes beyond

---

*While this chapter will not cover the subject, there are guidelines for the conduct of research involving animals. The research office at your school or employing agency should be consulted when animal experimentation is considered or encountered.

†It would be inappropriate for a nurse-midwife to conduct research on cancer clients. If these cancer clients were pregnant, then special consultation regarding cancer aspects should be sought. A researcher is often required to submit a curriculum vitae to the appropriate research review board to determine the expertise of the researcher in the field under study.

‡Several years ago this writer coauthored an article on the LeVeen shunt (Seybert, P.L., Gordon, K., and Jackson, B.S. [1979]. The LeVeen shunt: new hope for ascites patients, *Nursing '79*, **9**(1): 24-31, January). Dr. LeVeen wrote the authors to compliment them on the article but to also comment on his research. At the time of the study, clients with ascites were randomly assigned to one of two groups, those who received medical management and those who received surgical implantation of the LeVeen shunt. It was clear to the researchers partway into the study that the group receiving surgical intervention was faring much better. The experiment was terminated before assessing the number of subjects that had originally been planned. It would have been unethical and perhaps illegal, that is, malpractice or failure to provide the acceptable standard of care, to continue the experiment.

just this point. To safeguard the basic human right of self-determination, free and informed consent is expected to include the following: an explanation of the study; the procedures to be followed and their purposes; a description of physical and mental crisis or discomforts, any invasion of privacy, and any threat to dignity; and the methods used to protect anonymity and ensure confidentiality. The client should also be informed of alternate courses available (ANA Commission on Nursing Research, 1975 and Gargano, 1978, p.167).

While quite simplistically the tenets of informed consent make good sense, seem easy to follow, and everyone should, could, and does follow them, in fact that has not been the case. Before the 1970s there is essentially no mention of informed consent in the nursing research texts. The federal guidelines involving human subjects in research that will be discussed in this chapter were not developed until the mid-1970s, and in fact unethical research took place here in the United States even in the 1960s and 1970s. Some of the most atrocious and hence memorable are worth mentioning as sad reminders of our own tarnished research heritage, as well as some of the more difficult conundrums encountered when research involving human subjects is undertaken.

In the 1965 case of *Hyman v The Jewish Chronic Disease Hospital,* New York, it was revealed that aged and senile clients were subjected to live cancer cells to study their rejection responses. Effective consent had not been obtained. Fraud and deceit had been used in dealing with the subjects. The two physicians involved were placed on probation for 1 year. They claimed that they did not wish to evoke emotional reactions or refusals to participate by informing the subjects of the nature of the study.

In the infamous Milledgeville, Georgia case exposed in 1969, investigational drugs were used on mentally disabled children without first obtaining the opinion of a clinical psychiatrist, and there was no explicit review or institutional approval of the program before implementation.

It must be emphasized here, and it will be repeated later, that researchers themselves must not take the privilege nor are they vested with the privilege of determining such things as risk-benefit ratios and who is and who is not competent to give consent. From their expertise they may suggest such things, but then an objective panel of experts from the professional and public communities must review these plans before the research is ever conducted.

This final example draws from the 1973 suit of the infamous Tuskegee, Alabama syphilis study. For over 40 years the United States Public Health Service conducted a study using two groups of black males. One group consisted of those who had untreated syphilis and the second group consisted of about half as many who were judged to be free of the disease. During the study no treatment for syphilis was provided. Withholding treatment remained part of the study even after penicillin became generally available in the 1950s. Steps were even taken to keep the subjects from obtaining it. The charge that low-income and poorly educated people are used for research is hard to deny in this case.

While it seems clear that these three cases were clinical research studies, what constitutes *research versus clinical evaluation* is not always clear. When the formalities of the research review process should be pursued may seem vague at times. While it is advisable to err in the direction of conservatism and seek out a formal, objective review of the plan for informed consent, this is not always done. Sometimes the reason is naiveté, although this is less and less of an acceptable excuse, and sometimes the reason is because the investigator unilaterally determines that to do so would be less than expeditious.

PRODUCT TESTING

Nurses are often approached by manufacturers to test products on clients. Moore (1984) points out that all nurses should be aware of the Food and Drug Administration (FDA) guidelines and regulations for the *testing of medical devices* before initiating any form of clinical testing. Medical devices are classified under Section 513 in the Federal Food, Drug, and Cosmetic Act according to the extent of control necessary to ensure safety and effectiveness of each device. The classes are as follows:

Class I: General controls. Included in Class I are devices whose safety and effectiveness can be reasonably assured by the general controls of the Good Manufacturing Practices Regulations (GMP). The GMP part of the act ensures that manufacturers will follow specific guidelines for packaging, storing, and providing specific product instructions. An example of Class I devices is ostomy supplies.

Class II: Performance standards. General controls are insufficient in this class to ensure the safety and efficacy of the product, and the manufacturer must provide information to give this assurance. Devices included in Class II are cardiac pacemakers, sutures, surgical metallic mesh, and biopsy needs.

Class III: Premarket approval. This class includes devices whose safety and effectiveness are insufficiently ensured by general controls and performance standards. These products are represented to be life-sustaining, life-supporting, implanted into the body, or present a potential, unreasonable risk or illness or injury to the client. Devices in this class are required to have approved applications for premarket approval. Extensive laboratory, animal, and human studies, which often require 2 to 3 years to complete, are required for Class III devices. Examples include heart valves, bone cements, contact lenses, and implantables left in the body for 30 days or longer.

It is important for nurses to be aware of their own institution's policies toward product testing. The class of the device will obviously make a difference as to how the institution will react. If a nurse suspects that, for example, a Class II device is being tested in an ad hoc or unauthorized manner and without client consent, she should discuss this with her supervisor and other appropriate authorities.

Unauthorized Research

It is not unusual for ad hoc or informal and *unauthorized research* to go on. While it may seem to be harmless, again it is not the purview of the investigator to make that determination. Nurses must carefully avoid being involved in ad hoc research for the following reasons:

1. These treatments or methods of care are usually not monitored as closely for untoward effects, hence exposing the client to unwarranted risk
2. The clients' rights to informed consent in clinical trials are not protected
3. The success or failure of these unrecorded trials contribute nothing to the organized scientific knowledge of the efficacy or complications of the treatment
4. The lack of independent quality supervision allows deviations from the adopted experimental program that may eliminate the program's effectiveness (Hanks, 1984).

• • •

There are additional considerations that must be taken from an ethical perspective. Generally speaking, the public trusts caregivers, especially nurses and physicians. It sometimes puts the caregiver in an awkward role to ask the client to also permit her to perform research. There might be risks inherent in the research that do not exist in the care. Even when these risks are clearly identified, and they must be, is the caregiver comfortable when posing those risks? Is she convinced that the benefits outweigh the risks? Will the client feel comfortable in refusing to participate in the caregiver's research while continuing to require her care? Has it been made clear to the client, as it must, that he may refuse to participate or may withdraw from the study without consequence or compromise to his care or his relationship to the institution? What if harm occurs? Will the research cost the client additional money, is it warranted, and has he been apprised, as he must be?

Numbers of books and articles have been written on this subject. They are introduced here to illustrate that the legal and ethical concepts behind research and informed consent are rarely clear-cut. The nurse researcher or the nurse who is involved in any way with a research project must raise cogent questions for herself when evaluating the ethics and legal points of the research.

• Federal Guidelines Regarding Ethical and Legal Considerations of Research Involving Human Subjects

INSTITUTIONAL REVIEW BOARDS

The *National Research Act* (P.L. 93-348) was passed on July 12, 1974. The subject was *Institutional Review Boards,* (IRBs) *Ethics Guidance Program.* Quite simply it requires that any agency, such as a hospital or school, applying for a grant or contract for any project or program involving biomedical or behavioral research using human subjects must submit with its application assurances that it has established an institutional Review Board (IRB) to review the research and protect the rights of the human subjects of such research. At agencies where no federal grants or contracts have been awarded there is usually a review mechanism resembling the IRB system.

The IRB must have at least five members of various backgrounds to promote a complete and adequate project review. The members must be qualified through their expertise and experience and reflect a racial and cultural diversity. The IRB must have both men and women as members and may not consist of only one profession. The IRB must have one member whose concerns are primarily nonscientific, such as a lawyer, a member of the clergy, or an ethicist. At least one member must be from outside the agency.

The IRB's function is to review research and report any serious or continuing noncompliance by investigators. The IRB has the authority to approve research, require modifications, or disapprove research activities. A researcher must receive some form of IRB approval, such as expedited, exempt, emergency-compassionate, or full review, before beginning to conduct research.

To approve research, the IRB must determine that the following Code of Federal Regulations has been satisfied:

1. The risks to the subjects are minimized.
2. The risks to the subjects are reasonable in relation to the anticipated benefits.
3. The selection of the subjects is equitable.
4. Informed consent in one of several possible forms must and will be sought from each prospective subject or the subject's legally authorized representative.
5. The informed consent must be properly documented.
6. Where appropriate, the research plan makes adequate provision for monitoring the data collected to ensure the subjects' safety.
7. Where appropriate, there are adequate provisions to protect the privacy of the subjects and the confidentiality of the data.
8. Where some or all of the subjects are likely to be vulnerable to coercion or undue influence, such as persons with acute or severe physical or mental illness or persons who are economically or educationally disadvantaged, appropriate additional safeguards are included.

IRBs have the authority to suspend or terminate approval of research that is not conducted in accordance with IRB requirements or that has been associated with unexpected serious harm to the subjects.

IRBs have a mechanism for reviewing research in an expedited manner when there is minimal risk to the research subjects. Once again, it is worth mentioning that the researcher may determine that a project involves minimal risk, but the IRB makes the final determination and research may not be undertaken until then. An expedited review usually shortens the length of the review process. A full list of research categories eligible for an expedited review is available from any IRB office and includes the following:

1. The collection of hair and nail clippings in a nondisfiguring manner
2. The collection of excreta and external secretions including sweat
3. The recording of data from subjects 18 years of age or older, using noninvasive procedures routinely employed in clinical practice
4. Voice recordings
5. The study of existing data, documents, records, pathological specimens, or diagnostic data

Note that an expedited review does not automatically exempt the researcher from obtaining informed consent.

The *Federal Register* periodically contains updated information of federal guidelines for research involving human subjects. Every researcher should consult with an agency's research office to ensure that the application being prepared adheres to the most current requirements. A nurse involved in research, such as caring for research subjects, may consult the agency's research office to determine if the study is being conducted according to the most up-to-date regulations.

GUIDELINES FOR INFORMED CONSENT

There have been a number of references to informed consent already. This section deals with what informed consent is and what constitutes an acceptable informed consent form.

No investigator may involve a human being as a research subject before obtaining the legally effective informed consent of the subject or the subject's legally authorized representative. Prospective subjects must have time to decide if they want to participate, and the investigator must not coerce the subject into participating. The language of the consent form must be understandable. The subject in no way should be asked to waive his rights or to release the investigator or the institution from liability for negligence according to the Code of Federal Regulations.

The following are basic elements of an informed consent form:

1. A statement that the study involves research, an explanation of the purposes of the research, a delineation of the expected duration of the subject's participation, a description of the procedures to be followed, and an identification of any procedures that are experimental

2. A description of any reasonably foreseeable risks or discomforts to the subjects

3. A description of any benefits to the subject or to others that may reasonably be expected from the research

4. A disclosure of appropriate alternative procedures or courses of treatment, if any, that might be advantageous to the subject

5. A statement describing to what extent, if any, the confidentiality of the records identifying the subject will be maintained

6. For research involving more than minimal risk, an explanation as to whether any medical treatments are available if injury occurs and, if so, what they consist of, or where further information may be obtained

7. An explanation of who to contact for answers to pertinent questions about the research and research subjects' rights, and who to contact in the event of a research-related injury to the subject

8. A statement that participation is voluntary, that refusal to participate will not involve any penalty or loss of benefits to which the subject is otherwise entitled, and the subject may discontinue participation at any time without any penalty or loss of otherwise entitled benefits

ANONYMITY AND CONFIDENTIALITY

Anonymity and confidentiality in research are usually assured in writing. This is sometimes difficult in unique research situations that capture the public's attention, for example, Dr. Barney Clark, the first recipient of the artificial heart. *Anonymity* is the protection of the participant in a study so that even the researcher cannot link the subject with the information provided (Polit and Hungler, p.609). Often one will see written on an informed consent form a statement to the effect that the data are pooled, hence it is impossible to identify one research subject from an aggregate. That also makes it impossible for a subject to withdraw from a study once the data have been pooled. *Confidentiality* is slightly different from anonymity and protects the participants in a study so that their individual identities will not be linked to the information that they provided and publicly divulged.

There are exceptions to these guidelines and situations where the IRB might grant waivers or amend its process or guidelines. The researcher is advised to consult with the IRB in individual and unusual circumstances. The boxed material on pp. 38 and 39 provides a specific example of an informed consent.

Generally the signed informed consent form is given to the subject. The researcher may also wish to keep a copy. Some research, such as a retrospective chart audit, may not require informed consent. In some cases where minimal risk is involved, the investigator may only have to provide the subject with an information sheet. The IRB will give advice on these matters and make the final determination as to the most appropriate documentation format.

• Special Legal and Ethical Considerations in Research: Incompetent and Vulnerable People as Potential Research Subjects

This section serves as an overview to ethical and legal considerations that must be taken when particularly *vulnerable* or *incompetent populations* are identified as potential research subjects. Researchers are advised to consult their agency's RB for the most recent federal and state rules and guidelines when considering research involving the elderly, children, the mentally ill, prisoners, the deceased, the unborn, and students. In addition researchers should consult the IRB before planning research that potentially involves an oversubscribed research population. Such as organ transplant clients, or "captive" and convenient populations such as students.

It should be emphasized that special populations do not preclude the research being done; extra precautions must be taken, however, to protect their rights.

Davis (1981a) reminds us that a society can be judged by the way it treats its most vulnerable people, a point worth remembering in research that involves the elderly. In addition, Davis continues a cogent argument, "To insure continuing progress in pediatric research and practice, experimentation is necessary. If the consent requirement is taken seriously to the point of excluding research in children, then children themselves will be the ultimate sufferers" (1981b, p.247).

Mitchell cites the classic 1965 Darling case where physicians and nurses were found negligent in the care of a teenager who lost his leg because of poor cast

The Caldwell Medical Center
Code No. _____

Informed Consent

I understand that I am being treated with the drug *cis*-platin, which may cause the unpleasant side effects of nausea and vomiting. Treatment to control these side effects includes using various medications, reducing the intake of food and fluids before chemotherapy, maintaining a quiet environment, and accepting support from others. In addition, I understand that using various coping strategies is helpful to persons in similar situations.

I understand that the purpose of this study is to help clients learn some coping technques and evaluate how their use affects the occurrence of nausea and vomiting after *cis*-platin is administered. If I agree to participate in this research study, I understand that I will be randomly assigned to one of the following three nursing treatment programs:

1. I will meet with one of the investigators before I receive my chemotherapy. We will discuss my experience and the methods that other clients and I have found helpful.

or

2. I will meet with one of the investigators before I receive my chemotherapy. I will follow directions for practicing a technique that produces, under my own control, a state of altered consciousness called self-hypnosis. I will be asked to practice this technique during and after receiving my chemotherapy. I will be expected to practice this technique daily so that I may learn to use it without being directed by another person.

or

3. I will be given the customary nursing care that is rendered to every client taking the drugs that I am receiving.

In addition, if necessary I will receive only the medication Reglan to control nausea and vomiting.

I understand that in no case will I receive less than the customary standard and expected level of nursing care that I am already receiving.

I understand that if I am selected to be in Group 2, a simple test to determine my susceptibility to this technique will be performed. Most people are susceptible, but if I am not and wish to continue in the study, I will be randomly assigned to one of the two remaining groups.

I understand that this research study has been discussed with my physician and that he is aware of my participation. The treatments prescribed to control the side effects of nausea and vomiting will not be altered if I participate in this study.

I understand that a nurse investigator will be in my room while my chemotherapy is ending and for 4 hours after the treatment. I understand that nursing care will be provided by the nurses on the unit and not by the nurse investigator. The research nurse will be taking notes on my reactions to the chemotherapy. Once an hour she will ask me to rate my nausea. I can expect that this will only take a few minutes of my time and if I am sleeping, I will not be awakened.

I have been told that this routine will be followed for three courses of chemotherapy, during three separate hospitalizations.

I understand that the benefits from this treatment are that I may experience less nausea and vomiting or fewer of the feelings of being sick to my stomach that often occur with *cis*-platin. There are no side effects or risks from my participation.

My participation is voluntary and I may choose to not participate or withdraw at any time without jeopardizing my future treatment.

My identity will not be revealed in any way. My name will be encoded so that I will remain anonymous.

I also understand that if I believe I have sustained an injury as a result of participating in this research study, I may contact the investigators, Ms. B.J. Simon at 608-0011 or B.A. Smith at 124-6142, or the Office of the Institutional Review Board at 124-2500 so that I can review the matter and identify the medical resources that may be available to me.

I understand the following statements:

1. The Caldwell Medical Center will furnish whatever emergency medical care that the medical staff of this hospital determine to be necessary.

2. I will be responsible for the cost of such emergency care personally, through my medical insurance, or by another form of coverage.

3. No monetary compensation for wages lost as a result of an injury will be paid to me by the Caldwell Medical Center.

4. I will receive a copy of this consent form.

_____   _____
Date   Patient

_____   _____
Witness   Investigator

The Institutional Review Board of the Caldwell Medical Center has approved the solicitation of subjects for participation in this research proposal.

application and observation. "In addition to serving as advocates for the psychologic as well as physical welfare of children, nurses are legally accountable for protecting children's rights and reporting inappropriate actions of other health professionals" (Mitchell, 1984, p.9).

Mitchell discussed the National Commission's concept of assent versus consent in regard to pediatric research. Assent contains the following three fundamental elements: a basic understanding of what the child will be expected to do and what will be done to the child, a comprehension of the basic purpose of the research, and an ability to express a preference regarding participation. In contrast to assent, consent requires a relatively advanced level of cognitive ability. Informed consent reflects competency standards requiring abstract appreciation and reasoning regarding the information provided. The issue of assent versus consent is an interesting one when determining at what age can children make meaningful decisions about participating in research. Based on the work by Piaget regarding cognitive ability, children at age 6 and older can participate in giving assent. Children at age 14 and older, while they are not legally authorized to give sole consent unless they are emancipated minors, can make such decisions as capably as adults (Mitchell, 1984).

Federal regulations require parental permission whenever a child is involved in research unless otherwise specified, for example, child abuse or mature minors at minimal risk. If the research involves more than a minimal risk and does not offer direct benefit to the individual child, both parents must give permission. When an individual reaches maturity, at age 18 in cases of research, he may render his own consent. He may do so at a younger age if he has been legally declared an emancipated minor. Questions regarding this should be addressed to the IRB or research administration office and not left to the discrimination of the researcher to answer.

No vulnerable population may be singled out for study because it is simply convenient. For example, prisoners may not be studied simply because they are an available and convenient group. Prisoners may be studied if the study pertains, for example, to the effects and processes of incarceration. Students are often convenient groups of subjects to research. They must not be singled out as research subjects because of convenience, but the research questions must have some bearing on their status as students.

• The Nurse as Researcher and Client Advocate

This section addresses the concept of the *nurse as a client advocate* in her role as caregiver or researcher.

The American Nurses' Association Commission on Nursing Research affirmed the profession's obligation to support the advancement of scientific knowledge. The ANA supports two sets of human rights in this regard. One set is concerned with the rights of qualified nurses to engage in research and to have access to the resources necessary for implementing scientific investigations. The second set deals with the rights of all persons who are recipients of health care services or who are participants in research performed by investigators whose studies impinge on the care provided by nurses.

The relationship of trust between client and nurse is an essential element of the professional code of ethics. This trust between client-subject and investigator requires that the researcher assume a special obligation to safeguard the subject. The nurse as researcher or caregiver must assure the client of the following:

1. The subject's rights will not be violated without his voluntary and informed consent.
2. No risk, discomfort, invasion of privacy, or threat to dignity beyond that initially stated in describing the subject's role in the study will be imposed without further permission being obtained.
3. The subject is assured that if he does not wish to participate in the study, he will neither be subjected to harrassment, nor will the quality of his care be influenced by this decision *(ANA Human Rights Guidelines, 1975)*.

Upon employment, a nurse should ask about what is expected of her regarding research. Will she be required to collect data or provide medicines or treatments in double-blind studies? Is she free not to participate? Are written protocols available for reference? Has the IRB ruled on each protocol? Is she free to decline participation without jeopardizing her position?

The ANA Human Rights Guidelines for Nurses state that "conditions of employment in settings in which clinical and/or other research is in progress need to be spelled out in detail for all potential workers. As a corollary, it follows that anyone employed in work that carries the potential of risk to others needs to be advised as to the types of risks involved, the ways of recognizing when risk is present, and the proper actions to take to counteract harmful effects and unnecessary danger."

Ignorance and naiveté in the face of ethical and legal guidelines for the conduct of research must never be an excuse for a nurse's failure to be a client advocate in research situations.

• Reviewing Research Involving the Use of Human Subjects

It is customary today when presenting a research report at a meeting or in a publication to comment that before conducting the research the project was reviewed by the IRB and the following plans, which are then described, were approved for the use of human subjects. It is likely that a paper will not be accepted for publication without such a discussion. It is often brief, no more than two or three sentences, but it tells the reader that the ethical and legal guidelines that have been discussed throughout this chapter have been applied in the conduct of that particular project. This also makes it almost impossible to report on informal, ad hoc research as has been described earlier. In addition, the public's trust in nurses as client advocates will be reaffirmed in their researcher role if the concept of human rights is discussed as a basic tenet preempting any scientific investigation.

It should be apparent from the preceding sections that while the need for guidelines for the use of human subjects in research was quite evident, and the principles themselves are clear, there are many instances when the nurse must use her best judgment both as a client advocate and as a researcher when evaluating the ethical nature of a research project. In any research situation, the basic guiding principle of protecting the client must always apply. When conflicts arise, the nurse must feel free to raise suitable questions with the appropriate resources and personnel. These may include the nursing supervisor, the director of nursing research, and the chairman of the IRB. The nurse should pursue answers to her questions about the clients as research subjects and her role in the project until she is satisfied that the client's rights and her rights as a professional nurse are protected.

• Summary

Since the National Research Act was passed in 1974, the federal government has taken special precautions to protect the rights of human research subjects. Institutional Review Boards (IRBs) were established at agencies conducting research to review all proposed research involving human subjects before the project is initiated. Ethical and legal guidelines are the underlying principles used by researchers to design protocols and IRBs to review them. No investigator may unilaterally determine the risk-benefit ratios inherent in the project and then conduct it without IRB approval. In addition, ignorance of ethical and legal guidelines directing the conduct of human research is no excuse for not following the proper review system.

This chapter reviews the historical evolution of the concept of informed consent constructed at the Nuremburg Tribunals after World War II. The concept of informed consent in research was discussed, giving examples from relatively recent research in the United States that by current standards would be considered unethical. The point was emphasized throughout for determining whether research is ethical and beneficial.

The National Research Act of 1974 was described followed by IRBs, that were mandated in all institutions receiving federal funds. The IRBs objectively review research proposals for the involvement of human subjects and evaluate the risk-benefit ratio.

Guidelines for adequate informed consent were listed and examples were given. Special considerations for children, the elderly, and the incompetent were discussed.

Finally, the concept of the nurse as caregiver and researcher was discussed. Nurses are first and foremost client advocates. They must always work to assure that the clients' rights have been ethically and legally considered before they participate in research.

• References

American Nurses' Association (1975). Commission on Nursing Research, Human Rights Guidelines for Nurses in Clinical and Other Research-er, Kansas City, Missouri.

Code of Federal Regulations, 45 CFR 46, Protection of human subjects, OPRR Reports, Revised March 8, 1983.

Cook, R. (1981). *Brain*, New York, Signet.

Creighton, H. (1977). Legal concerns of nursing research, *Nursing Research*, 26(5):337-340.

Davis, A. (1981a). Ethical consideration in gerontological nursing research, *Geriatric Nursing*, pp.269-272.

Davis, A. (1981b). Ethical issues in nursing research, *Western Journal of Nursing Research*, 3(2):247-248.

Gargano, W.J. (1978). Cancer nursing and the law: informed consent, Part II, *Cancer Nursing*, 167-168.

Hanks, G.E. (1983). Implementing human research regulations: second biennial report on the adequacy and uniformity of federal rules and policies, and of their implementation, for the protection of human subjects. In President's Commission for the Study of Ethical Problems in Medicine and Biomedical and Behavioral Research. March, 1983.

Hanks, G.E. (1984). The dangers of ad hoc protocols, *Journal of Clinical Oncology,* **2**(10):1177-1178.

Mitchell, K. (1984). Protecting children's rights during research, *Pediatric Nursing,* p.9.

Moore, L. (1984). Conducting clinical trials, *Journal of Enterostomal Therapy,* **11**:229-232.

Polit, D.F., and Hungler, B.P. (1983). *Nursing research: Principles and methods,* 2nd ed., Philadelphia, J.B. Lippincott Co.

• Additional Readings

Annas, G.J., and Healey, J. (1974). The patient rights advocate, *Journal of Nursing Administration,* **4**:25-31.

Appelbaum, P.S., and Roth, L.H. (1982). Competency to consent to research, *Archives of General Psychiatry,* **39**:951-958.

Armiger, S.B. (1977). Ethics of nursing research: profiles, principles, perspective, *Nursing Research,* **26**(5):330-336.

Goldberg, R.J. (1984). Disclosure of information to adult cancer patients: issues and update, *Journal of Clinical Oncology,* **2**(8):948-955, August.

Levine, R.J. (1983). Research involving children: an interpretation of the new regulations, *IRB: A Review of Human Subjects Research,* **5**(4) A1-5.

May, K.A. (1979). The nurse as researcher: impediment to informed consent? *Nursing Outlook,* **27**(1):36-39.

Robinson, G., and Merav, A. (1976). Informed consent: recall by patients tested postoperatively, *The Annals of Thoracic Surgery,* **22**(3):209-212, September.

Wilcox, R., Gerber, R.M., and DeWalt, E. (1977). Clinical research in nursing homes, *Nursing Outlook,* **25**(4):255-257.

TWO

THE
RESEARCH
PROCESS

The following chapters will introduce you to the systematic and orderly conduction of the research process and its relationship to the establishment of nursing theory, practice, and education based on research studies. Understanding the step-by-step process that researchers use will assist you in judging the soundness of research investigations. As you proceed through the chapters, research terminology pertinent to each step will be identified and exemplified. The steps of the research process generally proceed in the order outlined in the text but may vary depending on the nature of the research problem. It is important to remember that a researcher may vary the order of the steps slightly, but the steps must still be addressed in an orderly and systematic manner.

4

The Problem Statement

Judith Haber

LEARNING OBJECTIVES

After reading this chapter, the student will be able to do the following:

- Describe the relationship of the problem statement to the other components of the research process.
- Describe the process of identifying and refining a research problem.
- Identify the criteria for determining the significance of a research problem.
- Identify the characteristics of a research problem.
- Formulate a problem statement.
- Identify the criteria for critiquing a problem statement.
- Apply the critiquing criteria to the evaluation of a problem statement in a research report.

KEY TERMS

dependent variable	testability
independent variable	theory
population	variable
problem statement	

Formulating a problem statement is one of the key steps in the research process. It is the starting point of any research study. But selecting and defining the problem is often a difficult task, particularly for those who are just becoming acquainted with the research process. The task is difficult for several reasons. One reason is the bewildering array of possible topics to study, even in just one area. There are so many aspects of a topic to study that it is difficult to choose just one piece of the pie. Another reason is that a beginning researcher often lacks familiarity with the previous research studies done in a specific area. Yet another difficulty is selecting a problem to study if the beginning researcher is unsure of what the research process entails and what constitutes a researchable problem.

The ability to critique a problem statement is as important as the ability to formulate such a statement. The beginning researcher must have a working knowledge of what a problem statement is, the standards for writing one, and a set of guidelines for its evaluation.

This chapter introduces the ways that researchers formulate a problem statement and the research consumer's criteria for evaluating the merit of a problem statement.

• Exploring A Problem Area

The researcher spends a great deal of time selecting a problem for study. This process should not be hurried because it is the crux of the research project and provides an orderly direction for the remainder of the endeavor. This phase of the research process involves both thoughtful reflection and creativity to arrive at a problem that is specific, significant, interesting, and researchable.

Students may wonder where ideas for research studies come from. They may be uncertain about how a topic is selected and may feel that their inexperience hampers their ability to develop or assess an appropriate problem for study. It is reassuring to find that a problem or topic is not pulled out of thin air. A research problem should indicate that practical experience, a critical appraisal of the scientific literature, or an interest in an untested theory has provided the basis for the germination of a research idea. Table 4-1 illustrates how each of the preceding areas can influence the generation of ideas for a research problem.

• *Table 4-1* **How Practical Experience, Scientific Literature, and Untested Theory Influence the Development of a Research Idea**

Area	Influence	Example
Practical experience	Clinical practice provides a wealth of experience from which research problems can be derived. The nurse may observe the occurrence of a particular event or pattern and become curious about why it occurs as well as its relationship to other factors in the client's environment.	A nurse working on an oncology unit observes that certain clients appear to have a delayed grief reaction after being diagnosed as having a recurring malignancy. They seem to mourn ineffectively and often end up angry or hopeless. On the other hand, other clients appear to go through the stages of grieving in a systematic way and usually emerge with a more positive philosophical attitude. The nurse notes the differences in the two groups of clients and speculates about other factors that might contribute to this difference, such as open family communication patterns.
Critical appraisal of the scientific literature	The critical appraisal of research studies that appear in journals may indirectly suggest a problem area by stimulating the reader's thinking. The nurse may observe a conflict or inconsistency in the findings of several related research studies and wonder which findings are most valid.	A nurse working on a medical-surgical unit reads two research articles on methods for promoting wound healing in decubitus ulcers. Both studies propose similar theoretical rationales for the method of treatment, yet both propose different treatment protocols. One study reports significant findings and the other does not. The nurse thinks, "There is a conflict in this literature. How do I evaluate the discrepancy in these findings?"

Continued.

• *Table 4-1* **How Practical Experience, Scientific Literature, and Untested Theory Influence the Development of a Research Idea—cont'd**

Area	Influence	Example
Gaps in the literature	A research idea may be suggested by a research report that offers other areas for future study. Research ideas can be generated by research reports that suggest the value of replicating a particular study to extend or refine the existing scientific knowledge base.	A nurse working on a pediatric unit observes that children on prolonged steroid therapy appear to have a significant change in their body image. However, when the literature is reviewed relative to this topic, no research studies in this area are uncovered that would provide a scientific basis for this nurse's observations.
Interest in untested theory	Verification of an untested nursing theory provides a relatively uncharted territory from which research problems can be derived. Inasmuch as theories themselves are not tested, a researcher may think about investigating a particular concept or set of concepts related to a particular nursing theory. The deductive process would be used to generate the research problem. The researcher would pose questions such as, "If this theory is correct what kind of behavior would I expect to observe in particular clients and under which conditions?" or, "If this theory is valid, what kind of supporting evidence would I find?"	A nurse researcher utilizes Orem's self-care model, which views the person as a self-care agent, as the basis of a research study designed to verify particular aspects of this theory. A study is designed to investigate factors influencing self-care abilities in diabetic clients. Orem's theory provides the conceptual framework for the study.

• Refining the Problem Statement

The problem statement should reflect a refinement of the researcher's thinking. The evaluator of a research study should be able to discern that the researcher has done the following:

1. Defined a specific problem area
2. Reviewed the relevant scientific literature
3. Examined the problem's potential significance to nursing
4. Pragmatically examined the research problem's feasibility

DEFINING THE PROBLEM AREA

Defining a problem area or topic is essentially a creative process. Unfortunately, the evaluator of a research study is not privy to this process since it occurred during the study's conceptualization. Since that is the case, let us provide you with a glimpse of what the process of defining a problem area may be like for a researcher.

The researcher may have started with a list of general topics such as mother-infant relationships, family communication patterns, factors contributing to pain, or pediatric anxiety-reducing techniques to implement before open-heart surgery. General areas of interest are narrowed and defined so that the topic is more specific and circumscribed. A good research problem must have a specific focus. Having a narrowly defined problem does not mean that the topic is trivial or insignificant.

Consultation with teachers, advisors, or colleagues may provide valuable feedback that helps the beginning researcher to focus on a specific problem area. For example, the researcher may have told a faculty advisor that the area of interest was mother-infant relationships. The advisor may have said, "What is it about the topic that specifically interests you?" Such a conversation may have initiated a chain of thought that resulted in a decision to explore mother-infant attachment. This example illustrates how a broad area of interest—mother-infant relationships—was narrowed to a specific research topic—mother-infant attachment.

BEGINNING THE LITERATURE REVIEW

The literature review should reveal that the scientific literature relevant to the problem area has been critically examined (see Chapter 5). In the previous example of mother-infant attachment the researcher may have conducted a preliminary review of books and journals for theories and research studies regarding factors apparently critical to the attachment process. These factors should be potentially relevant, of interest, and measurable. Possible relevant factors mentioned in the literature would include any measurable maternal attachment behaviors, the suggested importance of body contact immediately after an awake delivery, and the possibility that attachment is established by the third postpartum month. This information could then be used by the researcher to further define the research problem. At this point, the researcher could write the following tentative problem statement:

Is body contact immediately after delivery related to the mother's attachment to her newborn infant?

Although the problem statement is not yet in its final form, the reader can envision the interrelatedness between the initial definition of the problem area, the literature review, and the refined problem statement. The person reading a research report examines the end product of this formulation process and thus should have an appreciation for this time-consuming effort.

SIGNIFICANCE

Before proceeding to a final formulation of the problem statement, it is crucial for the researcher to have examined the problem's potential significance to nursing. The research problem should have the potential for contributing to and extending the scientific body of nursing knowledge. The problem does not have to be of prize-winning caliber to be significant. However, it should meet the following criteria:

- Clients, nurses, the medical community in general and society will potentially benefit from the knowledge derived from this study.
- The results will be applicable for nursing practice, education, or administration.
- The results will be theoretically relevant.
- The findings will lend support to untested theoretical assumptions, challenge an existing theory, or clarify a conflict in the literature.
- The findings will potentially formulate or alter nursing practices or policies.

If the research problem has not met any of these criteria, it would be wise to extensively revise the problem or discard it.

FEASIBILITY

The feasibility of a research problem needs to be pragmatically examined. Regardless of how significant or researchable a problem may be, pragmatic considerations such as time; the availability of subjects, facilities, equipment, and money; the experience of the researcher; and any ethical considerations may cause the researcher to decide that the problem is inappropriate because it lacks feasibility (see Chapters 3 and 8).

• The Final Problem Statement

The final problem statement consists of an interrogative sentence or statement about the relationship between two or more variables (Kerlinger, 1973). The problem is stated in question form because this is the most direct way to pose a problem. The answer to the question posed by the problem statement will be sought in the research study. An example of an interrogative problem statement is the following:

What is the relationship between early ambulation and wound healing?

A good problem statement exhibits the following four characteristics:

- It clearly and unambiguously identifies the variables under consideration.
- It clearly expresses the variables' relationship to each other.
- It specifies the nature of the population being studied.
- It implies the possibility of empirical testing.

Since each of these elements is crucial to the formulation of a satisfactory problem statement we will discuss the above criteria in greater detail.

THE VARIABLES

When concepts are operationalized, they are usually called variables. Researchers call the properties that they sutdy variables. Such properties take on different values. Thus, a *variable* is, as the name suggests, something that varies. Properties that differ from each other such as age, weight, height, religion, and ethnicity are examples of variables. Researchers attempt to understand how and why differences in one variable are related to differences in another variable. For example, a researcher may be concerned about the variable of cervical cancer in young women. It is a variable because not all young women have cervical cancer. A researcher may also be interested in what other factors can be linked to cervical cancer. It has been discovered that diethylstilbestrol (DES) use during pregnancy appears to be related to cervical cancer in daughters. Thus, DES use is also a variable, since not every mother has taken DES.

When speaking of relationships between variables, the researcher is essentially asking, "Is X related to Y? What is the effect of X on Y? How are X_1 and X_2 related to Y?" The researcher is asking a question about the relationship between one or more independent variables and a dependent variable.*

An *independent variable,* usually symbolized by X, is the *antecedent* or the variable that has the presumed effect on the dependent variable. In experimental research studies, the independent variable is manipulated by the researcher. For example, a nurse may study how different intramuscular injection sites affect the client's perception of pain. The researcher may manipulate the independent variable—intramuscular injection sites—by using different injection sites (see Chapter 9). In nonexperimental research, the independent variable is not manipulated and is assumed to have occurred naturally before or during the study. For example, the researcher may be studying the relationship between the level of anxiety and the perception of pain. The independent variable—the level of anxiety—is not manipulated; it is just presumed to occur and is observed and measured as it naturally happens (see Chapter 10).

The *dependent variable,* represented by Y, if often referred to as the *consequence* or the presumed effect that varies with a change in the independent variable. The dependent variable is not manipulated. It is observed and assumed to vary with changes in the independent variable. Predictions are made *from* the independent variable *to* the dependent variable. It is the dependent variable that the researcher is interested in understanding, explaining, or predicting. For example, it might be assumed that the perception of pain—the dependent variable—will vary with changes in the level of anxiety—the independent variable. In this case we are trying to explain the perception of pain in relation to the level of anxiety.

Although variability in the dependent variable is assumed to depend on changes in the independent variable, that does not imply that there is a causal relationship between X and Y, or that changes in variable X cause variable Y to change. Let us

---

*In cases where there are more than one independent or dependent variables, subscripts are used to indicate the number of variables under consideration.

look at an example where nurses' attitudes toward rape were studied. The researcher discovered that older nurses had a more negative attitude about rape than did younger nurses. The researcher did not conclude that the nurses' attitudes toward rape were *caused* by their age, but at the same time it is apparent that there is a direction of relationship between age and attitudes about rape. That is, as the nurses' age increases, their attitudes about rape become more negative. This example highlights the fact that causal relationships are not necessarily implied by the independent and dependent variables. Rather, only a relational statement with possible directionality is proposed.

Although one independent and one dependent variable are used in the examples just given, there is no restriction on the number of variables that can be included in a problem statement. However, remember that problems should not be unnecessarily complex or unwieldly, particularly in beginning research efforts. Problem statements that include more than one independent or dependent variable are generally broken down into subproblems that are more concise.

Finally, it should be noted that variables are not inherently independent or dependent. A variable that is classified as independent in one study may be considered dependent in another study. For example, a nurse may review an article about personality factors that are predictive of alcoholism. In this case alcoholism is the dependent variable. When reviewing another article about the relationship between alcoholism and marital conflict, alcoholism is the independent variable. Whether a variable is independent or dependent is a function of the role it plays in a particular study.

POPULATION

The nature of the population being studied needs to be specified in the problem statement. If the scope of the problem has been narrowed down to a specific focus and the variables have been clearly identified, the nature of the population will be evident to the reader of a research report. For example, a problem statement that poses the question, "Is there a relationship between mothers who have had rooming-in and preschool childrens' adjustment to hospitalization?" suggests that the population under consideration includes mothers and their hospitalized preschool children. It is also implied that some of the mothers will have had rooming-in, in contrast to other mothers who have not. The researcher or the reader will have an initial idea of the composition of the study population from the outset (see Chapter 14).

TESTABILITY

The statement of the research problem must imply that the problem is testable, that is, measurable by either qualitative or quantitative methods. For example, the problem statement, "Should nurses work with dying clients?" is incorrectly stated for a variety of reasons; one reason is that it is not testable. It represents a value statement rather than a relational problem statement. A scientific or relational problem must propose a relationship between an independent and dependent variable and do this in such a way that it indicates that the variables of the relationship can somehow be measured.

Many interesting and important questions are not valid research problems because they are not amenable to testing.

The question, "Should nurses work with dying clients?" *could* be revised from a *philosophical* question to a *research* question that implies testability. Two examples of the revised problem statement might be the following:

- Is there a relationship between nurses' attitudes toward dying clients and the quality of nursing care?
- What is the effect of nurses' attitudes about death and dying on empathic communication with terminally ill clients?

These examples illustrate the relationship between the variables, identify the independent and dependent variables, and imply the testability of the research problem.

Now that the elements of the formal problem statement have been presented in greater detail, this information can be integrated by formulating a formal problem statement about mother-infant attachment. Earlier in this chapter the following unrefined problem statement was formulated:

Is body contact immediately after delivery related to the mother's attachment to her newborn infant?

This problem statement was originally derived from a general area of interest—mother-infant relationships. The topic was more specifically defined by delineating a particular problem area—mother-infant attachment. The problem crystalized still further after a preliminary literature review, and emerged in the unrefined form just given. Utilizing the four criteria inherent in a satisfactory problem statement, it is now possible to propose a refined or formal problem statement. That is, one that specifically states the problem in question form, and specifies the relationship between the key variables in the study, the population being studied, and the empirical testability of the problem. Congruent with these four criteria, the following problem statement can then be formulated:

What is the effect of skin-to-skin contact between the mother and infant in the first hour after delivery on later maternal attachment behavior?

Table 4-2 identifies the components of this problem statement as they relate to and are congruent with the four problem statement criteria. Table 4-3 provides additional

---

• *Table 4-2* **Components of the Problem Statement and Related Criteria**

Variables	Population	Testability
Independent variable: skin-to-skin contact Dependent variable: maternal attachment behavior	Mothers Newborn infants	Comparison of skin-to-skin contact 1 hour after delivery versus no skin-to-skin contact Differential effect on maternal attachment behavior

• *Table 4-3*   **Examples of Unrefined and Refined Problem Statements**

Type of design suggested	Unrefined problem statement	Critique of problem statement	Refined problem statement
Nonexperimental	Do nurses's attitudes toward AIDS clients affect the emotional state of the client?	Not a concise relational statement. Testability is not implied	Is there a relationship between the nurse's attitudes toward AIDS and the emotional status of the AIDS client?
Experimental	How does client teaching influence maternal anxiety, post discharge by primiparas?	Not a concise relational statement. Testability is not implied. Variables are not clear	Is there a relationship between the amount of client teaching and the level of anxiety in primiparas after discharge?
Experimental	What is the effectiveness of health teaching for hospitalized cardiac clients in a group setting?	Population is not specific	What is the effect of post cardiac group health teaching on health behaviors of patients after an initial myocardial infarction?
Experimental	Does positioning have an effect on the occurrence of decubitus ulcers in unconscious clients?	Variables are not clear	What is the difference in the incidence of contractures in comatose clients in relation to frequency of repositioning?
Experimental	How do nurse-run client education classes impact on the housebound elderly?	Not a relational statement. Population is not defined adequately. Variables are not clearly defined. Testability is not implied	Is there a relationship between nurse-administered educational rehabilitation programs and independent behavior in chronically ill housebound elderly clients?
Nonexperimental	How does how you feel during pregnancy affect how the mother attaches to her baby?	Not a concise relational statement. Variables are not clearly defined	Is there a relationship between the physical symptoms of pregnancy and maternal-fetal attachment in primigravidas?

• *Table 4-3*   **Examples of Unrefined and Refined Problem Statements—cont'd**

Type of design suggested	Unrefined problem statement	Critique of problem statement	Refined problem statement
Experimental	Do hysterectomy patients need sexual counseling?	Not a relational statement Variables are not clearly specified Testability is not implied	Is there a relationship between sexual counseling and the postoperative adjustment of hysterectomy patients?
Nonexperimental	How does assertiveness relate to feelings of power in depressed women?	Not a clear relational statement Variables are not clearly specified	Is there a relationship between assertive behavior and the perception of power in depressed women?

examples of unrefined and refined problem statements. It is important to note that the process of moving from the general topic area to the unrefined problem and finally to the refined, formal problem statement often involves several intermediate steps.

• Critiquing the Problem Statement

The box on p. 58 offers critiquing criteria pertinent to the material discussed in this chapter.

Once the basics of developing a problem statement have been learned, a transition can be made from the development of a research problem to the critical appraisal of a research problem.

Several criteria for evaluating this initial phase of the research process—the problem statement—can be derived from the preceding discussion. Such criteria provide valid guidelines for critiquing this phase of the research process, regardless of whether the nurse is evaluating the potential merit of a researchable problem of his or her own or is critically evaluating a published research study that is potentially applicable in practice. Since this text focuses on the nurse as a critical consumer of research, the following discussion will pertain primarily to the evaluation of the problem statement in a research report.

Since the problem statement represents the basis for the study, it is essential that it be introduced at the beginning of the research report. This will indicate the focus and direction of the study to the readers, who will then be in a position to evaluate whether the rest of the study logically flows from its base. Often the author will begin by identifying the general problem area that originally represented some

---

Critiquing Criteria

prob statement state pg " ———— "

1. Has the problem been introduced promptly?
2. Is the problem stated clearly and unambiguously in question form?
3. Does the problem statement express a relationship between two or more variables, or at least between an independent and a dependent variable?
4. Does the problem statement specify the nature of the population being studied? *normal newborns → in general un begin. But sample criteria such as*
5. Does the problem statement imply the possibility of empirical testability? *more stated operationally measurable later,*
6. Has the problem been substantiated with adequate experiential and scientific background material?
7. Has the problem been placed within the context of an appropriate conceptual framework?
8. Has the purpose of the study, relative to the problem statement, been delineated?
9. Has the significance of the problem been identified?
10. Have pragmatic issues, such as feasibility, been addressed?

---

vague discontent or question regarding an unsolved problem. The experiential and scientific background that led to the specific problem is briefly summarized and the purpose of the study is identified. Finally, the formal problem statement and any related subproblems are proposed.

The purpose of the introductory summary of the experiential and scientific background is to provide the reader with a glimpse of how the author thought about the research problem's development. The introduction to the research problem places the study within an appropriate conceptual framework and sets the stage for the unfolding of the study. This introductory section should also include the *purpose* of the study, that is, why the investigator is doing the study. For example, the purpose may be to solve a problem encountered in the clinical area and thereby improve client care, or it may be to resolve a conflict in the literature regarding a clinical issue. The purpose of the study should not be confused with the *problem* of the study, which is the research question to be answered.

In reality, the reader will often find that the research problem is not clearly stated at the conclusion of this section. In fact, in some cases it is only hinted at and the reader is challenged to identify the problem under consideration. In other cases the problem statement is embedded in the introductory text. To some extent this will depend on the style of the particular journal. Nevertheless, the evaluator must remember that the main problem statement should be clearly delineated in the introductory section even if the subproblems are not.

After the quality of the problem statement has been evaluated, the reader looks for the presence of four key elements that were described and illustrated in an earlier section of this chapter. They are the following:

1. Is the problem stated clearly and unambiguously in question form?
2. Does the problem statement express a relationship between two or more variables, or at least between an independent and dependent variable?
3. Does the problem statement specify the nature of the population being studied?
4. Does the problem statement imply the possibility of empirical testing?

The reader will use these four elements as criteria for judging the soundness of a stated research problem. It is likely that if the problem is unclear in terms of the variables, the population, and the implications for testability the remainder of the study is going to falter. For example, a research study contained introductory material on anxiety in general, anxiety as it relates to the perioperative period, and the potentially beneficial influence of nursing care in relation to anxiety reduction. The author concluded that the purpose of the study was to determine whether or not selected measures of client anxiety could be shown to differ when different approaches to nursing care were used during the perioperative period. The author did not go on to state the research problems. However, the statement given seems to be the research problem rather than the purpose of the study and needs to be clearly stated as such. A restatement of the problem in question form might be the following:

$$(Y_1) \qquad\qquad (X_1, X_2, X_3)$$

What is the difference in client anxiety level in relation to different approaches to nursing care during the perioperative period?

If this process is clarified at the outset of a research study, all that follows in terms of the design can be logically developed. The reader will have a clear idea of what the report should convey, and can evaluate knowledgeably the material that follows.

CONCLUSION

The care that a researcher takes when formulating and stating a problem is often representative of the thoroughness of the overall design and conceptualization of the study. A methodically developed problem that is concisely and clearly stated provides both the researcher and the evaluator of the research with a firm foundation to depart from when conducting or critically appraising a research study. This may be a time-consuming and often frustrating endeavor for the researcher. But in the final analysis, the product, as evaluated by the consumer, has most often been worth the struggle.

• Summary

Formulating a problem statement is one of the key procedures in the research process. It is the starting point of any research study. A great deal of time is spent in selecting an appropriate problem for study. Practical experience, a critical appraisal of the scientific literature, or an interest in an ungrounded theory provides the basis for the germination of a research idea.

The research problem is refined through a process that proceeds from the identification of a general idea of interest to the definition of a more specific and circumscribed topic. A preliminary literature review reveals related factors that appear critical to the research topic of interest and aids in further definition of the research problem. The significance of the research problem must be identified in terms of its potential contribution to clients, nurses, the medical community in general, and society. Applicability of the problem for nursing practice as well as its theoretical relevance must be established. The findings should also have the potential for formulating or altering nursing practices or policies.

The feasibility of a research problem must be examined in light of pragmatic considerations such as time; availability of subjects, money, facilities, and equipment; experience of the researcher, and ethical issues.

The final problem statement consists of an interrogative statement about the relationship between two or more variables. The problem statement clearly identifies the relationship between the independent and dependent variables. It specifies the nature of the population being studied. The problem statement implies the possibility of empirical testing.

The critiquing process provides a set of criteria for the evaluation of the strengths and weaknesses of a problem statement as it appears in a research report. The critiquer assesses the clarity of the problem statement as well as the related subproblems, the specificity of the population, and the implications for testability. The interrelatedness between the problem statement, the literature review, the theoretical framework, and the hypotheses should be apparent. The appropriateness of the research design suggested by the problem statement is also evaluated. Finally, the purpose of the study, that is, *why* the researcher is doing the study, should be differentiated from the problem statement or the research question to be answered.

A clearly and concisely stated research problem provides a firm foundation to depart from when conducting or critically appraising a research study. The time-consuming process of developing a problem statement may often seem overwhelming or frustrating. However, the product, as evaluated by the research consumer, is most often worth the struggle.

• References

Curry, M.A. (1982). Maternal attachment behavior and the mother's self concept: the effect of early skin-to-skin contact, *Nursing Research,* **3112**:73-78.

Downs, F.S. and Newman, M.A. (1977). *A source book of nursing research,* 2nd ed., Philadelphia, F.A. Davis Co.

Fox, D.J. (1976). Critically evaluating the written research report, in Fox, J.D.: *Fundamentals of research in nursing,* 3rd ed., New York, Appleton-Century-Crofts, pp. 282-301.

Jaecox, A. and Prescott, R.A. (1978). Determining a study's relevance for clinical practice, *American Journal of Nursing,* **11**:1882-1889.

Kerlinger, F.N. (1973). *Foundations of behavioral research,* New York, Holt, Rhinehart & Winston, Inc.

Lim-Levy, F. (1982). The effect of oxygen inhalation on oral temperature, *Nursing Research,* **13**:(3), 150-152.

Polit, D.F. and Hungler, B.P. (1983). *Nursing research: Principles and methods,* 2nd ed., Philadelphia, J.B. Lippincott Co.

5

The Literature Review

Margaret Grey

LEARNING OBJECTIVES

After reading this chapter, the student should be able to do the following:
- Define the purposes of the literature review.
- List the most utilized sources of nursing and related literature.
- Critically evaluate literature reviews in selected research studies.

concept	primary source
conceptual literature	review of the literature
construct	secondary source
data-based literature	variables

• Overview

To critically evaluate literature reviews in published research papers, it is important for the student to understand how a review is conducted so that it can be judged whether an adequate review is presented.

Every research project should be an outcome of all previous thinking and research in the chosen area. Just how does this logical flow of ideas occur? It occurs through the conscious part of the research process that is known as the literature review. Now, you're probably thinking, "I know all about that because I've had to review published literature on a certain topic for term papers." While literature reviews for term papers are similar in that they must summarize what is known about an area, the literature review conducted for the purpose of supporting a research project is different in two important ways. First, the literature review places the current study in the context of previous research. As such, it includes both conceptual and data-based literature. *Conceptual literature* is published material dealing with the theory that underlies the research. *Data-based literature* is composed of all the published research studies dealing with the problem of interest. Second, this type of review requires a critical examination of the related literature. The review must identify the weaknesses, strengths, and gaps in the literature covering the topic area. Thus, it is not simply a narration of "so-and-so said." Rather, the literature review says what others said, how and why they said it, and with how much confidence the author views the findings.

Therefore, the literature review can be defined as an extensive, exhaustive, systematic, and critical examination of publications relevant to the research project (Seaman and Verhonick, 1982). As such, the literature review begins with locating as many relevant materials as possible and ends with writing a summary of the available knowledge.

By reviewing the literature, the researcher hopes to accomplish two main goals, that is, identifying and becoming familiar with all of the relevant published material, and composing this foundation so that it puts this study into the context of all of the previous research. These overall goals of the literature review are accomplished through the following five specific purposes of the review (Fox, 1983):

1. To develop the conceptual frame of reference for the study. This aspect of the literature review is discussed in detail in the next chapter. Primarily based on the conceptual literature, the development of the conceptual frame of reference for the study is especially important for the development of nursing and nursing research because it allows for the findings of research studies to contribute to the development of nursing theory. For this outcome to be possible, researchers must demonstrate familiarity with all points of view in the field, not just those that support their personal notions. It is particularly important that researchers distinguish between summaries of the work of others and their own views.

   2. To understand the status of research in the problem area. This is the most familiar purpose of the literature review. Here the researcher reviews the data-based literature and the reports of studies conducted in the area of interest. This step makes the gaps in our current understanding of a problem clear and helps to identify how this proposed research will fit into the study of the larger problem area. To understand the depth of this step the researcher should realize that the following four basic questions must be answered:

- *When* was this problem studied?
- *What* has been studied about this problem?
- *Where* has this problem been investigated?
- *Who* has been studied?

The answers to these four questions give the researcher an overall picture of the work that has been done in the topic area to date. Students who are new to the research process often ask how far back the literature review should go. This is not an easy question to answer. The basic decision depends on how much literature is new in an area and how much is older. If the researcher finds that there is nothing in the recent literature then she must go as far back as necessary to give a complete picture of what is known about the problem area, and the literature review might span 20 to 30 years. If, on the other hand, the topic is a new area of inquiry, the review may only span a few years. The only way the researcher knows the answer to this question, though, is to continue to go back in the literature until no new information is found.

   3. To provide clues to methodology and instrumentation. The third purpose of the literature review answers the following important question:

- *How* has this problem studied in the past?

This aspect of the literature review shows the researcher what has and has not been tried in regard to approaches and methods and what types of data gathering instruments exist.

   4. To estimate the potential for success of the proposed study. Having reviewed the work of others in the problem area, the researcher needs to assess at this stage whether or not the proposed study has potential for answering the research question. This assessment is based on the success others have had in studying the problem and the usefulness of their findings. As discussed in Chapter 3, the researcher has an ethical and legal oblication not to proceed with a study that has no potential for success. Therefore, the nurse must be willing to abandon or change the proposed research at this point, so that subjects are not enrolled in a useless study.

   5. To serve as a sounding board. Finally, the literature review helps the researcher to know when the problem has been specified enough. The researcher knows that a problem is well-specified when certain papers are clearly related to the problem and others are not directly related. Until the researcher can make this distinction, the review is not complete and the problem has not been specified enough. In other words, the literature discriminates which variables are important to the present investigation and which variables can be ignored for the contemplated study.

These purposes of the literature review and how they fit with the research process will become clearer as we study how a literature review is conducted. The process of conducting such a review is delineated so that you can assess the adequacy of a published review. You will need to see these steps reflected in the studies that you critique. In addition, the steps may be useful to you when writing term papers, care plans, and clinical reports.

• How the Literature Review is Conducted

As with any written work, the author of a research paper needs to define the scope of the problem to be addressed. For researchers, this step is the identification of the relevant concepts, constructs, and variables to be included in the review. This step goes hand-in-hand with the specification of the research problem discussed in the previous chapter. For instance, a researcher may be interested in the general problem of stress. One could undertake a review of the massive literature on stress from a number of angles, such as the physiology of the stress response, the effect of a particular stressful event such as hospitalization, or the effect of social support on people undergoing stressful experiences. If the problem is quite broad to begin with, the researcher may use the literature review to narrow the scope of the problem to one that is manageable. In so doing the researcher begins to define the important concepts and variables that need to be addressed.

If, on the other hand, the researcher comes to the literature review stage with a well-formulated problem that states all of the relevant variables and defines them, the literature review is already outlined.

Either way, the researcher needs to identify the related literature. Usually this is done by starting with the broad topic being studied and reading summary papers or reviews written by experts in the field. In this initial step the researcher becomes familiar with the previous research in the area and the views of others working in the area. Summary papers may be found in books or journals. Thus the logical place to begin a literature search is in the card catalogue of the library, looking under the topic area in question. For example, our researcher interested in some aspect of stress would look under "Stress" in the card catalogue. If the topic is well-studied, such as stress, many listings may be found and the process of refining the problem begins. Suppose the researcher has decided to study the problem of social support and stress; all of the books dealing with stress physiology would not be relevant and thus would not need to be reviewed. If books existed on social support and stress, the researcher would begin the review by reading them carefully to get an understanding of the major views on this problem.

By now you may be getting a mental picture of a researcher sitting in the library surrounded by books written on the chosen topic and are wondering how the researcher can keep it all straight. The age-old method of keeping bibliography cards is priceless in this regard. Bibliography cards can be quite detailed or they may merely provide notes to jog the memory about the piece reviewed. All cards should contain the following information: bibliographic information, including author's name(s), title of the book or article, publication information, and a summary of the major points made in the work. Keeping bibliography cards allows the researcher to know what literature has already been consulted, whether it was useful or not, and the appropriate sources to be cited when writing the research report.

Books provide only one source of literature. Since books are usually summaries of previous theory and research in an area, they provide a foundation for building the conceptual framework of the research. However, books take longer to publish than journal articles and so they are sometimes not up to date. In addition, books do not usually provide in-depth reports of individual research projects and thus cannot provide the data-based literature needed to build an understanding of the status of research in a specific problem area.

The search for published articles dealing with a specific problem begins by using either literature indexes or computerized data bases. Both serve the purpose of identifying articles dealing with a topic of interest. Several such indexes exist and help in our search. The most commonly used indexes in nursing research are listed in the box on p. 66. An index is a list of articles about topics. Computerized databases are also lists of published articles cross-referenced by author and subject, but these are available on-line rather than in hard copies in the library (see Chapter 17).

Whether generated by hand or by computer, the researcher eventually acquires a list of relevant articles. The task then is to locate and critically review these papers so that the researcher becomes totally familiar with all points of view in the problem area. The list may include both primary and secondary sources. *Primary sources,* for example, are first-hand accounts, research reports written by the researcher, or client records. *Secondary sources* are at least once removed from the primary author. Common secondary sources include summaries of research studies, textbooks, and biographies. While secondary sources are useful in guiding the researcher to all of the relevant work in the chosen area, literature reviews should be built chiefly on primary sources because secondary sources may be contaminated by the bias of the individual writing the summary. Since the purpose of the literature review is to place the study in the context of previous work, it should be as unbiased as possible.

Having read and summarized the conceptual and data-based literature available on a certain problem area, the researcher writes the review, clarifying for the reader what has been studied about the problem in the past, how it has been studied, and who has been studied. In addition, the review should make clear what is known about the problem or what is assumed to be known, what is not known, and how this particular piece of research will help to answer what is not known.

Indexes Commonly Used in Nursing Research

Nursing Indexes

1. The International Nursing Index

This index references articles from over 200 nursing journals and nursing articles from more than 2,000 nonnursing journals. References are listed alphabetically by author and subject and cover articles beginning with 1966.

2. The Nursing Studies Index

This annotated guide to reported studies, research methods, and historical and biographical materials covers English periodicals, books, and pamphlets. This index includes nursing literature for the period 1900 to 1959.

3. The Nursing Research Index

This index appears annually in the last issue of *Nursing Research* and contains alphabetical listings of research studies published in the last year by author and subject.

Nonnursing Indexes

1. The Indexus Medicus

This index includes over 2,000 biomedical journals published worldwide as well as several nursing journals. Entries are listed alphabetically by author and subject.

2. The Social Science Citation Index

This index covers all areas of the social sciences and includes over 1000 social science journals from history and economics to sociology. Many topics included are relevant to areas of nursing research.

3. The Science Citation Index

This index covers the technological and scientific references that may be useful in physiologic research in nursing.

4. The Educational Resources Information Center (ERIC)

ERIC publishes a monthly index called *The Current Index to Journals in Education* that references articles by subject and author from over 500 journals. Authors dealing with nursing education or client education might find this index useful.

5. Psychological Abstracts

This index publishes abstracts of more than 120 books and 800 journals yearly in the fields of psychology and behavioral science.

• Organization of the Literature Review

Both beginning researchers and readers of research articles are often troubled by questions about the depth and breadth of the literature review. How broad the review needs to be depends on a number of factors. One factor is the length of the report. Journal editors usually require the literature review to be brief so the report can concentrate on the findings of the particular study. The nature of the problem itself may dictate how many peripherally related studies need to be addressed. A problem that has been heavily studied may require the researcher to be familiar with many articles, each directly relevant to the problem. On the other hand, a new problem that has not been extensively studied may require the researcher to become familiar with articles that are only peripherally related to the problem so that a meaningful framework can be developed. The question of depth is also determined by the relevance of the article to the stated problem. In general, the more closely the article is related to the problem, the more detail needs to be presented. Studies that are indirectly related are often summarized quite briefly.

As with any written work, the organization of the literature review is of paramount importance. The review is written so that the development of the major concepts for study are made explicitly clear to the reader. Thus, the literature review should include an introduction, a summary of the related literature, and a summary of the current knowledge of the problem. Usually, the researcher begins with the broader topic area and progressively limits the problem to the one being studied with more detailed summaries of previous work in the area. The review should organize and summarize the literature so that it is clear to the reader how the researcher chose to study this particular aspect of a problem. Often the review of the literature is organized by variables of importance to the study. Thus the researcher may introduce the independent variable and summarize the literature relevant to it, then outline the dependent variables of interest and what is known about their relationship to the independent variable, and finally discuss any antecedent or intervening variables of importance. The summary would then indicate what the proposed relationships among these variables would be expected to be on the basis of the previous work in the field. In addition, the review should point out all of the contradictions and inconsistencies in the previous work. Summaries of each section should make clear that the researcher has thought about the results studied in the literature review and has not merely identified what is in the literature.

Although it is important that the literature review reflect the author's views on the topic as they relate to the literature available in the problem area, it is equally important that the review be objective. In other words, reports of studies that contradict the author's hypothesis should not be omitted; rather, such studies should be analyzed for the potential reasons for these discrepancies. Often these discrepancies form the basis of further research in an area.

• Critiquing the Literature Review

Evaluating a literature review is a difficult task. To a certain extent, it is difficult to evaluate a review if the reader is not familiar with the topic studied. However, there are several areas to consider when reading literature reviews in published research reports. Criteria for evaluating the literature review are summarized in the box on p. 68.

The first area to consider is the type of report. We have said that journals

---

Critiquing Criteria

1. What type of report is this? If it is abridged, the literature review is likely to be brief.
2. Does the review of the literature follow immediately after the introduction and the statement of the problem?
3. Are all relevant concepts and variables included in the review?
4. Does the review follow a logical sequence leading to the summary of the current knowledge of the problem?
5. Is there a summary of the literature reviewed, the gaps in current knowledge about the problem, and how this study intends to fill in those gaps?
6. Are both conceptual literature and data-based literature included?
7. Are the sources for the literature review mostly primary or mostly secondary sources?
8. Can you follow the logic of the author in building the literature review?
9. Is there evidence that the review is unbiased?

---

frequently require literature reviews to be brief and to the point. Thus the reviews found in journal articles are likely to be condensed. It is useful to page through the rest of the journal where the current article is found. Is this review similar to others? If so, the brevity of the review may reflect the requirements of the journal. If the report is a dissertation or thesis the reader should expect that the literature review will be complete and cover all relevant areas.

Next, the reader should determine if the literature review follows immediately after the introduction. Since the purpose of the literature review is to place the current work in the context of previous work, the review should follow the statement of the problem. In addition, this placement allows the reader to follow precisely the thinking of the researcher in the development of the specific hypotheses within the problem area.

Since the literature review's purpose is to inform the reader to what extent the researcher has placed the current investigation in the context of previous work, this thinking should be reflected in what you read. A good review builds a case for the need for this study to be conducted in light of what has previously been accomplished and how this study will extend current knowledge of the problem area. It should be very clear what the researcher is accepting as true for this study on the basis of previous work in the area. It should be equally clear what areas the researcher considers to be in need of further research. The specific study in question should then be designed around these gaps in current knowledge. In addition, if the study relates explicitly to a particular theory, that relationship should be stated.

Another purpose of the review is to demonstrate to the reader that the researcher

Weak	*Better*
Goebel and others (1984) studied the effectiveness of a postpartum educational program on infant car seat usage. Excerpts from their review are as follows: "Some parents say it is too much work to use safety belts for children. . . . "Even the strongest parents cannot safely restrain an infant sitting in the parent's lap. . . . "In addition to the safety of the child, the parents' psychological comfort is another incentive for the use of car seats."	Blouse and colleagues* demonstrated in a survey that parents feel that using safety belts for children is too much work. "Since previous work by Truck* has shown that a child's weight is multiplied by ten to twenty times during the impact of an automobile accident, it is clear that even the strongest parent will not be able to restrain an infant sitting in the parent's lap. "Other studies have suggested that the use of child restraints will increase the parents' psychological comfort as well."

*These references are fictitious.

Fig. 5-1   Excerpt from a weak literature review and how to improve it.

is familiar with *all* points of view in the topic area. The complete review covers all conceptual and data-based literature that is directly relevant to the specific problem under study. If, because of space restrictions, the review needs to be summarized, the reader should expect that this is reflected in the report. As much as possible, the sources referred to should be primary sources, rather than secondary sources. Fig. 5-1 illustrates how a written literature review should reflect the studies cited, and how the importance of the study should be based on previous data and not the opinion of the researcher.

Finally, the literature review should be judged by how well it shows the need for this study to have been conducted. It should be quite obvious to the reader exactly what the gaps in knowledge are, and how this study intends to contribute to filling in those gaps. This criterion requires that the review be written in a logical sequence, flowing from the general problem to the specific problem, and finally providing justification for the hypotheses generated.

Critiquing a literature review is difficult, but the reader should be able to see how the researcher built the study based on the previous work in the topic area. If there are areas that are not addressed, or if the review seems biased to the researcher's point of view, the review may be considered to be deficient. Since it is important that all research build on previous work, this step of the research process is critical to the overall worth of the study.

• Summary

The purpose of this chapter was to introduce the student to the process of the literature review so that the student can critically evaluate published research.

The literature review was defined as an extensive, exhaustive, systematic, and critical examination of publications relevant to the research project. Such literature reviews utilize both conceptual and data based literature to place the current work in the context of all previous research in the problem area. Reviews may utilize both primary and secondary sources, but should arise mostly from primary sources.

The literature review helps the researcher to identify and become familiar with all relevant published material in the problem area and to write this foundation so that the review places the study in the context of all previous research in the area. The literature review also serves the following five specific puposes: to develop the conceptual frame of reference for the study, to understand the status of research in the problem area, to provide clues to methodology and instrumentation, to estimate the potential for success of the proposed study, and to serve as a sounding board.

The chapter also presented information on how a literature search is conducted and written. This information and information on commonly used indexes relevant to nursing research was presented so that the student can begin to judge whether all the necessary steps are reflected in the written report.

Finally, suggestions for critically reading the review of the literature are given. In addition, examples of statements from one review and recommendations for change are given.

• References

Fox, D. (1982). *Fundamentals of research in nursing,* Norwalk, Conn., Appleton-Century Crofts.

Goebel, J.B., Copps, T.J., and Sulayman, R.F. (1984). Infant car seat usage: Effectiveness of a postpartum educational program, *Journal of Obstetrics and Gynecology Nursing,* **13**(1):33-36.

Polit, D, and Hungler, B. (1983). *Nursing research, Principles and methods,* 2nd ed., Philadelphia, J.B. Lippincott Co.

Seaman, C.C.H., and Verhonick, P.J. (1982). *Research methods for undergraduate students in nursing,* Norwalk, Conn., Appleton-Century-Crofts.

6

The Theoretical Framework

Harriet R. Feldman

LEARNING OBJECTIVES

After reading this chapter, the student should be able to do the following:
- Identify the purpose and the nature of a theoretical framework.
- Describe the process involved in developing a theoretical framework.
- Contrast the borrowed versus new theory approaches in the development of nursing science.
- Formulate conceptual and operational definitions.
- Describe how a theoretical framework guides research.
- Identify how hypotheses are generated.
- Define nursing theory.
- Identify the phenomena of concern to nursing.
- Describe the points of critical appraisal used to evaluate the appropriateness, cohesiveness, and consistency of a theoretical framework.

KEY TERMS

concept	operational definition
conceptual definition	proposition
construct	theoretical framework
hypothesis	theory

• Definition of a Theory

Theory has been defined in a number of ways. For example, Chinn and Jacobs (1983) broadly define *theory* as a "systematic abstraction of reality that serves some purpose" (p.2). They continue by describing each part of the definition; that is, *systematic* implies a specific organizational pattern, *abstraction* connotes that theory is a representation of reality, and *purposes* include description, explanation, and prediction of phenomena and control of some reality. Stevens (1979) defines theory as "a statement that purports to account for or characterize some phenomenon . . . it pulls out the salient parts of a phenomenon so that one can separate the critical and necessary factors (or relationships) from the accidental and unessential factors (or relationships)" (p.1). This definition implies purpose, because it differentiates critical from extraneous factors and accounts for phenomena. Neither a specific organizational pattern nor a relationship to reality is implied in Stevens' definition.

Reynolds (1971) approaches theory in yet another way, defining it as "abstract statements that are considered part of scientific knowledge in either the set-of-laws, the axiomatic, or the causal process forms" (p.11). Set-of-laws refers to "well-supported empirical generalizations or 'laws'" (p.10); axiomatic refers to an "interrelated set of definitions, axioms, and propositions" (p.10) derived from axioms; and causal process specifically means "a set of descriptions of causal processes" (pp.10-11). This definition encompasses the concepts of systematic process and abstraction; also, the emphasis is on scientific knowledge. It does not, however, make explicit the concept of purpose.

Our final definition of theory is perhaps the one most widely used. It takes a basic view of science, that is, the development of general explanations about natural phenomena via theories. To be more precise, "a theory is a set of interrelated constructs (concepts), definitions, and propositions that present a systematic view of phenomena by specifying relations among variables, with the purpose of explaining and predicting the phenomena" (Kerlinger, 1973, p.9). Abstraction expressed in the term *construct*, a systematic process, and a statement of purpose are included in this definition; furthermore, specific components of the process are identified.

This chapter addresses the nature and purpose of a theoretical framework in a research study and shows how to develop and critique a theoretical framework. The preceding definitions serve as a guide to the forthcoming discussion of these topics.

• Definition of a Theoretical Framework

A *theoretical framework* provides a context for examining a problem, that is, the theoretical *rationale* for developing hypotheses. It is also a frame of reference that is a base for observations, definitions of variables, research designs, interpretations, and generalizations. When reporting research, the investigator is obliged to clearly articulate the theoretical basis for hypothesis formulation, study findings, and outcome interpretations.

• Purpose of Having a Theoretical Framework in a Research Study

You may be wondering why you need a theoretical framework in a research study. You may ask, "Why can't I just match any two variables that make sense to me and look at their relationship?" As an analogy, consider the first time you traveled by car to an unfamiliar place. How did you get to your destination? Did you use a map? Did you follow someone's directions? Did you stick to the prescribed route, or did you try a shortcut? Did you turn left instead of right because it seemed logical, or did you use known information to make that decision? The map served as a guide to your destination, and when conducting research, a theoretical rationale serves as a guide or map to systematically identify a logical, precisely defined relationship between variables. Other purposes of a theoretical rationale include providing clear descriptions of variables, suggesting ways or methods to conduct the study, and guiding the interpretation, evaluation, and integration of study findings.

• How to Develop a Theoretical Framework

Although in the role of research consumer you will not be expected to develop a theoretical framework, an understanding of the process will assist you in critiquing this aspect of the research study. Therefore the basis for and intricacies of developing a theoretical framework will be discussed and numerous examples provided.

BORROWED VERSUS NEW THEORY

When developing a theoretical framework for nursing research studies, knowledge is acquired using two approaches. It is either developed primarily in disciplines other than nursing and borrowed for the purpose of answering nursing questions, or it is derived by identifying and asking questions about phenomena that are unique to nursing. There are pros and cons to both approaches, and these views will be briefly described.

To date, most nursing research has been based on theories borrowed from other disciplines. Phillips (1977) sees this as a problem and states, "The process of borrowing theories and models from other disciplines has hampered nurses in learning how to ask questions which are of specific concern to nursing or in conceptualizing how the borrowed knowledge is to be used to generate theory to expand nursing science" (p.4). Further concerns expressed by Feldman (1980) are whether or not "such theories have been substantially supported in other disciplines" (p.87) and whether or not they are "generalizable to nursing" (p.87). The advantages of using a borrowed theory are that many of the theories of other disciplines are well-developed and have been supported by substantial hypothesis testing, and that nursing science will be advanced if the overall research effort demonstrates the synthesis of borrowed knowledge to reflect a nursing focus.

Theories of learning and self-esteem can be used to illustrate how to "borrow" theories from other disciplines for the purpose of asking nursing questions. Adult learning theories take a self-directed approach to learning. A nursing question that uses this theory is, "Do diabetics who use self-directed learning techniques perform foot care more frequently and more correctly than diabetics who do not use self-directed learning techniques?" Self-esteem theory involves the evolution of a sense of identity so that the individual develops a self-evaluation, that is, in terms of approval/disapproval, adequate/inadequate, acceptable/unacceptable, and capable/incapable parameters. This self-evaluation is intended to influence interactions with others and with the environment. A nursing question that uses this theory is, "What is the relationship between self-esteem and engagement in social interactions in the retired older population?"

A case can be made for developing new theories that are unique to nursing. Having a knowledge base specifically created to reflect a nursing focus helps nursing define its uniqueness, hence its difference from other disciplines. Nursing theory development is in its infancy and is far from being refined and tested enough to be able to rely on its validity. The following are examples of theories that have been derived from nursing models. Nursing research is currently being conducted to test their validity.

Orem's model of self-care (1980) has generated theories of self-care, self-care deficits, and nursing systems. King's (1981) model of personal, interpersonal, and social systems has generated a theory of goal attainment. Roger's (1970) life process, interactive person-environment model has generated a theory of complementarity. These theories contribute to the development of nursing as a unique scientific discipline. In contrast, you may wonder if all of nursing's knowledge base should be unique. You may ask if it is even useful to have such a base. Answers to these questions are controversial, and you are referred to the readings of Johnson (1968), Phillips (1977), Feldman (1980), and Fawcett (1983) to view various perspectives.

To summarize, the growth of nursing science has been evidenced through the development of borrowed and new theories. The contribution made using borrowed theories is most appropriate when data are related specifically to nursing; new theories based on nursing models, while not abundant at this time, are steadily increasing. As a consumer of nursing research, it is important for you to evaluate the theoretical rationale of research studies in terms of relevance to nursing. You should ask if the investigator states the relevance of the problem to nursing, if the borrowed theories and the reported studies from other disciplines are related to nursing data, and if the findings are related to nursing, that is, nursing practice, nursing education, and/or nursing administration.

SELECTION OF CONCEPTS

A *concept* is an image or symbolic representation of an abstract idea. It is formed by generalizing from particular characteristics. For example, health is a concept formed

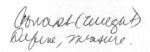

by generalizing from particular behaviors, for example, being mobile, being free of infection, and communicating appropriately. Other concepts include pain, intelligence, weight, grieving, self-concept, and achievement. Concepts facilitate the delineation of ideas so that systematic inquiry can proceed. Some concepts are directly observable, such as a chair or rain, and others are indirectly observable, for example, anxiety or intelligence.

Since concepts are the basis for refining ideas and developing theory, it is important to select those concepts that clearly reflect the subject matter being pursued. In evaluating a piece of research, you must consider whether or not the concepts or variables as defined are examined both in general and specifically in the context of the problem under investigation (see Chapters 7 and 13). Furthermore, consider if they are being measured with the appropriate instruments (see Chapter 13).

IDENTIFYING THE INTERRELATIONSHIPS AMONG CONCEPTS

In the process of examining the concepts or variables that guide the research effort, relationships emerge. For example, from a review of the literature in a particular area such as stress, information about related variables can be found, for example, onset of illness, certain physiological responses, and learning ability. Relationships can also be identified through systematic observation and experience. A relationship may be invariable, tentative, or inconclusive. An example of an invariable relationship is a law. In this case, no known contradiction has been observed. A tentative or inconclusive relationship is a hypothesis, which expresses a relationship between two or more variables and does not convey truth or falsity. Both laws and hypotheses are types of propositions.

The literature review is the part of the research report that generally specifies the theoretical rationale and should explicitly identify propositions in relation to the individual variables described. The hypotheses should express relationships between variables in an unambiguous, precise manner, and they should be based on the propositions that evolved from the theoretical framework (see Chapter 5).

• Formulating Definitions

As stated earlier, concepts are representations of abstract ideas. To develop a theoretical framework that can generate and test hypotheses, concepts must be clearly defined. If you think back to the earlier illustration about traveling to an unfamiliar place, how do you think you would have arrived if the directions simply read, "First you take one road, then turn at another and proceed to three more roads?" Without a clear conception of which road, what direction to turn, and how far to proceed, you would probably get lost. The same process applies to any concept. For example, how would you define pain? anxiety? or intelligence? In addition to knowing the names of the roads to travel, other specifics are clearly needed, such as what type of vehicle will you use, what town you will travel through, how you will know when you've arrived, and how far you will travel. These parameters delineate the procedure to follow by identifying what *operations* must occur to make the trip. When defining concepts for the purpose of systematic examination, you must include both conceptual and operational information.

CONCEPTUAL DEFINITIONS

Concepts, no matter what their level of abstraction, must be defined as unambiguously as possible, so that they can be easily communicated to others. Even the word "can" is open to varied interpretations, for example, a container, being able to, or a commode. A *conceptual definition* conveys the general meaning of the concept, as does a dictionary definition. It reflects the theory used in the study of that concept. The following are examples of conceptual definitions:

Recovery: the process of healing that takes place after an injury.

Concept: an image or symbolic representation of an abstract idea.

Postoperative pain: discomfort an individual experiences after a surgical procedure.

Mothering: "an interaction between a human adult and a child that conveys a positive affect and is reciprocal in nature. The interaction involves reciprocal contact, touching, and vocalization" (Chinn and Jacobs, 1983, p.93).

Fear: "an escape or avoidance response in relation to a specific object or situation" (Swanson, 1977, p.178).

Sociability: "the tendency to desire friendly interaction with others" (Rogers, 1977, p.171).

Since these are general definitions, they do not include an indication of how the concepts will be measured.

OPERATIONAL DEFINITIONS

Operationalization adds another dimension to the conceptual definition by delineating the procedures or operations required to measure the concept. It supplies the information needed to collect data on the problem being studied. Some concepts are easily defined in operational terms, for example, pulse can be measured numerically. Other concepts are more difficult to operationally define, such as anxiety, leaving it up to the investigator to locate and select an instrument that best measures the concept. The following are examples of operational definitions:

Sensation pain rating: the periodic self-report of the intensity of the sensation component of the pain experience, reported by subjects using the Pilowsky and Kaufman (1965) visual analogue scale.

Extended skin-to-skin contact: "at least half of the infant's naked body touching the mother's naked trunk for 15 minutes or more during the first hour following delivery" (Curry, 1982, p.74).

Articulation of body concept: the "extent to which the body is experienced as having definite limits or 'boundaries,' and the 'parts' within these boundaries experienced as describe, yet joined into a definite structure" (Witkin, Dyk, Faterson, and others, 1974, p.116). Articulation of the body concept is measured using the Figure Drawing Test.

Time of day: "a specific morning and afternoon hour span, namely, 8:30 to 9:30 AM and 2:30 to 3:30 PM" (Rodgers, 1977, p.172).

Ventilatory function: "the mechanics of breathing measured by tests of vital capacity and expiratory flow rate" (Lindeman and VanAernam, 1977, p.45).

Preferred rate of walking: "the rate which an individual assumes when instructed to walk in his most comfortable, natural manner. This rate is measured in miles per hour and steps per minute" (Newman, 1977, p.141).

Each of these examples has a conceptual definition and at least one index of measurement that makes it operational. To summarize, an operational definition provides specificity and direction for the concept to guide the development of the research study. Once the concept is operationalized it is termed a *variable*, and at that point it begins to play a significant role in formulating the theoretical rationale. In the role of research consumer you are responsible for evaluating whether or not variables are clearly defined, both conceptually and operationally. If the meaning of the variable is vague or if the measurement used does not reflect the same meaning as the variable, comparisons of the research with other investigations will not be valid and the research will be impossible to replicate (see Chapter 7).

Some research reports present conceptual definitions followed by a description of measurement in another section, such as methodology or instrumentation. Other reports present operational definitions; still others may present no definitions, leaving interpretations about the meaning of the variables to the reader. Of course in the latter instance it is easy to get lost.

• Formulating the Theoretical Rationale

Once a general problem area has been isolated, the literature has been reviewed, and the variables have been defined, a theoretical rationale for the relationship between variables can be articulated. The internal structures, such as concepts, definitions, and theoretical rationale, must have clarity and continuity so that the investigator can advance a hypothesis, and thereby state expectations concerning the relationship of the variables under study. Both *clarity* and *continuity* are hallmarks you should be looking for when critiquing research. For example, you should inquire about the breadth and depth of the literature review, the unambiguous definitions of concepts and variables, and the advancement of a logical and explicit theoretical rationale firmly based on these structures.

• How to Use a Theoretical Framework as a Guide in Research Study

The theoretical framework of a research study places the problem in a theoretical context, bringing meaning to the problem and study findings. It summarizes the existing knowledge in the field of inquiry and identifies the linkages among the concepts, thereby establishing a basis for predicting specific outcomes or generating hypotheses (Fig. 6-1). These linkages or *propositions* spell out how defined concepts are interrelated and lay a foundation for the development of methods that test the validity and strength of identified relationships. The examples that follow will clarify how theory guides the research process.

Suppose you were interested in alternatives to medication for the treatment of postoperative pain. An examination of the literature might lead you to relaxation training as an intervention. The following series of questions might occur to you:

- On what basis has a linkage between pain and relaxation been established?
- What is the nature of the linkage?
- How can this linkage or relationship be tested?
- What methods can be used for the purpose of testing?

To answer these questions, you must begin with an exploration of the theoretical framework that is most suitable for pursuing the research problem.

Wells (1982) examined the relationship between relaxation and postoperative pain. In establishing a theoretical explanation for linking these variables she alluded to the gate control theory of pain, citing two components of the pain experience, physiological and psychological, and the interaction of these components. Citing Melzack and Wall (1970), she stated, "The physiological component involves adequate stimulus initiating neural transmission to higher centers in the brain. Localization and integration with motivational and affective input occurs in the cortical and subcortical structures. Descending control from the higher centers alters the transmission of additional impulses from the periphery" (p.236). She further stated that the "psy-

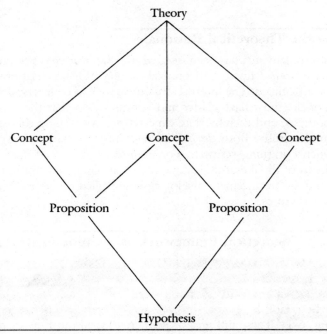

Fig. 6-1   Process of hypothesis generation.

chological component involves the interaction of many factors: focus of attention; coping style; cultural background; previous experience with pain; anxiety; and perceived control" (p.236). Specific aspects of the postoperative pain experience for adult cholecystectomy patients, such as abdominal muscle tension and neural input from structures affected by the incision, were identified. In describing the relaxation response, she referred to both physiological and psychological effects of this technique. She explicitly concluded that "a relaxation technique applied to postoperative pain may reduce the physiological input due to secondary reflex muscle contraction as well as alter the psychological variables of focus of attention, anxiety, and perceived control" (p.236).

Fig. 6-2 illustrates that the various linkages between the proposed variables, that is, relaxation, by influencing certain psychological and physiological components of the pain experience, were expected to alter that experience. Taking this rationale a step further, the following hypotheses can be generated:

1. Clients who practice a relaxation technique will experience reduced postoperative muscle tension in involved muscle groups as compared with clients who do not practice a relaxation technique.
2. Clients who practice a relaxation technique will experience reduced intensity of postoperative pain as compared with clients who do not practice a relaxation technique.
3. Clients who practice a relaxation technique will experience reduced postoperative pain distress as compared with clients who do not practice a relaxation technique.
4. Clients who practice a relaxation technique will report reduced postoperative anxiety.

The first hypothesis evolved from the theoretical linkage between relaxation and physiological factors associated with pain. The second and third hypotheses evolved from the theoretical linkage between relaxation and physiological and psychological factors, respectively, associated with pain. The fourth hypothesis evolved from the theoretical linkage between relaxation and psychological factors associated with pain.

Once hypotheses are generated, they are tested. This involves selecting the individual subjects to participate in the study, using instruments that will validly and reliably measure the variables, developing a method of systematically collecting the information needed to test hypothesized relationships, and selecting statistical measures that will determine the extent and meaning or significance of the relationships. Furthermore, the outcomes of the study must be viewed in terms of their support or nonsupport of the chosen theoretical rationale.

As you can see, the theoretical framework plays an important role in guiding the entire process of the research study. If the framework is logically sound and substantiated by previous research studies, there is a strong possibility that the hypotheses evolving from that framework will be supported; however, if the hypotheses are not based firmly on a theoretical rationale, there can be no confidence in the findings.

How the theoretical rationale provides a basis for hypothesis development in a research study may not always be made explicit in the research report. For example,

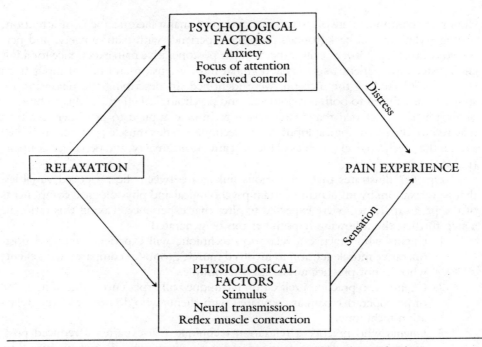

Fig. 6-2   Inventory of relationship between relaxation and pain.

Heidt (1981), in her study of therapeutic touch and anxiety, indicated, "the potential of this intervention (therapeutic touch) for eliciting in the subject a state of physiological relaxation" (p.32). She further discussed repatterning energy fields and the use of self therapeutically as two facets of therapeutic touch. Nowhere in the discussion of the theoretical background of the study did she state how therapeutic touch relates to anxiety reduction or how relaxation might form a connecting link between these two variables. Fig. 6-3 illustrates how this relationship might have been conceived. Study hypotheses were not explicitly substantiated in the investigator's presentation of the theoretical rationale, leaving theoretical interpretations to the reader.

In some cases, the theoretical rationale is inappropriately used. For example, a theory designed to explain a particular behavior in infants may not be appropriate for the study of those behaviors in adults. Similarly, a theory developed from Rogers' interactive conceptual model (1970) is not appropriate for the study of cause and effect relationships. The inappropriate use of theory, aside from being logically unsound, leads to erroneous conclusions about the problem being studied.

In other cases the theoretical rationale may be weak; perhaps it was not sufficiently tested, the assumptions were incompatible, the concepts were ill-defined, or the terms were inconsistent.

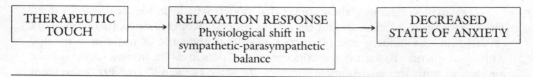

| THERAPEUTIC TOUCH | → | RELAXATION RESPONSE Physiological shift in sympathetic-parasympathetic balance | → | DECREASED STATE OF ANXIETY |

Fig. 6-3   Inventory of relationship between therapeutic touch and anxiety.

• The Contribution of Nursing Models to Research

In the previous discussion of *borrowed versus new theory,* it was pointed out that theories unique to nursing help nursing define how it is different from other disciplines. Nursing theories reflect particular views of the person, health, and other concepts that contribute to the development of a body of knowledge specific to nursing's concerns. But what is *nursing* theory? What are nursing's phenomena of concern? Where do nursing theories come from if they are not borrowed from other disciplines?

Fawcett (1978) defines *nursing theory* as "a set of propositions consisting of defined and interrelated units which presents a systematic view of the person, the environment, health, and nursing by specifying relations among relevant variables" (p.25). The phenomena of concern to nursing are the person, the environment, health, and nursing. Therefore theories that deal with these phenomena are termed *nursing* theories. These phenomena, as stated, are not conceptualized or operationalized. Clearly, terms must be defined before relationships among them can be specified. The next logical question is, "How are these phenomena defined?" The *person,* for example, can be viewed as active or waiting to be acted upon, inherently good or inherently bad, an energy field (Rogers, 1970), or an integrated whole (Orem, 1971). The answer to the question of defining phenomena lies in the *conceptual models* that form the bases for constructing nursing theories.

"A conceptual model is a highly abstract umbrella of related multidimensional concepts . . . [it] . . . provides a perspective for a science, telling the scientist what to look at" (Fawcett, 1978, pp.18-19). A conceptual model is developed inductively, using unsystematic observations, intuition, and other unstructured approaches. Theoretical models on the other hand, postulate relationships based on available theories, empirical research findings, and other structured approaches.

There are several well-known conceptual models in nursing that have served as a basis for theory development. Among them are Rogers' life process interactive person-environment model (1970); King's model of personal, interpersonal, and social systems (1980); Orem's model of self-care (1980); and Roy's adaptation model (1976). Each of these models addresses the four phenomena of concern to nursing but from different perspectives. For example, Rogers' conceptual model views the person and the environment as energy fields coextensive with the universe, that is, person-environment interactions are mutual and simultaneous. King's conceptual model, however, views the person and the environment as separate and interactions as cause and effect processes.

You may wonder how these conceptual models actually guide the research effort. The following description should clarify this process. Rogers' conceptual framework (1970) guided Goldberg and Fitzpatrick (1980) in their use of movement therapy with aged clients. Based on the concept of the person as "a holistic being whose interaction with the environment changes the state of being" (p.339), movement therapy was described as a positive integrating force or an integrated and holistic intervention. This intervention was proposed to be associated with positive changes in self-esteem, morale, agitation, attitude toward the individual's own aging, and lonely dissatisfaction. Study hypotheses, methods used to measure the variables such as self-esteem and morale, and the procedure for collecting data about the variables were based on Rogers' interactive framework. Among other findings, Goldberg and Fitzpatrick reported a significant improvement in total morale and attitude toward the client's own aging for the group who received movement therapy. It was concluded that movement therapy is a holistic, effective nursing intervention that adds support to the validity of Rogers' conceptual framework.

With this background on what nursing models are, what the phenomena of concern to nursing are, and how nursing theories develop, we can summarize the contribution of a nursing model to research. Chapter 2 focused on the scientific approach to the research process, including the philosophy of science, the sources of human knowledge, and the characteristics of the scientific approach. The development of nursing knowledge was said to depend upon both philosophy and science. Additionally, the individual researcher's own philosophy of human behavior and other related phenomena was said to guide the intent of the research effort. Similarly a nursing conceptual model serves as the philosophical view of specific phenomena of concern to nursing, from which nursing theories come. As such, it is instrumental in guiding the nursing research effort.

• Critiquing the Theoretical Framework

The criteria for critiquing a theoretical framework are found in the box on p. 83. The theoretical framework provides the context that clarifies and specifies problems, develops and tests hypotheses, evaluates research findings, and makes generalizations. As research consumers, it is important for nurses to know how to critically appraise the conceptual and theoretical bases for research. The following discussion is intended to assist you in this process.

Initially, you will probably focus on the concepts being studied. Concepts should clearly reflect the area of investigation. Using the general concept of stress when anxiety is more appropriate to the research focus creates difficulties in defining variables and delineating hypotheses.

Next, you must evaluate the completeness and appropriateness of the operational definitions of each concept. Once they are defined, you must consider whether or not the variables are examined in general and specifically in the context of the problem under investigation. The literature review is the source for this kind of discussion.

Critiquing Criteria

1. Is the theoretical framework clearly identified?
2. Are the concepts clearly and operationally defined?
3. Does the operationalization adequately reflect each conceptual definition?
4. Was sufficient literature reviewed to support the proposed relationships?
5. Is the theoretical basis for hypothesis formulation clearly articulated? Is it logical?
6. Are the relationships among propositions clearly stated? *only 1 or 2*
7. Is the conceptual framework consistent throughout, that is, is the basic philosophical view of the phenomena of concern maintained throughout the study?
8. If the theory is borrowed from a discipline other than nursing, are the data related specifically to nursing?
9. Are the study findings related to the theoretical rationale?

Finally, it is important to appraise the instruments used to measure the variables in terms of appropriateness, for example, does the instrument measure the variables as defined and is the instrument consistent with the theoretical framework? How do they hold up when compared with other instruments? Are all of the subparts consistently measuring the same characteristics? Are the instruments maintaining their stability when repeatedly used over time?

A second aspect of appraising the theoretical rationale relates to the interrelationships among concepts, or *hypotheses*. Briefly stated, hypotheses should express relationships between variables precisely and unambiguously. They should be based on the propositions that come from the theoretical framework and directly answer the research problem identified early in the report. A more detailed discussion of critiquing hypotheses appears in Chapter 7.

When you evaluate the theoretical framework itself, it is important to examine both the depth and breadth of the literature review. Has the investigator included sufficient information "so that the reader could be assured that the investigator had considered a broad spectrum of possibilities for investigating the problem?" (Downs and Newman, 1977, p.4). Is there consistency throughout in terms of the philosophical view of phenomena? Are previous studies sufficiently described so that their validity can be determined? Is there a firm basis for linking the variables and determining the direction of hypotheses? Can the theory be empirically tested? Does the research contribute to the understanding of the phenomena of interest? Are the findings discussed in relation to the theoretical framework? In summary, you must evaluate whether or not the theoretical framework or the map led you to your findings of destination in a logical and systematic way.

• Summary

This chapter provides information about the nature and purpose of a theoretical framework. It addresses the relationship between theory and research, emphasizing the importance of theory as a guide to systematically identify and study the logical, precise relationships between variables.

A concept is an image or symbolic representation of an abstract idea. Concepts help us refine the ideas that form the basis for developing theory. To facilitate the process of refinement, concepts must be clearly defined. Additionally, operationalization of the definitions serves to delineate the procedures or operations required to measure the concept.

Theory is defined as "a set of interrelated constructs, definitions, and propositions that present a systematic view of phenomena by specifying relations among variables, with the purpose of explaining and predicting the phenomena" (Kerlinger, 1973, p.9). A theoretical rationale provides a road map or context for examining problems and developing and testing hypotheses. It brings meaning to the problem and study findings by summarizing existing knowledge in the field of inquiry and identifying linkages among concepts.

In developing a theoretical framework for nursing, knowledge may be acquired from other disciplines or directly from nursing. In either case, that knowledge is used to specifically answer nursing questions. Nursing conceptual models provide a context for constructing theories that deal with phenomena of concern to nursing, that is, the person, the environment, health, and nursing. They help nursing define how it is different from other disciplines.

Of significance to the research consumer is the evaluation or critique of the theoretical rationale of a research study. It is important to consider not only the clarity and logic of the theoretical rationale itself, but also whether or not the operational definitions, measurement instruments, methods of carrying out collection of data about the variables, hypotheses, and findings are consistent with the theory.

• References

Chinn, P., and Jacobs, M. (1973). *Theory and nursing: A systematic approach,* St. Louis, The C.V. Mosby Co.

Cleland, V. (1967). The use of existing theories, *Nursing Research,* **16**:118-121.

Downs, F., and Newman, M. (1977). A sourcebook of nursing research, 2nd ed., Philadelphia, F.A. Davis Co.

Fawcett, J. (1978). The "what" of theory development. In National League for Nursing, *Theory development: what, why, how?* New York.

Fawcett, J. (1983). Hallmarks of success in nursing theory development. In Chinn, P.: *Advances in nursing theory development,* Rockville, Md., Aspen Systems Corp., pp. 3-17.

Feldman, H. (1980). Nursing research in the 1980s:

Issues and implications, *Advances in Nursing Science,* **3**:85-92.

Goldberg, W., and Fitzpatrick, J. (1980). Movement therapy with the aged, *Nursing Research,* **29**:339-346.

Heidt, P. (1981). Effects of therapeutic touch on anxiety level of hospitalized patients, *Nursing Research,* **30**:32-37.

Johnson, D. (1968). Theory in nursing: Borrowed and unique, *Nursing Research,* **17**:206-209.

Kerlinger, F. (1973). *Foundations of behavioral research,* New York, Holt, Rinehart & Winston, Inc.

King, I. (1981). *A theory for nursing: Systems, concepts, process,* New York, John Wiley & Sons, Inc.

Lindeman, C., and VanAlrnan, B. (1977). Nursing

intervention with the presurgical patient—the effects of structured and unstructured preoperative teaching. In Downs, F. and Newman, M., eds.: *A sourcebook of nursing research,* 2nd ed., Philadelphia, F.A. Davis Co.

Newman, M. (1972). Nursing's theoretical revolution, *Nursing Outlook,* **20:**449-453.

Newman, M. (1977). Movement tempo and the experience of time. In Downs, F. and Newman, M., eds.: *A sourcebook of nursing research,* 2nd ed., Philadelphia, F.A. Davis Co.

Orem, D. (1971). *Nursing: Concepts of practice,* New York, McGraw-Hill Book Co.

Orem, D. (1980). *Nursing: Concepts of practice,* 2nd ed., New York, McGraw-Hill Book Co.

Phillips, J. (1977). Nursing systems and nursing models, *Image,* **9:**4-7.

Pilowsky, I., and Kaufman, A. (1965). An experimental study of a typical phantom pain, *British Journal of Psychiatry,* **3:**1185-1187.

Reynolds, P. (1971). *A primer in theory construction,* Indianapolis, The Bobbs-Merrill Co., Inc.

Rodgers, J. (1977). Relationship between sociability and personal space preference at two different times of day. In Downs, F. and Newman, M., eds.: *A sourcebook of nursing research,* 2nd ed., Philadelphia, F.A. Davis Co.

Rogers, M. (1970). *An introduction to the theoretical basis of nursing,* Philadelphia, F.A. Davis Co.

Roy, Sr., C. (1976). *Introduction to nursing: An adaptation model,* Englewood Cliffs, N.J., Prentice-Hall, Inc.

Stevens, B. (1979). *Nursing theory: Analysis, application, evaluation,* Boston, Little, Brown & Co.

Swanson, A. (1977). Fearfulness of children in relation to maternal anxiety, self-differentiation and accuracy of perception. In Downs, F. and Newman, M., eds.: *A sourcebook of nursing research,* 2nd ed., Philadelphia, F.A. Davis Co.

Wells, N. (1982). The effect of relaxation on postoperative muscle tension and pain, *Nursing Research,* **31:**236-238.

Witkins, H., Dyk, R., Faterson, H., and others. (1974). *Psychological differentiation,* Potomac, Md. Erlbaum.

• Suggested Readings

Benoliel, J. (1977). The interaction between theory and research, *Nursing Outlook,* **25:**108-113.

Ellis, R. (1968). Characteristics of significant theories, *Nursing Research,* **17:**217-222.

Jacox, A. (1974). Theory construction in nursing: An overview, *Nursing Research,* **23:**4-13.

National League for Nursing. (1978). *Theory development: What, why, how?* New York.

Newman, M. (1979). *Theory development in nursing,* Philadelphia, F.A. Davis Co.

Quint, J. (1967). The case for theories generated from empirical data, *Nursing Research,* **16:**109-114.

Walker, L. (1971). Toward a clearer understanding of nursing theory, *Nursing Research,* **20:**428-435.

7

The Hypothesis

Judith Haber

LEARNING OBJECTIVES

After reading this chapter, the student will be able to do the following:

- Identify the characteristics of a hypothesis.
- Discuss the relationship of the hypothesis to the other research process components.
- Describe the advantages and disadvantages of directional and nondirectional hypotheses.
- Compare and contrast the use of statistical versus research hypotheses.
- Discuss the appropriate use of research questions in a research study.
- Formulate a hypothesis.
- Identify the criteria used for critiquing a hypothesis.
- Apply the critiquing criteria to the evaluation of a hypothesis in a research report.

KEY TERMS

conceptual definitions	operational definitions
dependent variable	research hypothesis
directional hypothesis	statistical hypothesis
hypothesis	testability
independent variable	theory
nondirectional hypothesis	

A hypothesis attempts to answer the question posed by the research problem. It is a vehicle for testing the validity of the theoretical framework's assumptions. Actually, a hypothesis is a bridge between theory and the real world. In the scientific realm, researchers derive hypotheses from theories and subject the hypotheses to empirical testing. As such, a hypothesis is an integral component of the scientific method (see Chapter 2). The theory's validity is not directly examined. Instead, it is through the hypothesis that the merit of a theory can be evaluated. The hypothesis of a research study is analogous to a compass that indicates which direction the research study will proceed.

This chapter will present the purpose and characteristics of the hypothesis, its interrelationship with the research process, and the criteria for critiquing hypotheses.

• Definition

Hypotheses flow from the problem statement, literature review, and theoretical framework. Fig. 7-1 illustrates this flow. A *hypothesis* is an assumptive statement about the relationship between two or more variables. A hypothesis converts the question posed by the research problem into a declarative statement that predicts an expected outcome.

Each hypothesis represents a unit or subset of the research problem. For example, a research problem might pose the question: Is there a relationship between maternal-infant sleep rhythms, maternal social support systems, and postpartum blues? This problem can be broken down into the following two subproblems:

1. Is there a relationship between maternal-infant sleep rhythms and postpartum blues?
2. Is there a relationship between maternal social support systems and postpartum blues?

A hypothesis can then be generated for each unit of the research problem, the subproblems. The hypotheses of the research problem mentioned before might be stated in the following way:

Hypothesis 1:   Synchrony in maternal-infant sleep rhythms will be negatively related to postpartum blues.

Hypothesis 2:   Perception of positive maternal social support systems will be negatively related to postpartum blues.

The critiquer of a research report will want to evaluate whether the hypotheses of the study represent subsets of the main research problem as illustrated by the examples just given.

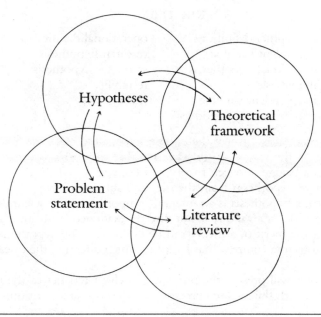

Fig. 7-1   Interrelationship between problem statement, literature review, theoretical framework, and hypothesis.

Hypotheses are formulated before the study is actually conducted because they will provide direction for the collection, analyses, and interpretation of data. Hypotheses have three purposes. Their first purpose is to provide a bridge between theory and reality and in this sense they unify the two domains. Their second purpose is to be powerful tools for the advancement of knowledge, since they enable the researcher to objectively enter new areas of discovery. Their third purpose is to provide direction for any research endeavor by tentatively identifying the anticipated outcome.

• Characteristics

Nurses who are conducting research or nurses critiquing published research studies must have a working knowledge about what constitutes a "good" hypothesis. Such knowledge will enable them to have a standard for evaluating their own work or the work of others. The following discussion about the characteristics of hypotheses will present criteria to be used when formulating or evaluating a hypothesis.

THE RELATIONSHIP STATEMENT

The first characteristic of a hypothesis is that it is a declarative statement that identifies the predicted relationship between two or more variables. This implies that there is a systematic relationship between an independent and a dependent variable. The direction of the predicted relationship is also specified in this statement. Phrases such as *greater than, less than, positively, negatively,* or *curvilinearly related* (U- or ∩-shaped), and *difference in* connote the directionality that is proposed in the hypothesis. It is not unusual for a beginning researcher to generate a hypothesis that omits one of the two required variables or that fails to make a prediction about the direction of the relationship. For example, the following prediction, "Children who have asthma will respond favorably to postural drainage treatments," is not a scientifically acceptable hypothesis. There is only one stated variable, postural drainage treatments. This statement could be revised to make it an acceptable hypothesis containing two variables and a relational statement. The hypothesis could then be stated in the following manner: "Asthmatic children who receive postural drainage treatments (independent variable) will have less bronchial congestion (dependent variable) than children with no postural drainage." In this hypothesis the two variables are explicitly identified, and the relational aspect of the prediction is contained in the phrase *less than*.

The nature of the relationship, either causal or associative, is also implied by the hypothesis. A causal relationship is one where the researcher is able to predict that the independent variable *(X)* causes a change in the dependent variable *(Y)*. It is rare in research that one is in a firm enough position to take a definitive stand about a cause-and-effect relationship. Variables are more commonly related in noncausal ways. That is, the variables are systematically related, but in an associative way. This means that there is a systematic movement in the associated values of the two phenomena. For example, there is increasing evidence that cigarette smoking is related to lung cancer. It is tempting to state that there is a causal relationship between cigarette smoking and lung cancer. However, do not overlook the fact that not all cigarette smokers develop lung cancer, and not all of those who develop lung cancer are cigarette smokers. Consequently, it would be scientifically unsound to take a position advocating the presence of a causal relationship between these two variables. Rather, one can only say that there is an associative relationship between the variables of cigarette smoking and lung cancer, a relationship where there is a strong systematic association between the two phenomena.

TESTABILITY

The second characteristic of a hypothesis is its *testability*. This means that the variables of the study must lend themselves to observation, measurement, and analysis. The hypothesis is either supported or not supported after the data have been collected and analyzed. The predicted outcome proposed by the hypothesis will or will not be congruent with the actual outcome when the hypothesis is tested. Hypotheses advance scientific knowledge by confirming or disconfirming theories.

Hypotheses may fail to meet the criteria of testability because the researcher has not made a prediction about the anticipated outcome, the variables are not observable or measurable, or the hypothesis is couched in terms that are value laden. Table 7-1 illustrates each of these points and provides a remedy for each problem.

• *Table 7-1*   Hypotheses That Fail to Meet the Criteria of Testability

Problematic hypothesis	Problematic issue	Revised hypothesis
Anxiety is related to learning.	No predictive statement about the relationship is made, therefore the relationship is not verifiable.	Anxiety is curvilinearly (∩-shaped) related to problem solving behavior.
Clients who receive pre-operative instruction have less postoperative stress than clients who do not.	The "postoperative stress" variable must be specifically defined so that it is observable or measurable or the relationship is not testable.	Clients who attend preoperative education classes have less postoperative emotional stress than clients who do not.
Small group teaching will be better than individualized teaching for dietary compliance in diabetic clients.	"Better than" is a value-laden word that is not objective. Moral and ethical questions containing words such as "should," "ought," "better than," and "bad for" are not scientifically testable.	Dietary compliance will be greater in diabetic clients receiving diet instruction in small groups than in diabetic clients receiving individualized diet instruction.

THEORY BASE

A sound hypothesis is consistent with an existing body of theory and research findings. Regardless of whether a hypothesis is arrived at inductively or deductively (see Chapter 2), it must be based on a sound scientific rationale. The reader of a research report should be able to identify the flow of ideas from the problem statement to the literature review, to the conceptual framework, and through the hypotheses (see Chapters 5 and 6). Fig. 7-2 illustrates this process in relation to the problem statement, "What is the effect of skin-to-skin contact between the mother and the infant in the first hour after delivery on later maternal attachment behavior?" It is clear that there is an explicitly developed, relevant body of scientific data that provides the theoretical grounding for the study. The hypotheses, as stated in Fig. 7-2, are logically derived from the framework.

WORDING THE HYPOTHESIS

As you read the scientific literature and become more familiar with it, you will observe that there are a variety of ways to word a hypothesis. Regardless of the specific format used to state the hypothesis, the statement should be worded in clear, simple, and concise terms. If this criterion is met, the reader will understand the following:
1. The variables of the hypothesis
2. The population being studied
3. The predicted outcome of the hypothesis

Problem statement	Literature review	Conceptual framework	Hypotheses
What is the effect of skin-to-skin contact between the mother and the infant in the first hour after delivery on later maternal attachment behavior?	1. Animal studies related to mother-infant separation 2. Human Contact Studies and their effect on mother-infant attachment 3. Attachment behaviors 4. Labor and delivery experience 5. Maternal life experience	1. Infants are born with unique characteristics that affect the development of maternal attachment 2. Before and after delivery the mother's individual characteristics and life history had and would continue to have an effect on her feelings of attachment 3. The first hour after delivery is a sensitive period and the interactions that occur at this time are potentially critical experiences 4. By 3 months after delivery, most mothers develop an attachment to their infants	1. Mothers who had extended skin-to-skin contact with their infants during the first hour after delivery would display significantly more maternal attachment behaviors 36 hours after delivery than mothers who did not have skin-to-skin contact with their infants 2. Mothers who had extended skin-to-skin contact with their infants during the first hour after delivery will have significantly more maternal attachment behaviors 3 months after delivery than mothers who did not have initial skin-to-skin contact with their infants

Fig. 7-2   Flow of data between problem statement, literature review, theoretical framework, and hypothesis.

• *Table 7-2*   **Examples of How Hypotheses are Worded**

Hypothesis	Variables*	Type of hypothesis	Type of design suggested
1. There will be a relationship between self-concept and suicidal behavior	*IV:* Self-concept *DV:* Suicidal behavior	Nondirectional research	Nonexperimental
2. Oxygen inhalation by nasal cannula of up to 6 L/min. does not affect oral temperature measurement taken with an electronic thermometer	*IV:* Oxygen inhalation by nasal cannula *DV:* Oral temperature	Directional Statistical	Experimental
3. Synchrony of maternal and newborn sleep rhythms will be negatively related to postpartum blues	*IV:* Synchrony of maternal and newborn sleep rhythms *DV:* Postpartum blues	Directional Research	Nonexperimental
4. Structured preoperative education is more effective than structured postoperative education in reducing the client's perception of pain	*IV:* Preoperative education *IV:* Postoperative education *DV:* Perception of pain	Directional Research	Experimental
5. The incidence of adolescent pregnancy in girls attending birth control education classes will not differ from that of girls who do not attend birth control education classes	*IV:* Birth control education classes *DV:* Adolescent pregnancy	Directional Statistical	Experimental
6. Clients on home dialysis treatment will demonstrate more self-care behavior than clients on hospital-based dialysis treatment	*IV:* Home dialysis treatment *IV:* Hospital-based dialysis treatment *DV:* Self-care behavior	Directional Research	Nonexperimental

*IV, independent variable; *DV*, dependent variable.

• *Table 7-2*   Examples of How Hypotheses are Worded—cont'd

Hypothesis	Variables*	Type of hypothesis	Type of design suggested
7. Progressive relaxation will be more effective in reducing indices of physiological arousal than hypnotic relaxation or self-relaxation in cardiac rehabilitation patients	*IV:* Progressive relaxation *IV:* Hypnotic relaxation *IV:* Self-relaxation *DV:* Physiological arousal indices	Directional Research	Experimental
8. There will be a negative relationship between the age of the nurse and her attitude toward rape	*IV:* Age of the nurse *DV:* Attitude toward rape	Nondirectional Research	Nonexperimental
9. There will be a positive relationship between trust and self-disclosure in marital relationships	*IV:* Trust *DV:* Self-disclosure	Directional Research	Nonexperimental
10. There will be a greater decrease in posttest state anxiety scores in subjects treated with noncontact therapeutic touch than in subjects treated with contact therapeutic touch	*IV:* Noncontact therapeutic touch *IV:* Contact therapeutic touch *DV:* State anxiety	Directional Research	Experimental

This information may be further clarified by the definition section of a study (see Chapters 6 and 13).

DIRECTIONAL VERSUS NONDIRECTIONAL HYPOTHESES

Hypotheses can be formulated directionally or nondirectionally. A *directional hypothesis* is one that specifies the expected direction of the relationship between the independent and dependent variable. The reader of a directional hypothesis may observe that the existence of a relationship is proposed as well as the nature or direction of that relationship. The following is an example of a directional hypothesis: "Nurse positive reinforcement will have a greater effect on client learning of self-care tasks than nurse negative reinforcement." Examples of directional hypotheses can also be found in Table 7-2 in examples 2 through 7, 9, and 10.

In contrast, a *nondirectional hypothesis,* while indicating the existence of a relationship between the variables, does not specify the anticipated direction of the relationship. The following is an example of a nondirectional hypothesis: "There is a relationship between perception of self-competence and breast-feeding behavior." Other examples of nondirectional hypotheses are illustrated in Table 7-2, examples 1 and 8.

Nurses who are learning to critique research studies should be aware that both the directional and nondirectional forms of hypotheses statements are acceptable. However, also be aware that there are definite pros and cons pertaining to each one.

Proponents of the nondirectional hypothesis state that this format is more objective and impartial than the directional hypothesis. It is argued that the directional hypothesis is potentially biased, because the researcher, in stating an anticipated outcome, has demonstrated a commitment to a particular position.

On the other side of the coin, proponents of the directional hypothesis argue that researchers naturally have hunches, guesses, or expectations concerning the outcome of their research. It was the hunch, the curiosity, or the guess that initially led them to speculate about the problem. The literature review and the conceptual framework provided the theoretical foundation for deriving the hypothesis. Consequently, it might be said that a deductive hypothesis derived from a theory will almost always be directional (see Chapter 6). The theory will provide a critical rationale for proposing that relationships between variables will have particular outcomes. When there is no theory or related research to draw on for rationale, or findings in previous research studies are ambivalent, the nondirectional hypothesis may be appropriate.

In summary, the evaluator of a hypothesis should know that there are several advantages to directional hypotheses, making them appropriate for use in most studies. The advantages are the following:

1. They indicate to the reader that a theory base has been used to derive the hypotheses and that the phenomena under investigation have been critically thought about and interrelated. The reader should realize that nondirectional hypotheses may also be deduced from a theory base. However, because of the exploratory nature of many studies utilizing nondirectional hypotheses, the theory base may be less developed.
2. They provide the reader with a specific theoretical frame of reference within which the study is being conducted.
3. They suggest to the reader that the researcher is not sitting on a theoretical fence, and as a result, the analyses of data can be accomplished in a statistically more sensitive way.

The important thing for the critiquer to keep in mind regarding directionality of the hypotheses is whether or not there is a sound rationale for the choice the researcher has proposed regarding directionality.

STATISTICAL VERSUS RESEARCH HYPOTHESES

Readers of research reports may observe that a hypothesis is further categorized as either a research or a statistical hypothesis. A *research hypothesis,* also known as a scientific hypothesis, consists of a statement about the expected relationship between the variables. A research hypothesis indicates what the outcome of the study is expected to be. Examples 1, 3, 4, and 6 through 10 of Table 7-2 represent research hypotheses.

A *statistical hypothesis,* also known as a null hypothesis, states that there is no relationship between the independent and dependent variable. Examples 2 and 5 in Table 7-2 illustrate statistical hypotheses. If in the data analysis a statistically significant relationship emerges between the variables at a specified level of significance, the null hypothesis is rejected. Rejection of the statistical hypothesis is equivalent to acceptance of the research hypothesis. Some researchers refer to the null hypothesis as a statistical contrivance that obscures a straightforward prediction of the outcome. Others state that it is more exact and conservative statistically; that failure to reject the null hypothesis implies that there is insufficient evidence to support the idea of a real difference.

Readers of research reports will note that, in general, research hypotheses are more commonly stated than statistical hypotheses. It is more desirable to state the researcher's actual expectation. The reader then has a more precise idea of the proposed outcome. In any actual study that involves statistical analysis the underlying null hypothesis is usually assumed without being explicitly stated.

• Research Questions

Research studies do not always contain hypotheses. As you become more familiar with the scientific literature, you will notice that exploratory studies usually do not have hypotheses. This is particularly common where there is a dearth of literature or related research studies in a particular area that is of interest to the researcher. The researcher, interested in finding out more about a particular phenomenon, may engage in a fact-finding or relationship-finding mission guided only by research questions. The outcome of the exploratory study may be that data about the phenomenon is amassed and the researcher is then able to formulate hypotheses for a future study.

Research questions tend to be more general than the research problems discussed in Chapter 4. However, the more specific they are, the more they provide direction for the study. The following are some examples of research questions:

1. What are the factors that produce success on state board exams for associate degree nursing students?
2. What are the hospital unit organizational factors that contribute to quality nursing care?
3. How does the use of nursing diagnosis improve client care?
4. What are the community resources that homebound elderly clients need to remain in the community?

In other studies, research questions are formulated in addition to hypotheses to answer questions related to ancillary data. Such questions do not directly pertain to the proposed outcomes of the hypotheses. Rather, they may provide additional and sometimes serendipitous findings that are enriching to the study and valuable in providing direction for further study. Sometimes they are the kernels of new or future hypotheses.

The evaluator of a research study needs to determine whether or not it was appropriate to formulate a research question rather than a hypothesis, given the nature and context of the study.

• Critiquing the Hypothesis

Hypotheses represent the core of an empirical research study. As such, it is important that nurses not only understand how to formulate hypotheses, but they must also know how to critically appraise them. Consequently, we will now turn our attention to the evaluation of hypotheses in research reports.

When reviewing a research report, several criteria for critiquing the hypothesis should be used as a standard for evaluating the strengths and weaknesses of the hypotheses.

1. The hypothesis should directly answer the research problem that was posed at the beginning of the report. Its placement in the research report logically follows the problem statement, the literature review, and the theoretical framework because the hypothesis should reflect the culmination and expression of this conceptual process. It should be consistent with both the literature review and the theoretical framework. The flow of this process, as depicted in Fig. 7-2, should be explicit and apparent to the reader. If this criterion is met, the reader feels reasonably assured that the basis for the hypothesis is theoretically sound.

2. As the reader examines the actual hypothesis several aspects of the statement should be critically appraised. First, the hypothesis should consist of a declarative statement that objectively and succinctly expresses the relationship between an independent and dependent variable. In wording a complex versus a simple hypothesis, there may be more than one independent and dependent variable.

Second, the reader can expect that often there will be more than one hypothesis, particularly if there is more than one independent and dependent variable. If you recall, an earlier section of the chapter indicated that each hypothesis should be specific to one relationship. Consequently, if there are multiple variables in the problem or if the problem statement is broken down into subproblems, the reader may anticipate that there should be several hypotheses.

Third, the variables of the hypothesis should be understandable to the reader. Often in the interest of formulating a succinct hypothesis statement, the complete meaning of the variables is not apparent. The critiquer must realize that sometimes a researcher is caught between the "devil and the deep blue sea" on that issue. It may be a choice between having a complete but verbose hypothesis paragraph, or a less complete but concise hypothesis. The solution to this dilemma is for the researcher to have a definition section in the research report. The inclusion of conceptual and operational definitions (see Chapters 6 and 13) provides the complete explication of the variables. The critiquer is then able to examine the hypothesis side by side with the definitions and determine the exact nature of the variables under consideration. An excellent example of this process appears in a research article by Trainor (1982). The researcher hypothesized that

Visitors would demonstrate a significantly greater level of acceptance of their own ostomy than nonvisitors.

This is an appropriately worded hypothesis. However, it is not completely clear what the variable "visitor" implies. It is only when one examines the definition of "visitor" and "nonvisitor" that the exact nature of the variable becomes clear to the reader.

> *Visitor:* a person with an ostomy who is a member of a local United Ostomy Association chapter and who has visited other ostomates.
>
> *Nonvisitor:* a person with an ostomy who is a member of a local United Ostomy Association chapter but who has neither trained as a visitor nor visited other ostomates.

The context of the variables is now revealed to the evaluator.

Fourth, although a hypothesis can legitimately be nondirectional, it is preferable to indicate the direction of the relationship between the variables in the hypothesis. The reader will find that when there is a dearth of data available for the literature review; that is, the researcher has chosen to study a relatively undefined area of interest, the nondirectional hypothesis may be appropriate. There simply may not be enough information aviable to make a sound judgment about the direction of the proposed relationship. All that could be proposed is that there will be a relationship between two variables. Essentially, the critiquer wants to determine the appropriateness of the researcher's choice regarding directionality of the hypothesis.

3. The notion of testability is central to the soundness of a hypothesis. One criterion related to testability is that the hypothesis should be stated in such a way that it can be clearly supported or not supported. While the previous statement is very important to keep in mind, the reader should also understand that ultimately, neither theories nor hypotheses are ever proved beyond the shadow of a doubt through hypothesis testing. Researchers who claim that their data have "proven" the validity of their hypothesis should be regarded with grave reservation. The reader should realize that at best, findings that support a hypothesis are considered tentative. If repeated replication of a study yields the same results, greater confidence can be placed in the conclusions advanced by the researchers. An important thing to remember about testability is that while hypotheses are more likely to be accepted with increasing evidence, they are never ultimately proven.

Another point about testability for the consumer to consider is that the hypothesis should be objectively stated and devoid of any value-laden words. Value-laden hypotheses are not empirically testable. Quantifiable words such as *greater than, less than, decrease, increase,* and *positively, negatively,* and *curvilinearly related* convey the idea of objectivity and testability. The reader should be immediately suspicious of hypotheses that are not stated objectively.

4. The evaluator of a research study should be cognizant of the fact that the way that the proposed relationship of the hypothesis is phrased suggests the type of research design that will be appropriate for the study. For example, if a hypothesis proposes that treatment X_1 will have a greater effect on Y than treatment X_2, an experimental or quasi-experimental design is suggested (see Chapter 9). If a hypothesis proposes that there will be a positive relationship between variables X and Y, a

nonexperimental design is suggested (see Chapter 10). A review of Table 7-2 will provide you with additional examples of hypotheses and the type of research design that is suggested by each hypothesis. The reader of a research report should evaluate whether or not the selected research design is congruent with the hypothesis. This factor has important implications for the remainder of the study in terms of the appropriateness of sample selection, data collection, data analysis, interpretation of findings, and ultimately the conclusions advanced by the researcher.

5. If the research report contains research questions rather than hypotheses, the reader will want to evaluate whether or not this is appropriate to the study. The criterion for making this decision, as presented earlier in this chapter, is whether or not the study is of an exploratory nature. If it is, then it is appropriate to have research questions rather than hypotheses. Ancillary research questions should be evaluated as to whether or not they answer additional questions secondary to the hypotheses. Sometimes the substance of an additional research question is more appropriately posed as another hypothesis in that it relates in a major way to the original research problem.

CONCLUSION

After you have explored the scientific literature and evaluated enough hypotheses, you will have an appreciation for how carefully a hypothesis must be worded. The hypothesis represents the core of the scientific method. The remainder of a study revolves around testing the hypothesis. To determine the merit of a hypothesis that has been formulated or reviewed in the literature, the reader must have and use criteria to objectively evaluate it.

• Summary

Criteria for critiquing the hypothesis are given in the box on p. 99.

A hypothesis attempts to answer the question posed by the research problem. When testing the validity of the theoretical framework's assumptions, the hypothesis bridges the theoretical and real worlds.

A hypothesis is a declarative statement about the relationship between two or more variables that predicts an expected outcome. Characteristics of a hypothesis include a relationship statement, implications regarding testability, and consistency with a defined theory base. Hypotheses can be formulated in a directional or a nondirectional manner. Hypotheses can be further categorized as either research or statistical hypotheses.

Research questions may be utilized instead of hypotheses in exploratory research studies. Research questions may also be formulated in addition to hypotheses to answer questions related to ancillary data.

The critiquing process provides a set of criteria for the evaluation of the strengths and weaknesses of a hypothesis as it is presented in a research report. The reader

Critiquing Criteria

1. Does the hypothesis directly answer the research question?
2. Is the hypothesis concisely stated in a declarative form?
3. Are the independent and dependent variables identified in the statement of the hypothesis?
4. Are the variables measurable or potentially measurable?
5. Are each of the hypotheses specific to one relationship so that each hypothesis can either be supported or not supported?
6. Is the hypothesis stated in such a way that it is testable?
7. Is the hypothesis stated objectively, without value-laden words?
8. Is the direction of the relationship in each hypothesis clearly stated?
9. Is each hypothesis consistent with the literature review?
10. Is the theoretical rationale explicit?
11. Are the research questions stated in relation to the auxiliary data except in the case of an exploratory study?

evaluates the wording of the hypothesis in terms of the clarity of the relational statement, the implications for testability, and its congruence with a theory base. The appropriateness of the hypothesis in relation to the type of research design suggested by the design is also examined. The appropriate use of research questions is also evaluated.

The hypothesis represents the core of a research study. The remainder of the study revolves around the testing of the hypothesis. The hypothesis must be as accurate as possible because it is analogous to a compass inidcating the direction for the research endeavor to proceed.

• References

Campbell, D.T. and Stanley, J.C. (1963). *Experimental and quasi-experimental designs for research,* Chicago: Rand-McNally College Publishing Co.

Curry, M.A. (1952). Maternal attachment behavior and the mother's self-concept: the effect of early skin-to-skin contact, *Nursing Research,* **31**(2): 73-78.

Downs, F.S. and Newman, M.A. (1977). *A source book of nursing research,* Philadelphia, F.A. Davis Co.

Kerlinger, F.N. (1973). *Foundations of behavioral research,* New York, Holt, Rinehart & Winston.

Newman, M.A. (1979). *Theory development in nursing,* Philadelphia, F.A. Davis Co.

Polit, D.F. and Hungler, B.P. (1983). *Nursing research: Principles and methods,* 2nd ed., Philadelphia, J.B. Lippincott Co.

Trainor, M.A. (1982). Acceptance of ostomy and the visitor role in a self-help group for ostomy patients, *Nursing Research,* **31**(2):102-106.

Van Dalen, D.B. (1979). *Understanding educational Research,* New York, McGraw-Hill Book Co.

8

Introduction to Design

Geri LoBiondo-Wood

LEARNING OBJECTIVES

After reading this chapter, the student should be able to do the following:
- Define research design.
- Identify the purpose of the research design.
- Describe the concepts that affect the research design.
- Define control as it affects the research design.
- Compare and contrast the elements that affect control.
- Begin to evaluate what degree of control should be exercised in the design.
- Define internal validity.
- Identify the threats to internal validity.
- Define external validity.
- Identify the conditions that affect external validity.
- Evaluate the design using the critiquing questions.

KEY TERMS

constancy	homogeneity
control	instrumentation
control group	internal validity
design	maturation
ecological validity	mortality
experimental group	population validity
external validity	randomization
extraneous variable	selection bias
history	testing

The word *design* implies the organization of elements into a masterful work of art. In the world of art and fashion, design conjures up images of processes and techniques that are used to express a total concept. When an individual creates, process and form are employed. The form, process, and degree of adherence to structure depend on the aims of the creator. The same can be said of the research process. The research process and the development of research design need not be a sterile procedure, but one where the researcher develops a masterful work within the limits of a problem and the related theoretical basis.

Nursing is concerned with a variety of structures that require varying degrees of process and form, such as the administration of holistic and quality client care, staff organization, student education, and continuing education. When client care is administered, the nursing process based on assessment, planning, intervention, and evaluation is utilized. Before these four steps can be accomplished, a certain level of knowledge is required. This knowledge is derived from theory, practice, and experience. Validation of these areas is derived from research. To understand and utilize research, it is necessary to have knowledge of the process and an equally important in-depth knowledge of the content of the subject area being studied. Previous chapters have stressed the importance of theory and subject matter knowledge. How a researcher structures, implements, or designs an investigation affects the results of a research project.

For the consumer to understand the implications of research and to utilize research, a basic knowledge of the central issues in the design of a research project should be understood. This chapter will provide an overview of the meaning, purpose, and importance of research design while the following chapters will present specific types of designs.

• Purpose of Research Design

The purpose of the research design is to provide the scheme for answering specific research questions. The design then becomes the vehicle for the hypothesis. To answer research questions, the principles of scientific inquiry are utilized. Therefore the design involves a plan, structure, and strategy. These three concepts of design guide a researcher when writing the hypothesis, during the operationalization, or the carrying out of the project, and in the analysis and evaluation of the data. The overall purpose of the research design is twofold: to aid in the solution of research questions and to maintain control. All research attempts to answer questions. The design is coupled with the methods and procedures and together they are the mechanisms for finding solutions to research questions. *Control* is defined as the measures that the researcher utilizes to hold the conditions of the investigation uniform. By holding the conditions uniform, the researcher avoids possible bias impinging on the dependent variable that may affect the outcome. A variety of considerations, including the type of design chosen, affect the accomplishment of this end. These considerations include objectivity in the conceptualization of the problem, accuracy, economy, control of the experiment, internal validity, and external validity. There are statistical principles behind the many forms of control, but a clear conceptual understanding is of greater importance to the consumer of research.

OBJECTIVITY IN THE CONCEPTUALIZATION

Objectivity in the conceptualization of the problem is derived from a review of the literature and development of a theoretical framework (Fig. 8-1). Using the literature, the researcher assesses the depth and breadth of available knowledge concerning the problem. The literature review and theoretical framework should demonstrate to the reader that the researcher reviewed the literature with a critical and objective eye (see Chapters 2 and 5), as this affects the type of design chosen. For example, a question regarding the relationship of the length of a breast-feeding teaching program may suggest either a correlational or experimental design (see Chapters 9 and 10), while a question regarding the growth in size of a woman's body during pregnancy and maternal perception of the unborn child may suggest a survey or case study (see Chapters 10 and 11). Therefore, it should be obvious how the researcher's literature review reflects the following:

- When the problem was studied
- What aspects of the problem were studied
- Where it was investigated
- By whom it was investigated

The review that incorporates these aspects allows the consumer to judge the objectivity of the problem area and, therefore, if the design chosen matches the problem.

ACCURACY

Accuracy is also accomplished through the theoretical framework, review of the literature, and as a result of the researcher's preparation (see Chapters 5 and 6). Accuracy means that all aspects of a study systematically and logically follow from the identified problem statement. The beginning researcher is wise to answer a question involving few variables that do not require the use of sophisticated designs. The simplicity of a research project does not render it useless or of a lesser value for practice. Although the project is simple, the researcher should not forego accuracy. The consumer should feel that the investigator used the appropriate type of design that answered the research question with a minimum of contamination. The issues of contamination or control will be discussed later in this chapter. Also, many clinical problems have not yet been researched. Therefore a primary or pilot study would be a wise approach. The key is the accuracy, validity, and objectivity used by the researcher in attempting to answer the question. Accordingly, the researcher should read various levels of studies and assess how and if the criteria for each step of the research process were followed. Consumers of research will find that many nursing journals publish not only sophisticated clinical research projects, but also smaller clinical studies that can be applied to practice.

ECONOMY

When critiquing the research design, the evaluator also needs to be aware of the pragmatic consideration of economy. Sometimes the reality of this does not truly sink in until one does research. It is important to consider economy when reviewing a study, including availability of the subjects, timing of the research, time required for the subjects to participate, cost in terms of such items as reproduction, and analysis of the data (Table 8-1). These pragmatic considerations are not presented as a step in the research process as are the theoretical framework or methods, but they do affect every step of the process. As such, the reader of a study should consider these when assessing the investigation. The student researcher may or may not have monies or accessible services. When critiquing an investigation, note the credentials of the author and if the investigation was part of a student project or part of a fully granted project. If the project was a student project, the standards of critiquing are applied more liberally than for a prepared, experienced researcher or clinician. Finally, the pragmatic issues raised affect the scope and breadth of an investigation and therefore its generalizability.

CONTROL

A researcher attempts to use a design to maximize the degree of control over the tested variables. *Control* involves holding the conditions of the study constant. An efficient design can maximize results, decrease errors, and control preexisting or impaired conditions that may affect outcome. To maximize efforts, the researcher should maximize control. To accomplish these tasks, the research design and methods should demonstrate the researcher's efforts at control. For example, in a study by Farr, Keene, Samson, and Michael (1984), the researchers attempted to determine if a relationship existed between the degree of circadian alteration and the subject reentrainment to typical circadian profiles. Their hypotheses were the following:

   I. Normal circadian rhythms are altered in response to surgical trauma.

  II. Normal circadian rhythms uncouple in response to surgical trauma.

 III. Alterations in normal circadian rhythms are an additional stress to that of surgical trauma and therefore should affect reentrainment, or return to normal rhythmic state.

• *Table 8-1* **Pragmatic Considerations in Determining Feasibility of a Research Problem**

Factor	Pragmatic consideration
Time	The research problem must be one that can be studied within a realistic period of time. All researchers have deadlines for completion of a project. It is essential that the scope of the problem be circumscribed enough to provide ample time for the completion of the entire project. Research studies generally take longer than anticipated to complete.
Subject availability	The researcher needs to determine whether or not a sufficient number of eligible subjects will be available and willing to participate in the study. If one has a captive audience, like students in a classroom, it may be relatively easy to enlist their cooperation. When a study involves the subjects' independent time and effort, they may be unwilling to participate when there is no apparent reward for doing so. Other potential subjects may have fears about harm or confidentiality and may be suspicious of the research process in general. Subjects with unusual characteristics are often difficult to locate. In general, people are fairly cooperative about participating, but a researcher must consider meeting a larger subject pool than will actually participate. At times, when reading a research report it may be noted how the procedures were liberalized or the number of subjects was altered. This was probably a result of some unforeseen pragmatic consideration.
Facility and equipment availability	All research projects require some kind of equipment. The equipment may be questionnaires, telephones, stationery, stamps, technical equipment, or other apparatus. Most research projects require the availability of some kind of facility. The facility may be a hospital site for data collection or laboratory space, or a computer center for data analyses.
Money	Research projects require some expenditure of money. Before embarking on a study, the researcher probably itemized the expenses and projected the total cost of the project. This provides a clear picture of the budgetary needs for items like books, stationery, postage, printing, technical equipment, telephone and computer charges, and salaries. These expenses can range from about $50 for a small-scale student project to hundreds of thousands of dollars for a large-scale federally funded project.
Researcher experience	The selection of the research problem should be based on the nurse's realm of experience and interest. It is much easier to develop a research study related to a topic that is either theoretically or experientially familiar. Selecting a problem that is of interest to the researcher is essential for maintaining enthusiam when the project has its inevitable ups and downs.
Ethics	Research problems that place unethical demands on subjects may not be feasible for study. Researchers must take ethical considerations seriously. The consideration of ethics may affect the choice between an experimental or nonexperimental design.

To test these hypotheses and apply control, the investigators included in their study individuals who were active in the daytime, in relatively good health, free of renal problems, hypertension, and endocrine disorders, and taking no medications known to interfere with catecholamine secretion, adrenal cortical secretions, or electrolyte excretion. Subjects were also excluded if postoperative complications developed. This study illustrates how investigators in one study planned their design to apply controls. Control is important in all designs. When critiquing various research designs, the issue of control is always raised but with varying levels of flexibility. The issues to be discussed here will become clearer as you review the various types of designs discussed in later chapters (see Chapters 9 to 11). Control is accomplished by ruling out *extraneous variables* that compete with the independent variables as an explanation for the relationship or outcome of the study. Extraneous variables are variables that interfere with the operations of the phenomena being studied, such as age and sex. Means of controlling extraneous variables include the following:

- Use of a homogeneous sample
- Use of consistent data collection procedures
- Manipulation of the independent variable
- Randomization

The following example will be used to illustrate and define these concepts:

> An investigator might be interested in how a new stop-smoking program (independent variable) affects smoking behavior (dependent variable). The independent variable is assumed to affect the outcome or dependent variable. But the investigator needs to be relatively sure that the decrease in smoking is truly related to the stop-smoking program rather than to some other variable, such as motivation. The design of the research study alone does not inherently provide control. But an appropriately designed study with the necessary controls built in can increase the researcher's ability to answer this research question.

Homogeneous Sampling

In the stop-smoking study, extraneous variables may affect the dependent variable. The characteristics of a study's subjects are a common extraneous variable. Age, sex, and even newer smoking laws may affect the outcome in the stop-smoking example. These variables may therefore affect the outcome, even though they are extraneous or outside of the study's design. As a control for these and other similar problems, the researcher's subjects should demonstrate *homogeneity* or similarity with respect to the extraneous variables relevant to the particular study (see Chapter 14). These extraneous variables are not fixed, but need to be reviewed and decided on, based on the specific problem and its theoretical base. By using a sample of homogeneous subjects, the researcher has used a straightforward step of control. This step limits the *generalizability* or the application of the outcomes to other populations when analyzing and discussing the outcomes (see Chapter 18). Results can then only be generalized to a similar population of individuals. You may say that this is limiting. This is not necessarily so because no treatment or program may be applicable to all populations, and the consumer or utilizer of research findings needs to take the differences in populations into consideration. It is better to have a "clean" study that can be used to make generalizations about a specific population than a messy one that can be used to generalize little or nothing.

If the researcher feels that one of the extraneous variables is important, then it may be included in the design. In the smoking example, if individuals are working in an area where smoking is not allowed and this is considered to be important, then the researcher could build it into the design and set up a control for it. This can be done by comparing two different work areas, one where smoking is allowed and one where it is not. The important concept to keep in mind is that before the data are collected the researcher should have identified, planned for, or controlled the important extraneous variables.

Constancy in Data Collection

Another basic, yet critical, component of control is constancy in data collection conditions or procedures. *Constancy* refers to the notion that the data collection procedures should reflect to the consumer a cookbooklike recipe of how the researcher controlled the conditions of the study. This means that environmental conditions, timing of data collection, data collection instruments, and data collection procedures used to gain the data are the same for each subject. An example of a well-controlled laboratory experiment was done by Lim-Levy (1982) (see Appendix B). Lim-Levy's study was performed to determine the effect of oxygen inhalation by nasal cannula on oral temperatures. To control conditions, one electronic thermometer was used, subjects were requested verbally and in writing to refrain from vigorous activity, eating, drinking, and smoking for 1 hour before the procedure, mouth breathers were excluded, subjects were requested to sit quietly for at least 15 minutes before the experiment, and a comfortable sitting area was provided for the subjects. This type of control aided the researcher's ability to draw conclusions, discuss, and cite the need for further research in this area. For the consumer, it demonstrates a clear, consistent, and specific means of data collection. Another method of assuring constancy of data collection methods is training the data collectors similarly.

Not all of the problems nurses wish to research are amenable to laboratory study. Studies set in clinical settings also need constancy of data collection procedures to demonstrate to the consumer the efforts taken to address the concept of control.

Manipulation of Independent Variable

A third and very effective means of control is manipulation of the independent variable. This refers to administration of a program, treatment, or intervention to only one group within the study but not to the other subjects in the study. The first group is known as the *experimental group,* and the other group is known as the control group. In a *control group* the phenomena under study are held at a constant or comparison level. For example, suppose a researcher wishes to study the level of infection rates between a new type of surgical dressing and an old type. The older method represents the control group and the new method the experimental group. Experimental designs use manipulation. Nonexperimental designs do not manipulate the independent variable. This does not decrease the usefulness of a nonexperimental design, but the use of a control group in an experimental design is related to the level of the problem and again its theoretical framework. But if the problem is amenable to a design that incorporates manipulation of the independent variable, it can increase the theoretical and statistical power of the researcher to draw generalizable results, that is, if all of the other considerations of control are equally addressed (see Chapters 9 and 10). Again the reader should be cautioned that the lack of manipulation of the independent variable does not mean a weaker study. The level of the problem, the amount of theoretical work, and the research that has preceded a project, all affect the researcher's choice of a design.

Randomization

Researchers may also choose other forms of control such as randomization. *Randomization* is when the required number of subjects from the population are obtained in such a manner that each subject in a population has an equal chance of being selected. Randomization eliminates bias, aids in the attainment of a representative sample, and can be employed in various designs (see Chapters 9 and 14). Curry (1982) used one method of randomization when assigning primiparous women to receive or not to receive extended skin-to-skin contact with their newborns in the immediate postpartum period to assess if there were differences in various maternal attachment behaviors and self-concept.

Randomization can also be done with paper and pencil type instruments. By randomly ordering items on the instruments the investigator can assess if there is a difference in response that can be related to the order of the items. This may be especially important in longitudinal studies where bias from giving the same instrument to the same subjects on a number of occasions can be a problem (see Chapters 10 and 14).

CONTROL AND FLEXIBILITY

The same level of control cannot be exercised in all types of designs. The various types of designs that will be introduced to you in the following chapters will fully illuminate the issues that are being introduced to you within this chapter. At times, when a researcher wishes to explore a new area where little or no literature on the concept exists, the researcher will probably use an exploratory design. In this type of study, the researcher is interested in describing or categorizing a phenomenon in a group of individuals. Rubin's (1967a, 1967b) early work on the development of maternal tasks during pregnancy is an example of exploratory research. In this research, she attempted to categorize conceptually the various maternal tasks of pregnancy. Rubin interviewed women throughout their pregnancies and from these extensive interviews developed a framework of the maternal tasks of pregnancy. In critiquing this type of study, the issue of control should be applied in a highly flexible manner because of the preliminary nature of the work.

If it is determined from a review of a study that the researcher intended to conduct a correlational study, or a study that looks at the relationship between or among the variables, then the issue of control takes on more importance (see Chapter 10). Control needs to be strictly exercised as far as it is possible. At this intermediate level of design, it should be clear to the reviewer that the researcher considered the extraneous variables that may have accounted for the outcomes.

All aspects of control are strictly applied to studies that utilize an experimental design (see Chapter 9). The reviewer should be able to locate in the research report how the researcher met the following criteria: the conditions of the research were constant throughout the study, assignment of subjects was random, and an experimental group and control group were utilized. The Lim-Levy study (1982) is an example where all the aspects of control were addressed. Because of the control exercised by Lim-Levy, the reviewer can see that the highest level of control was applied and that extraneous variables were thereby considered.

INTERNAL AND EXTERNAL VALIDITY

When reading research, one needs to feel that the results of a study are valid, based on precision, and faithful to what the researcher wished to measure. For a study to form the basis of further research, practice, and theory development, it must be believable and dependable. There are two important criteria for evaluating the credibility and dependability of the results: internal validity and external validity.

Internal Validity

Internal validity asks if the independent variable really made the difference. This requires the researcher to rule out other factors or threats as rival explanations of the relationship between the variables. Thus internal validity refers to the causal relationship. Internal validity problems revolve around the issues of control. Six major threats to internal validity are defined by Campbell and Stanley (1966). These should be considered by the researcher in planning the design and by the consumer before implementation of results in practice. If these threats are not considered, they could negate the results of the research. How these threats my affect specific designs will be addressed in the following chapters. The following are threats to internal validity:

1. *History*. In addition to the independent variables, another specific event that may have an effect on the dependent variable may occur either inside or outside the experimental setting; this is referred to as history. For example, in a study of the effects of a breast-feeding teaching program on the length of time of breast-feeding, an event such as government-sponsored advertisements on the importance of breast-feeding featured on television and newspapers may be a threat of history.
2. *Maturation*. Maturation refers to the developmental, biological, or psychological processes that operate within an individual as a function of time and are external to the events of the investigation. For example, suppose one wishes to evaluate the effect of a specific teaching method on baccalaureate

students' achievements on a skills test. The investigator would record the students' abilities before and after the teaching method. Between the pretest and posttest, the students have grown older and wiser. This growth or change is unrelated to the investigation and may explain differences between the two testing periods.

3. *Testing*. Testing is defined as the effect of taking a pretest on the score of a posttest. The effect of taking a pretest may sensitize an individual and improve the score of the posttest. Individuals generally score higher when they take a test a second time regardless of the treatment. The differences between posttest and pretest scores may not be a result of the independent variable, but rather of the experience gained through testing.

4. *Instrumentation*. Instrumentation threats are changes in the measurement of the variables or observational techniques that may account for changes in the obtained measurement. Lim-Levy's use (1982) of the same equipment and procedures for each data collection session is an example of how a researcher took steps to avoid the threat of instrumentation. Another example that fits into this area is related to techniques of observation. If an investigator has several raters collecting observational data, they must all be trained in a similar manner. If they are not similarly trained, a lack of consistency may occur in their ratings and therefore a major threat to internal validity will occur.

5. *Mortality*. Mortality is the loss of study subjects from the first data collection point (pretest) to the second data collection point (posttest). If the subjects who remain in the study are not similar to those who dropped out, the results could be affected. In a study of how a media campaign affects the incidence of breast-feeding, if most dropouts were non-breast-feeding women, the perception given could be that exposure to the media campaign increased the number of breast-feeding women, whereas it was the effect of experimental mortality that lead to the observed results.

6. *Selection bias*. If the precautions are not used to gain a representative sample, a bias of subjects could result from the way the subjects were chosen. Selection effects are a problem in studies where the individuals themselves decide whether or not to participate in a study. Suppose an investigator wishes to assess if a new breast-feeding program contributes to the incidence and length of time of breast-feeding. If the new program is offered to all, chances are that women who are more motivated to learn about breast-feeding will take part in the program. Assessment of the effectiveness of the program is problematic because the investigator cannot be sure if the new program increased the number of women who breast-fed their newborns, or if only highly motivated individuals joined the program.

External Validity

External validity deals with possible problems of generalizability of the investigation's findings to additional populations and to other environmental conditions. External validity questions under what conditions and with what types of subjects the same results can be expected to occur. The goal of the researcher is to select a design that maximizes both internal and external validity. At times this is not always possible; if this is the case, then the researcher needs to establish a minimum requirement of meeting the criteria of external validity.

External validity is classified into two types: population validity and ecological validity. *Population validity* refers to the generalization of results to other populations. An example of a threat to population validity occurs when the researcher is not able to attain the ideal sample population. At times, numbers of available subjects may be low or not accessible by the researcher, and the researcher may then need to choose a nonprobability method of sample over a probability method (see Chapter 14). This may affect generalizability or external validity.

Ecological validity refers to the generalization of results to other settings or environmental conditions. An example of a threat to ecological validity occurs when the investigator has not described in detail the method or procedures used in the research project. The lack of explanation may lead the reviewer to use or generalize the results to a population that is dissimilar to the one being studied. This lack of explanation may also then affect the replication or repetition of the same research procedures in a second study. If replication of a study can be accomplished with similar results, the utility of the first study increases. Without an explanation of the methods or the sample used, the reviewer may be left in a quandry as to where and how to apply the findings. There are other additional threats to external validity that are dependent on the type of design utilized by the researcher, but these are beyond the scope of this textbook. A detailed coverage of the issue is offered in Campbell and Stanley (1963).

• Critiquing the Research Design

Criteria for critiquing the research design are given in the box on p. 111.

Critiquing the design of a study requires one to first have knowledge of the overall implications that the choice of a particular design may have for the study as a whole. The concept of the research design is an all-inclusive concept parallel to the concept of the theoretical framework. The research design is similar to the theoretical framework in that it deals with a piece of the research study that affects the whole. For one to knowledgeably critique the design in light of the entire study, it is important to understand the factors that influence the choice and the implications of the design. In this chapter, the meaning, purpose, and important factors of design choice as well as the vocabulary that accompanies these factors have been introduced.

Several criteria for evaluating the design can be drawn from the preceding chapter. One should remember that these criteria are applied differently with various designs. Different application does not mean that the consumer will find a haphazard approach to design. It means that each design has particular criteria that allow the evaluator to classify the design as to type, such as experimental or nonexperimental. These criteria need to be met and addressed in conducting an experiment. The par-

---

Critiquing Criteria

1. Is the type of design employed appropriate to the structured question?
2. Does the researcher utilize the various concepts of control that are consistent with the type of design chosen?
3. Does the design utilized seem to reflect the issues of economy?
4. Does the design utilized seem to flow from the proposed problem statement, theoretical framework, literature review, and hypothesis?
5. Does the design have controls for the threats of internal validity at an acceptable level?
6. Does the design have controls for the threats to external validity at an acceptable level?

---

ticulars of specific designs will be addressed in Chapters 9 through 11. The following discussion pertains primarily to the overall evaluation of a research design.

The research design should reflect that an objective review of the literature and the establishment of a theoretical framework guided the choice of the design. There is no explicit statement researching this in a research study. A consumer can evaluate this by critiquing the theoretical framework (see Chapter 6) and literature review (see Chapter 5). Is the problem new and not researched extensively, has a great deal been done on the problem, or is it a new or different way of looking at an old problem? Depending on the level of the problem, certain choices are made by the investigators. Manderino and Bzdek (1984) conducted a study to examine the efficacy of videotaped information and modeling as pain-reducing techniques for women during labor and delivery. They utilized various theory and research studies to design their study as objectively and accurately as possible. Before the study began, the investigators identified methodological problems in the research that they cited and built various design controls into their study (Manderino and Bzdek, 1984, p.10).

The consumer should be alert for the means used by investigators to maintain control, such as homogeneity in the sample, consistent data collection procedures, how or if the independent variable was manipulated, and whether randomization was utilized. As you will see in Chapter 9, all of these criteria must be met for an experimental design. As you begin to understand the types of designs and levels of research, namely, quasi-experimental and nonexperimental designs such as survey and interrelationship designs, you will find that these concepts are applied in varying degrees, or as in the case of a survey study, the independent variable is not manipulated at all (see Chapter 10). The level of control and its applications presented in Chapters 9 and 10 will provide you with the remaining knowledge to fully critique the aspects of the design in a study.

Once it has been established whether the necessary control or uniformity of conditions has been maintained, the evaluator needs to determine if the study is believable or valid. The evaluator should ask if the findings are the result of the variables tested and internally valid or if there could be another explanation. To assess this aspect, the threats to internal validity should be reviewed. If the investigator's study was systematic, well grounded in theory, and followed the criteria for each of the process, then you will probably conclude that the study is internally valid.

In addition, the critical reader needs to know if a study has external validity or generalizability to other populations or environmental conditions. External validity can be claimed only after internal validity has been established. If the credibility of a study (internal validity) has not been established, then a study could not be generalized (external validity) to other populations. Determination of external validity goes hand in hand with the sampling frame (see Chapter 14). If the study is not representative of any one group or phenomena of interest, then external validity may be limited or not present at all. The evaluator will find that establishment of internal and external validity needs not only knowledge of the threats to internal and external validity, but also a knowledge of the phenomena being studied. A knowledge of the phenomena being studied allows critical judgments to be made regarding the linkage of theories and variables for testing. The critical reader should find that the design follows from the theoretical framework, literature review, problem statement, and hypotheses. The evaluator should feel, based on clinical knowledge as well as the knowledge of the research process, that the investigators in a study are not comparing apples to oranges.

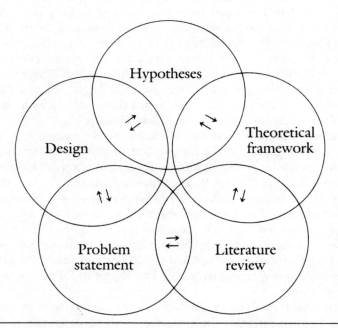

Fig. 8-1   Interrelationship between design, problem statement, literature review, theoretical framework, and hypothesis.

• Summary

The purpose of the design is to provide the format of a masterful and creative piece of research. As you will find in the following chapters, there are many types of designs. No matter which type of design the researcher uses, the purpose always remains the same. The consumer of research should be able to locate within the study a sense of the question that the researcher wished to answer. The question should be proposed with a plan or scheme for the accomplishment of the investigation. Depending on the question, the consumer should be able to recognize the steps taken by the investigator to ensure control.

The choice of the specific design depends on the nature of the problem. To specify the nature of the problem requires that the design reflects the investigator's attempts to maintain objectivity, accuracy, pragmatic considerations, and, most importantly, control. Control not only affects the outcome of a study, but also its future utility. The design should also reflect how the investigator attempted to control threats to both internal and external validity. Internal validity needs to be established before external validity can be. Both are considered within the sampling structure.

No matter which design the researcher chooses, it should be evident to the reader that the choice was based on a thorough examination of the problem within its theoretical framework. The design, problem statement, literature review, theoretical framework, and hypothesis should all interrelate to demonstrate a woven pattern (see Fig. 8-1). It should also be kept in mind that the choice of the design is affected by pragmatic issues and, at times, two different designs may be equally valid for the same problem. The main issues of control have been only minimally addressed here and will be covered in depth as they pertain to specific designs.

• References

Campbell, D., and Stanley, J. (1966). *Experimental and Quasi-experimental designs for research*, Chicago, Rand McNally.

Curry, M.A. (1982). Maternal-attachment behavior and the mother's self-concept, *Nursing Research*, **31**:73.

Farr, L., Keene, A., Samson, D., and Michael, A. (1984). Alterations in circadian excretion of urinary variables and physiological indicators of stress following surgery, *Nursing Research*, **33**:140-146.

Lim-Levy, F. (1982). The effect of oxygen inhalation on oral temperature, *Nursing Research*, **31**:150-153.

Mandarino, M.A., and Bzdik, V.M. (1984). Effects of modeling and information on reactions to pain: a childbirth-preparation analogue, *Nursing Research*, **33**:9-14.

Rubin, R. (1967a). Attainment of the maternal role, part I: processes, *Nursing Research*, **16**:237-245.

Rubin, R. (1967b). Attainment of the maternal role, part II: models and referents, *Nursing Research*, **16**:342-346.

• Additional Readings

Cook, T.D., and Campbell, D.T. (1979). *Quasi-experimentation: design analysis issues for field settings*, Boston, Houghton-Mifflin Co.

Huck, S.W., Cormier, W.H., and Bounds, Jr., W.G. (1974). *Reading Statistics and Research*, New York, Harper & Row, Publishers.

Judd, C.M., and Kenny, D.A. (1981). *Estimating the effects of social interventions*, Cambridge, Cambridge University Press.

Kerlinger, F.N. (1973). *Foundations of behavioral research*, New York, Holt, Rinehart & Winston, Inc.

Schantz, D., and Linderman, C.A. (1982). The research design, *The Journal of Nursing Administration*, **82**(2):35-38.

·

———————————————————

9

Experimental and Quasi-experimental Designs

Margaret Grey

———————————————

·

LEARNING OBJECTIVES

After reading this chapter, the student should be able to do the following:
- List the criteria necessary for inferring cause-effect relationships.
- Distinguish the differences between several experimental and quasi-experimental designs.
- Define internal validity problems associated with several experimental and quasi-experimental designs.
- Critically evaluate the findings of selected studies that test cause-effect relationships.

KEY TERMS

antecedent variable	intervening variable
control	manipulation
dependent variable	quasi-experimental design
experimental design	randomization
independent variable	

The purpose of this chapter is to acquaint you with the issues involved in interpreting studies that utilize experimental and quasi-experimental designs. One of the fundamental purposes of scientific research in any profession is to determine cause-effect relationships. In nursing, for example, we are concerned with developing effective approaches to maintaining and restoring wellness. Testing such nursing interventions to determine how well they actually work is accomplished by using experimental and quasi-experimental designs. These designs differ from nonexperimental designs in one important way: the researcher actively brings about the desired effect, and does not passively observe behaviors or actions. In other words, the researcher is interested in making something happen, not merely observing the routine.

Experimental designs are particularly suitable for testing cause-effect relationships because they help to eliminate potential alternative explanations for the findings. To infer causality requires that the following three criteria be met: the causal variable and effect variable must be associated with each other, the cause must precede the effect, and the relationship must not be explainable by another variable. When the reader critiques studies that utilize experimental and quasi-experimental designs, the primary focus will be on the validity of the conclusion that the experimental treatment, or the independent variable, caused the desired effect on the outcome, or dependent, variable. The validity of the conclusion depends on just how well the researcher has controlled the other variables that may explain the relationship studied. Thus the focus of this chapter will be to explain how the various types of experimental and quasi-experimental designs control these extraneous variables.

It should be made clear, however, that most research in nursing is not experimental. This is because nursing, unlike the physical sciences, is just beginning to identify the content and theory that is the exclusive province of nursing science. In addition, an experimental design requires that all of the relevant variables have been defined so that they can be manipulated and studied. In most problem areas in nursing, this requirement has not been met. Therefore nonexperimental designs utilized in identifying variables and determining their relationship to each other often need to be done before experimental studies.

• The True Experimental Design

An *experiment* is a scientific investigation that makes observations and collects data according to explicit criteria. True experiments, long considered the "ideal of science," have three identifying properties—randomization, control, and manipulation. These properties allow for other explanations of the phenomenon to be ruled out and thereby provide the strength of the design for testing cause-effect relationships.

RANDOMIZATION

Randomization involves the assignment of subjects to either the experimental or control group on a purely random basis. That is, each subject has an equal chance of being assigned to either group. Random assignment to group allows for the elimination of any systematic bias in the groups with respect to attributes that may affect the dependent variable being studied. The procedure for random assignment assumes that any important intervening variables will be equally distributed between the groups, and, as discussed in Chapter 8, minimizes variance.

CONTROL

By *control* we mean the introduction of one or more constants into the experimental situation. Control is acquired by manipulating the causal or independent variable, by randomly assigning subjects to a group, by very carefully preparing experimental protocols, and by using comparison groups. In experimental research the comparison group is the control group, or the group that receives the usual treatment, rather than the innovative experimental one.

MANIPULATION

We have said that experimental designs are characterized by the researcher "doing something" to at least some of the involved subjects. This "something," or the independent variable, is *manipulated* by giving it to some participants in the study and not to others, or by giving different amounts of it to different groups. The independent variable might be a treatment, a teaching plan, or a medication. It is the effect of this manipulation that is measured to determine the effect of the experimental treatment.

• • •

To see how these properties allow for other explanations of a phenomenon to be ruled out so that causal inferences can be made, let us examine the use of these properties in one such report. Wolfer and Visintainer (1975) studied the effect of stress-point preparation in reducing the stress of hospitalization and surgery on children (see Appendix A). The authors manipulated their independent variable of stress-point preparation. The children in their experiment were randomly assigned to two groups. One group received stress-point preparation and the other group received routine preoperative care. In addition, the independent variable was carefully controlled so that all of the children in the experimental group had exactly the same preparation. Thus by manipulating the independent variable, by introducing careful controls on the sample and the experimental protocol to minimize variance, and by randomly assigning the children to experimental or control groups, the authors were able to test and support their hypothesis that the children in the stress-point preparation group would demonstrate less upset behavior postoperatively than the children in the control group. The use of this design allowed the investigators to rule out possible threats to the validity of the findings such as selection, maturation, and history and avoided potential problems with interpreting the results. One possible alternative explanation might have been that the groups were different in a way that might have caused the experimental preoperative preparation to look as if it worked because the children in the experimental group were better adjusted before the study. Another possible threat controlled by the design was that some of the children may have had rooming-in with their parents and others did not, and those children who had rooming-in were less upset after surgery. Both of these potential threats to the validity of the findings are controlled by the use of the experimental design, because the properties of the experiment assure that the groups are equivalent before the introduction of the experimental treatment.

The strength of the true experimental design lies in its ability to help the researcher and the reader to control the effects of any extraneous variables that might constitute threats to internal validity. Such extraneous variables may either be antecedent or intervening. *Antecedent variables* are variables that occur before the study but may affect the dependent variable and confuse the results. Factors such as age, sex, socioeconomic status, and health status might be important antecedent variables in nursing research, because they may affect dependent variables such as recovery time and ability to integrate health care behaviors. *Intervening variables* are variables that occur during the course of the study and are not part of the study, but affect the dependent variable. Suppose a new head nurse who was not supportive of the Wolfer and Visintainer study (1975) came to the experimental floor while the study was being conducted. It is conceivable that the head nurse could undermine the study and possibly reduce the effect of the stress-point preparation. Then the authors would not have found that their new procedure worked better than the usual way. This result, however, would not be a true result; it would merely reflect the effect of the intervening variable.

TYPES OF EXPERIMENTAL DESIGNS

There are several different experimental designs (Campbell and Stanley, 1966). Each is based on the classic design called the *true experiment* diagrammed in Fig. 9-1. In this and the following illustrations, a simple notation will be used to describe the design. R stands for random assignment of subjects to group, X is the experimental treatment, and O stands for the observations or measurements made of the dependent

$$R \quad O1 \quad \times \quad O2$$
$$R \quad O1 \qquad O2$$

Fig. 9-1   The true experiment.

variable. All true experimental designs have subjects randomly assigned to groups, have an experimental treatment introduced to some of the subjects, and have the effects of the treatment observed. Designs vary primarily in the number of observations that are made.

As shown, subjects are randomly assigned to the two groups, experimental and control, so that antecedent variables are controlled. Then pretest measures or observations are made so that the researcher has a baseline for determining the effect of the independent variable. The researcher then introduces the experimental variable to one of the groups and measures the dependent variable again to see if it has changed. The control group gets no experimental treatment but is also measured later to compare with the experimental group. The degree of difference between the two groups at the end of the study indicates the confidence that the researcher has that a causal link exists between the independent and dependent variables. Because random assignment and the control inherent in this design minimize the effects of many threats to internal validity, it is a strong design for testing cause-effect relationships. However, the design is not perfect. Some threats cannot be controlled in true experimental studies (see Chapter 8). Mortality effects are often a problem in such studies, because people tend to drop out of studies that require their participation over a period of time. If there is a difference in the number of people who drop out of the experimental group from that of the control group, a mortality effect might explain the findings. When reading such a work, examine the sample and the results carefully to see if mortality occurred. Testing is also a problem in these studies, because the researcher is usually giving the same measurement twice, and subjects tend to score better the second time just by learning the test. Researchers can get around this problem in one of two ways. They might use different forms of the same test for the two measurements, or they might use a more complex experimental design called the Solomon four-group design.

The *Solomon four-group design,* shown in Fig. 9-2, has two groups that are identical to those utilized in the classic experimental design, plus two additional groups, an experimental after-group and a control after-group. As the diagram shows, all four groups have randomly assigned subjects as with experimental studies, but the addition of these last two groups helps to rule out testing threats to internal validity that the before and after groups may experience. Suppose a researcher is interested in the effects of some counseling on chronically ill clients' self-esteem, but just taking a measure of self-esteem may influence how the subjects report themselves. For example, the items might make the subjects think more about how they view themselves, so that the next time they fill out the questionnaire, their self-esteem might look as if it has improved. In reality, however, their self-esteem may be the same as it was

$$R \quad 01 \quad \times \quad 02$$
$$R \quad 01 \quad \quad 02$$
$$R \quad \quad \times \quad 02$$
$$R \quad \quad \quad 02$$

Fig. 9-2   The Solomon four-group design.

before, it just looks different because they took the test before. The use of this design, with the two groups that do not receive the pretest, allows for evaluating the effect of the pretest on the posttest in the first two groups. While this design helps to evaluate the effects of testing, the threat of mortality remains a problem as with the classic experimental design.

Another frequently utilized experimental design is the *after only design*, shown in Fig. 9-3. This design is composed of two randomly selected groups and neither group is pretested or measured. Again, the independent variable is introduced to the experimental group and not the control group. The process of randomly assigning the subjects to groups is assumed to be sufficient to assure a lack of bias, so that the researcher can still determine if the treatment created significant differences between the two groups. This design is particularly useful when testing effects are expected to be a major problem and the number of available subjects is too limited to use a Solomon four-group design. Many examples of this design can be found in the nursing literature (see Kruszewski and others, 1979).

FIELD AND LABORATORY EXPERIMENTS

Experiments can also be classified by setting. Field experiments and laboratory experiments share the properties of control, randomization, and manipulation, and utilize the same design characteristics, but they are conducted in various environments. Laboratory experiments take place in an artificial setting that is created specifically for the purpose of research. In the laboratory the researcher has almost total control over the features of the environment, such as temperature, humidity, noise level, and subject conditions. On the other hand, field experiments are exactly what the name implies—experiments that take place in some real, existing social setting such as a hospital or clinic where the phenomenon of interest usually occurs. Since most experiments in the nursing literature are field experiments and control is such an important element in the conduction of experiments, it should be obvious that studies conducted in the field are subject to treatment contamination by factors specific to the setting that the researcher cannot control. However, studies conducted in the laboratory are by nature "artificial," because the setting is created for the purpose of research. Thus laboratory experiments, while stronger in relationship to internal validity questions than field work, suffer more from problems with external validity. For example, a subject's behavior in the laboratory may be quite different from the person's behavior in the real world, a dichotomy that presents problems in generalizing findings from the laboratory to the real world. When reading research reports, then, it is important to consider the setting of the experiment and what impact it might have on the findings of the study.

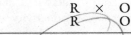

Fig. 9-3 The after only experimental design.

• Advantages and Disadvantages of the Experimental Design

As we have said, experimental designs are the most appropriate for testing cause-effect relationships. This is because of the design's ability to control the experimental situation. Therefore it offers better corroboration that, *if* the independent variable is manipulated in a certain way, *then* certain consequences can be expected to ensue. Such studies are important because one priority in the development of nursing and nursing research is the development of prescriptive theory (see Chapter 1). Wolfer and Visintainer (1975) were able to conclude from their study that the children who received the stress-point preparation, provided in a carefully controlled manner, showed the effect of this preparation by adjusting better postoperatively. This study, and others like it, allow nurses to anticipate in a scientific manner the probable effects of their nursing actions.

Still, experimental designs are not the ones most commonly utilized. There are several reasons that most nursing research studies are not experimental. First, experimentation assumes that all of the relevant variables involved in a phenomenon have been identified. For many areas of nursing research, this simply is not the case, and descriptive studies need to be completed before experimental interventions can be applied. Second, there are some significant disadvantages to these designs.

One problem with an experimental design is that many variables important in predicting outcomes of nursing care are not amenable to experimental manipulation. It is well known that health status varies with age and socioeconomic status. No matter how careful a researcher is, no one can assign subjects randomly by age or a certain level of income. In addition, some variables may be technically manipulable, but their nature may preclude actually doing so. For example, the ethics of a researcher who tried to randomly assign groups for a study of the effects of cigarette smoking and asked the experimental group to smoke two packs of cigarettes a day would be seriously questioned. It is also potentially true that such a study would not work, since nonsmokers randomly assigned to the smoking group would be unlikely to comply with the research task.

Another problem with experimental designs is that they may be difficult or impractical to perform in field settings. It may be quite difficult to randomly assign clients on a hospital floor to different groups when they might talk to each other about the different treatments. Experimental procedures may also be disruptive to the usual routine of the setting. If several different nurses are involved in administering the experimental program, it may be impossible to assure that the program is administered in the same way to each subject.

Finally, just being studied may influence the results of the study. This is called the *Hawthorne effect*. Named for the study at the Hawthorne plant of the General Electric Company where it was first noted, this effect means that just because subjects know they are participating in a study they may answer questions or perform differently. In the Hawthorne experiment, the researchers were trying to determine the effect of environmental factors on workers' productivity. Many different changes were made in the environment, and their effects on productivity were measured. No matter what the researchers did—improved the lighting or dimmed it, piped in music loudly or softly, or made no change—once the study began, productivity increased with each change. The increase in productivity was not a result of the environmental changes, but rather was caused by the attention being paid to the workers!

Because of these problems in carrying out true experiments, researchers frequently turn to another type of research design to evaluate cause-effect relationships. Such designs, because they look like experiments but lack some of the control of the true experimental design, are called quasi-experiments.

• Quasi-experimental Designs

In a quasi-experimental design full experimental control is not possible. *Quasi-experiments* are research designs where the researcher initiates an experimental treatment but some characteristic of a true experiment is lacking. Control may not be possible because of the nature of the independent variable or the nature of the available subjects. Usually what is lacking in a quasi-experimental design is the element of randomization. In other cases, the control group may be missing. However, like experiments, quasi-experiments involve the introduction of an experimental treatment.

In comparison to the true experimental design, quasi-experiments are quite similar in their utilization. Both types of designs are used when the researcher is interested in testing cause-effect relationships. However, the basic problem with the quasi-experimental approach is a weakened confidence in making causal assertions. Because of the lack of some controls in the research situation, quasi-experimental designs are subject to contamination by many, if not all, of the threats to internal validity discussed in Chapter 8.

There are many different quasi-experimental designs. We will discuss only the ones most commonly utilized in nursing research. Again we will use the notation introduced earlier in the chapter.

Refer back to the true experimental design shown in Fig. 9-1 and compare it to the *nonequivalent control group design* shown in Fig. 9-4. You should note that this design looks exactly like the true experiment except that subjects are not randomly assigned to groups. Suppose a researcher is interested in the effects of a new diabetes education program on the physical and psychosocial outcome of newly diagnosed clients. If conditions were right, the researcher might be able to randomly assign subjects to either the group receiving the new program or the group receiving the usual program, but for any number of reasons, that design might not be possible. For example, nurses on the floor where clients are admitted might be so excited about the new program that they cannot help but include the new information for all clients. So the researcher has two choices, to abandon the experiment or to conduct a quasi-experiment. To conduct a quasi-experiment, the researcher might find a similar unit

$$O1 \quad \times \quad O2$$
$$O1 \qquad \quad O2$$

Fig. 9-4   The nonequivalent control group design.

that has not been introduced to the new program and study the newly diagnosed diabetic clients who are admitted to that floor as a comparison group. The study would then involve this type of design.

The nonequivalent control group design is very commonly used in nursing research studies conducted in field settings. The basic problem with the design is the weakened confidence the researcher can have in assuming that the experimental and comparison groups are similar at the beginning of the study. Threats to internal validity such as selection, maturation, testing, and mortality are possible with this design. However, the design is relatively strong because the gathering of the data at the time of the pretest allows the researcher to compare the equivalence of the two groups on important antecedent variables before the introduction of the independent variable. In our example, the motivation of the clients to learn about their diabetes might be important in determining the effect of the new teaching program. The researcher could include in the measures taken at the outset of the study some measure of motivation to learn. Then differences between the two groups on this variable can be tested, and if significant differences exist, they can be controlled statistically in the analysis. Nonetheless, the strength of the causal assertions that can be made on the basis of such designs depends on the ability of the researcher to identify and measure or control possible threats to internal validity.

Now suppose that the researcher did not think to measure the subjects before the introduction of the new treatment, but afterward decides that it would be useful to have data demonstrating the effect of the program. Perhaps, for example, a third party asks for such data to determine whether the extra cost of the new teaching program should be paid. The study that could then be conducted would look like that drawn in Fig. 9-5.

This design, the *after only nonequivalent control group design*, is similar to the after only experimental design, but randomization is not utilized to assign subjects to group. This design makes the assumption that the two groups are equivalent and comparable before the introduction of the independent variable. Thus the soundness of the design and the confidence that we can put in the findings depends on the soundness of this assumption of preintervention comparability. Often it is very difficult to support the assertion that the two nonrandomly assigned groups are comparable at the outset of the study because there is no way of assessing its validity. In our example of the teaching program for newly diagnosed diabetic clients, measuring the subjects' motivation after the teaching program would not tell us whether their motivations differed before they received the program, and it is possible that the teaching program would motivate individuals to learn more about their health problem. Therefore the researcher's conclusion that the teaching program improved physical status and psychosocial outcome would be subject to the alternative conclusion that the

×   O

O

Fig. 9-5   The after only nonequivalent control group design.

01   ×   02

Fig. 9-6   The one group pretest-posttest design.

results were an effect of preexisting motivations (selection effect) in combination with greater learning in those so motivated (selection-maturation interaction). Nonetheless, this design is frequently utilized in nursing research because there often are limited opportunities for data collection and because it is particularly useful when testing effects may be problematic.

(3) A *preexperimental design* that is commonly employed in clinical nursing studies is the *one group pretest-posttest design*. This design is similar to the nonequivalent control group design except for the absence of the control group. It can be diagrammed as in Fig. 9-6.

The one group pretest-posttest design is employed when the researcher does not have access to an equivalent group and cannot use random assignment. The design then loses two important characteristics of experimentation, randomization and control over extraneous variables. While this design is better than not studying the effect of nursing care, it suffers from many problems in interpreting the results. In our diabetes example, how would the reader know if the improvement in the clients' physical status and psychosocial adjustment were not the result of the clients that happened to be admitted over the study period (selection)? Perhaps some event occurred on the study unit during the time of the project that would cause the researcher to conclude that the program had no impact (history). Any number of alternative conclusions could be drawn from these and similar data.

One approach that is utilized by researchers when only one group is available is to study that group over a longer period of time. This quasi-experimental design (4) is called a *time series design* and is pictured in Fig. 9-7.

To rule out some alternative explanations for the findings of a one group pretest-posttest design, researchers can measure the phenomenon of interest over a longer period of time and introduce the experimental treatment sometime during the course of the data collection period. Even with the absence of a control group, the broader number of data collection points helps to rule out such threats to validity as history effects. Obviously our problem with teaching diabetic clients will not lend itself to this design because we do not have access to them before the diagnosis.

An excellent example of how a time series design would strengthen causal conclusions is provided by Perry (1981). Perry studied the effect of a rehabilitation program on a group of clients with chronic lung disease, but she had only the one group to study. Thus it is difficult to be confident that the changes she found and

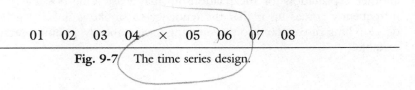

01   02   03   04   ×   05   06   07   08

Fig. 9-7   The time series design.

attributed to the rehabilitation program might not have happened without the program. On the other hand, the use of the time series design would have allowed Perry to follow the clients for a longer period of time and to be more confident that the program worked. This is because the time series weakens the alternative explanation that the program worked because of something else that happened during the study period. However, the testing threat to validity looms large in these designs, since measures are repeated so many times.

ADVANTAGES AND DISADVANTAGES OF QUASI-EXPERIMENTAL DESIGNS

Given the problems inherent in interpreting the results of studies utilizing quasi-experimental designs, you may be wondering why anyone would use them. The fact that quasi-experimental designs are used very frequently is because they are practical, feasible, and generalizable. These designs are more adaptable to the real world practice setting than the controlled experimental designs. In addition, for some hypotheses, these designs may be the only way to evaluate the effect of the independent variable of interest.

The weaknesses of the quasi-experimental approach involve mainly the ability to make clear cause-effect statements. However, if the researcher can rule out any plausible alternative explanations for the findings, such studies can lead to furthering knowledge about causal relationships. Researchers have several options for ferreting out these alternative explanations. They may control them a priori by design, control them statistically, or in some cases, common sense or knowledge of the problem and the population can suggest that a particular explanation is not plausible. Nonetheless, it is very important to replicate such studies to support the causal assertions developed through the use of quasi-experimental designs.

The literature on cigarette smoking is an excellent example of how findings from many studies, experimental and quasi-experimental, can be linked to establish a causal relationship. A large number of well-controlled experiments with laboratory animals randomly assigned to smoking and nonsmoking conditions has documented that smoking animals will develop lung disease. While such evidence is suggestive of a link between smoking and lung disease in humans, it is not directly transferable because animals and humans are different. But we cannot randomly assign humans to smoking and nonsmoking groups for ethical and other reasons. So researchers interested in this problem have to use quasi-experimental data to test their hypotheses about smoking and lung disease. Several different quasi-experimental designs have been used to study this problem and all had similar results, that there is a causal relationship between cigarette smoking and lung disease. Despite this massive evidence, the tobacco associations continue to insist that because the studies are not experimental, another explanation for the relationship may exist. One possible explanation that infrequently comes up is that the tendency to smoke is linked to the tendency to develop lung disease, and so the smoking itself is merely an unimportant intervening variable!

• Critiquing Experimental and Quasi-experimental Designs

We have said that various designs for research studies differ in the amount of control the researcher has over the antecedent and intervening variables that may impact the results of the study. True experimental designs offer the most possibility for control, and preexperimental designs offer the least. Quasi-experimental designs lie somewhere between. Research designs must balance the need for internal validity and external validity to produce useful results. In addition, judicious use of design requires that the chosen design be appropriate to the problem, free from bias, and capable of answering the research question.

Questions that the reader should pose when reading studies that test cause-effect relationships are listed in the box below. All of these questions should help the reader to judge whether it can be confidently believed that a causal relationship exists.

For studies where either experimental or quasi-experimental designs are utilized, first try to determine the type of design that was used. Often a statement describing

---

Critiquing Criteria

1. What design is used in the study?
2. Is the design experimental or quasi-experimental?
3. Is the problem one of a cause-effect relationship?
4. Is the method used appropriate to the problem?
5. Is the design suited to the setting of the study?

Experimental Designs

1. What experimental design is used in the study?
2. Is it clear how randomization, control, and manipulation were applied?
3. Are there any reasons to believe that there are alternative explanations for the findings?
4. Are all threats to validity, including mortality, addressed in the report?
5. Whether the experiment was conducted in the laboratory or a clinical setting, are the findings generalizable to the larger population of interest?

Quasi-experimental Designs

1. What quasi-experimental design is used in the study?
2. What are the most common threats to the validity of the findings of this design?
3. Have all plausible alternative explanations been addressed?
4. Are the author's explanations of threats to validity acceptable?
5. What does the author say about the limitations of the study?
6. Are there other limitations related to the design that are not mentioned?

the design of the study appears in the abstract and in the methods sections of the paper. If such a statement is not present, the reader should examine the paper for evidence of the following three characteristics: control, randomization, and manipulation. If all are discussed, the design is probably experimental. On the other hand, if the study involves the administration of an experimental treatment, but does not involve the random assignment of subjects to groups, the design is quasi-experimental.

Then try to identify which of the various designs within these two types of designs was used. Determining the answer to these questions gives you a head start because each design has its inherent threats to validity and this step makes it a bit easier to critically evaluate the study. The next question to ask is whether the researcher's problem required a solution to a cause-effect problem. If so, the study is suited to these designs. Finally, think about the conduct of the study in the setting. Is it realistic to think that the study could be conducted in a clinical setting without some contamination?

The most important question to ask yourself as you read experimental studies is, "What else could have happened to explain the findings?" Thus it is important that the author provide adequate accounts of how the procedures for randomization, control, and manipulation were carried out. The paper should include a description of the procedures for random assignment to such a degree that the reader could determine just how likely it was for any one subject to be assigned to a particular group. The description of the independent variable should also be detailed. The inclusion of this information helps the reader to decide if it is possible that the treatment given to some subjects in the experimental group might be different from what was given to others in the same group. In addition, threats to validity such as testing and mortality should be addressed. Otherwise, there is the potential for the findings of the study to be in error and less believable to the reader.

This question of potential alternative explanations for the findings is even more important when critically evaluating a quasi-experimental study because quasi-experimental designs cannot possibly control many plausible alternative explanations. A well-written report of a quasi-experimental study will systematically review potential threats to the validity of the findings. Then the reader's work is to decide if the author's explanations make sense.

As with all research, studies using these designs need to be generalizable to a larger population of people than those actually studied. Thus it is important to decide whether the experimental protocol eliminated some potential subjects and whether this impacted not only on internal validity, but also on external validity.

• Summary

This chapter has reviewed two types of design commonly used in nursing research to test hypotheses about cause-effect relationships. Experimental and quasi-experimental designs are useful for the development of nursing because they test the effects of nursing actions and leads to the development of prescriptive theory.

True experiments are characterized by the ability of the researcher to control extraneous variation, to manipulate the independent variable, and to randomly assign subjects to research groups. Experiments conducted either in clinical settings or in the laboratory provide the best evidence in support of a causal relationship because the following three criteria can be met:

1. The independent and dependent variable are related to each other.
2. The independent variable chronologically precedes the dependent variable.
3. The relationship cannot be explained by the presence of a third variable.

However, there are many times when experimental designs are impractical or unethical, so researchers will frequently turn to quasi-experimental designs to test cause-effect relationships. Quasi-experiments may lack either the randomization or comparison group characteristics of true experiments or both of these factors. Their usefulness in studying causal relationships depends on the ability of the researcher to rule out plausible threats to the validity of the findings, such as history, selection, maturation, and testing effects.

Finally, questions for the student to ask regarding the findings of experimental and quasi-experimental designs were presented. The overall purpose of critiquing such studies is to assess the validity of the findings and to determine if they are worth incorporating into the nurse's personal practice.

• References

Campbell, D., and Stanley, J. (1966). *Experimental and quasi-experimental designs for research,* Chicago, Rand McNally.

Fox, D.J. (1982). *Fundamentals of research in nursing,* Norwalk, Conn., Appleton-Century-Crofts.

Kruszewski, A.Z., Long, S.H., and Johnson, J.E. (1979). Effect of positioning on discomfort from intramuscular injections in the dorsogluteal site, *Nursing Research,* **28**(2):103-105.

Perry, J.A. (1981). Effectiveness of teaching in the rehabilitation of patients with chronic bronchitis and emphysema, *Nursing Research,* **30**(4):219-222.

Polit, D.F., and Hungler, B.P. (1983). *Nursing research: Principles and methods,* 2nd ed., Philadelphia, J.B. Lippincott.

Selltiz, C., Wrightsman, L.S., and Cook, S.W. (1976). *Research methods in social relations,* New York, Holt, Rinehart, & Winston.

Wolfer, J., and Visintainer, M.A. (1975). Pediatric surgical patients' and parents' stress responses and adjustment as a function of psychological preparation and stress-point nursing care, *Nursing Research,* **24**(4):244-255.

10

Nonexperimental Designs

Geri LoBiondo-Wood
Judith Haber
Christine Tassone Kovner

LEARNING OBJECTIVES

After reading this chapter, the student should be able to do the following:
- Describe the overall purpose of nonexperimental designs.
- Describe the characteristics of nonexperimental surveys and interrelationship research designs.
- Define the differences between surveys and interrelationship designs.
- List the advantages and disadvantages of each type of survey and interrelationship research design.
- Discuss relational inferences versus causal inferences as they relate to nonexperimental designs.
- Identify the criteria used to critique nonexperimental research designs.
- Apply the critiquing criteria to the evaluation of nonexperimental research designs as they appear in research reports.

KEY TERMS

correlational studies   nonexperimental research
cross-sectional studies   prediction studies
developmental studies   prospective studies
ex post facto studies   retrospective data
interrelationship studies   retrospective studies
longitudinal studies   survey research

Nonexperimental research designs are used in studies where the researcher wishes to construct a picture of a phenomenon or make account of events as they naturally occur. In experimental research the independent variable is manipulated; in nonexperimental research it is not. This is because experimental researchers are interested in looking at cause-effect relationships, but nonexperimental researchers are interested in finding meaning in observable phenomena. Thus in nonexperimental research the independent variables have already occurred, so to speak, and the investigator cannot directly control them by manipulation (Pedhazur, 1982, p.98). So an experimental researcher actively manipulates one or more variables, but a nonexperimental researcher observes events.

The reader of research reports will find that the majority of studies that are conducted and reported utilize a nonexperimental design. Many phenomena that are of interest and relevance to nursing do not lend themselves to an experimental design. For example, nurses studying the phenomena of pain may be interested in the amount of pain, variations in the amount of pain, and client responses to postoperative pain. To study the pain experience from any one of these perspectives, the investigator would not design an experimental study that would potentially intensify a client's pain just to study the phenomenon of pain. Instead, the researcher would perhaps examine the factors that contribute to the variability in a client's postoperative pain experience. A nonexperimental research design would then be utilized to help answer such questions.

Nonexperimental research also requires a clear, concise problem statement that is based on a theoretical framework. Even though the researcher does not actively manipulate the variables, the concepts of control introduced in Chapter 8 should be followed as much as possible.

Researchers are not in agreement on how to classify nonexperimental studies. For purposes of discussion, this chapter will divide nonexperimental designs into survey studies and interrelationship studies. An overall schema of research design is presented in Fig. 10-1. These categories are somewhat flexible, and other sources may classify nonexperimental studies in a different way. Some studies fall exclusively within one of these categories, whereas other studies have characteristics of more than one category. This chapter will introduce the reader to the various types of nonexperimental designs, the advantages and disadvantages of nonexperimental designs, the use of nonexperimental research, the issues of causality, and the critiquing process as it relates to nonexperimental research.

EXPERIMENTAL ⟶ QUASIEXPERIMENTAL ⟶ NONEXPERIMENTAL

Fig. 10-1   Continuum of research design.

• Survey Studies

The broadest category of nonexperimental research is the survey study. Survey studies collect detailed descriptions of existing phenomena and use the data to justify and assess current conditions and practices or to make more intelligent plans for improving them. Data may be collected by using either a structured questionnaire or a structured or unstructured interview (see Chapters 12 and 13). Survey researchers study either small or large samples of subjects drawn from defined populations. The units of analysis can be either broad or narrow and made up of people or institutions. For example, if a primary care rehabilitation unit was to be established in a hospital, a survey might be taken of the prospective applicant's attitudes with regard to primary nursing before selecting the staff of this unit. In a broader example, if a hospital were contemplating converting all client care units to primary nursing, a survey might be conducted to determine the attitudes of a representative sample of nurses in hospital X toward primary nursing. These data may then be the basis for projecting in-service needs of nursing regarding primary care. The scope and depth of a survey is then a function of the nature of the problem.

Surveys are descriptive and exploratory in nature. In descriptive surveys investigators attempt only to relate one variable to another and do not attempt to determine the cause. The investigators merely search for accurate information about the characteristics of particular subjects, groups, institutions, or situations, or the frequency of a phenomenon's occurrence. The variables of interest can be classified as opinions, attitudes, or facts. An example of an opinion or attitude variable might be the responses of nurses at different educational levels toward abortion (Littlefield-Derby, LoBiondo-Wood, and Olney-Springer, 1981). Another example of a survey is the study conducted by Brodie (1974). In this study, the researcher surveyed school-age children to describe the views of healthy children toward illness.

Examples of facts might include attributes of individuals that are a function of their membership in society such as gender, income level, political and religious affiliations, ethnic group, occupation, and educational level. Classic examples of survey research may be found in the surveys conducted during political campaigns to determine voter trends. Researchers commonly use demographic variables such as gender, economic status, and geographic location to provide an assessment of voter preference.

There are both advantages and disadvantages of survey research. Two major advantages are that a great deal of information can be obtained from a large population in a fairly economical manner and that survey research information can be surprisingly accurate. If a sample is representative of the population (see Chapter 14), a relatively small number of respondents can provide an accurate picture of the target population.

There are several disadvantages of survey studies. First, the information obtained in a survey tends to be superficial. The breadth rather than the depth of the information is emphasized. Second, conducting a survey requires a great deal of expertise in a variety of research areas. The survey investigator must know sampling techniques, questionnaire construction, interviewing, and data analysis to produce a reliable and valid study. Third, large-scale surveys can be time-consuming and costly, although the use of on-site personnel can reduce costs.

Research consumers should recognize that a well-constructed survey can provide a wealth of data about a particular phenomenon of interest even though relationships between variables are not being examined.

• Interrelationship Studies

In contrast to investigators who use survey research, other investigators who use nonexperimental designs endeavor to trace interrelationships between variables that will provide a deeper insight into the phenomenon of interest. These studies can be classified as interrelationship studies. The following types of interrelationship studies will be discussed: correlational, ex post facto, prediction, and developmental studies.

CORRELATIONAL STUDIES

The research consumer will find that an investigator utilizes a correlational design to examine the relationship between two or more variables. The researcher is not testing whether one variable causes another variable, but whether the variables covary, that is, as one variable changes does a related change occur in the other variable? The researcher utilizing this design is interested in quantifying the magnitude or strength of the relationship between the variables. In addition, the positive or negative direction of the relationship is also a central concern of the researcher (see Chapter 16 for a complete explanation of the correlation coefficient). For example, Newman and Gaudiano (1984) conducted a correlationship study that focused on depression as an explanation for the experience of decreased subjective time in the elderly. Newman defined subjective time as a ratio of awareness to the content of events in an individual's life $\left(\text{Subjective time} = \dfrac{\text{Awareness}}{\text{Content}} \right)$. An analysis of the data showed that there was a positive correlation ($r = 0.35$) between depression and subjective time estimates. This correlation was suggestive to the investigators that higher levels of depression were positively related to decreased subjective time estimation.

It should be remembered that the researchers were not testing a cause-effect relationship. All that is known is that the researchers found a relationship and that one variable (depression) varied in a consistent way with another variable, (subjective time estimate) for the particular sample studied. When reviewing a correlational study it is important to remember what relationship the researcher is testing and to notice whether the researcher implied a relationship that is consistent with the theoretical framework and hypotheses being tested.

Correlational studies offer researchers and research consumers the following advantages:
- An increased flexibility when investigating complex relationships among variables
- An efficient and effective method of collecting a large amount of data about a problem area
- A potential for practical application in clinical settings
- A potential foundation for future, more rigorous research studies
- A possible framework for investigating the relationship between variables that are inherently not manipulable

The reader will find that the correlational design has a quality of realism about it and is particularly appealing because it suggests the potential for practical solutions to clinical problems.

The following are disadvantages of correlational studies:
- The variables of interest are beyond the researcher's control.
- The researcher is unable to manipulate the variables of interest.
- The researcher does not employ randomization in the sampling procedures because of dealing with preexisting groups.
- The researcher is unable to determine a causal relationship between the variables because of the lack of manipulation, control, and randomization.

One of the most common misuses of a correlational design is the researcher's conclusion that a causal relationship exists between the variables. In the Newman and Guadiano investigation (1984), the researchers appropriately concluded that a relationship existed between the variables, but not that depression in the elderly caused a change in subjective time. The inability to draw causal statements should not lead the research consumer to think that a nonexperimental correlational study utilizes a weak design. It is a very useful design for clinical research studies because many of the phenomena of clinical interest are beyond the researcher's ability to manipulate, control, and randomize. For instance, a researcher interested in studying the grief experiences of women who have recently miscarried could not randomly assign subjects to grief and nongrief groups. Also, the experience of a miscarriage is a naturally occurring process and, as such, cannot be manipulated.

EX POST FACTO STUDIES

When scientists wish to explain causality or the factors that determine the occurrence of events or conditions, they prefer to employ an experimental design. However, they cannot always manipulate the independent variable X or utilize random assignments. In cases where experimental designs cannot be employed, ex post facto studies may be utilized. *Ex post facto* literally means "from after the fact." Ex post facto studies are also known as explanatory, descriptive studies (Van Dalen, 1979), causal-comparative studies (Van Dalen, 1979), or comparative surveys (Fox, 1982). As we discuss this design further, the reader will see that many elements of ex post facto research are similar to quasi-experimental designs (Campbell and Stanley, 1963).

• *Table 10-1*   **Paradigm for the Ex Post Facto Design**

Groups (not randomly assigned)	Independent variable (not manipulated by investigator)	Dependent variable
Exposed group	X	Y_E
Cigarette smokers	Cigarette smoking	Lung cancer
Control group		Y_C
Nonsmokers		No lung cancer

In ex post facto studies the consumer will find that the researcher hypothesizes, for instance that X (cigarette smoking) is related to and a determinant of Y (lung cancer), but X, the presumed cause, is not manipulated nor are subjects randomly assigned to groups. Rather, a group of subjects who have experienced X (cigarette smoking) in a normal situation is located and a control group of subjects who have not is chosen. The behavior, performance, or condition (lung tissue) of the two groups is compared to determine whether the exposure to X had the effect predicted by the hypothesis. Table 10-1 illustrates a paradigm for the ex post facto design. Examination of Table 10-1 reveals that while cigarette smoking appears to be a determinant of lung cancer, the researcher is still not in a position to conclude that there is a causal relationship between the variables because there has been no manipulation of the independent variable not random assignment of subjects to groups.

The advantages of the ex post facto design are similar to those inherent in the correlational design. The additional benefit of the ex post facto design is that it offers a higher level of control than the correlational design. Unlike the correlational design, the ex post facto design introduces the element of comparison groups, which provides an index of control not present in correlational studies. For example, in the cigarette smoking study, a group of nonsmokers' lung tissue samples are compared to samples of smokers' lung tissue. This comparison enables the researcher to establish that there is a differential effect of cigarette smoking on lung tissue. However, the researcher remains unable to draw a causal linkage between the two variables, and this inability is the major disadvantage of the ex post facto design.

Another disadvantage of ex post facto research is the problem of an alternative hypothesis being the reason for the documented relationship. If the researcher obtains data from two existing groups of subjects, such as one that has been exposed to X and one that has not, and the data support the hypothesis that X is related to Y, the researcher cannot be sure whether X or some extraneous variable is the real cause of the occurrence of Y. Finding naturally occurring groups of subjects who are similar in all respects except for their exposure to the variable of interest is very difficult. There is always the possibility that the groups differ in some other way, such as exposure to some other lung irritants, which can affect the findings of the study and produce spurious results. Consequently, the critiquer of such a study needs to cautiously evaluate the conclusions drawn by the investigator.

PREDICTION STUDIES

Researchers and particularly educators at times wish to make a forecast or prediction about how successful individuals will be in a particular setting, field of specialty, or circumstance. In this case, *prediction studies* are employed. For example, in a study conducted by Bello, Haber, King, and King (1980), an attempt was made to decrease the attrition rate of nursing students in an associate degree nursing program. Retrospective data of past students were used to establish the criteria for success or failure of students as measured by success on the state boards. Data utilized as criteria were verbal and math scores on the Comparative Guidance and Place (CGP) examination, high school algebra, biology, and chemistry grades, as well as demographic factors such as age, marital status, number of children, and related work experience. The goal of the study was to identify preexisting characteristics of the individual that were predictive of a relationship to the dependent variable, success on the state boards. The research consumer will find, as in this study, that prediction studies utilize retrospecitve data from one group to make predictions about similar group of students who are most likely to succeed in the future. This type of design generally employs sophisticated statistical techniques when exploring the relationships among variables in one group to make predictions about the behavior of another group.

The major advantage of predictive studies is that they facilitate intelligent decision making because objective criteria are available to guide the process. This can be particularly important in situations where critical choices, such as student selection, are made. The major disadvantage or limitation of prediction studies is that the design does not imply a cause-effect relationship between the chosen independent predictor variables and the dependent criterion variable. In addition, if the predictor variables were not chosen with a sound rationale, then a study may not be valid.

DEVELOPMENTAL STUDIES

There are also classifications of nonexperimental designs that use a time perspective. Investigators who utilize *developmental studies* are concerned with not only the existing status and interrelationship of phenomena but also with changes that result from the elapsing of time. The following four types of developmental study designs will be discussed: cross-sectional, longitudinal, retrospective, and prospective.

Cross-sectional and Longitudinal Studies

Cross-sectional studies examine data at one point in time. That is, the data are collected on only one occasion with the same subjects rather than on the same subjects at several points in time. An example of a cross-sectional study is Deets and Frobee's study of nurses' perceived incentives for employment (1984). Nurses were asked about their perceptions regarding employment incentives at one point in time, that is, when they filled out the questionnaire.

Another cross-sectional study approach is to simultaneously collect data on the variables of interest from different cohort groups. For example, if an investigator wishes to look at the development of maternal-fetal attachment in relationship to quickening in primiparas, the designated data collection periods may be the twelfth, twenty-fourth, and thirty-sixth weeks of pregnancy. The researcher would then select equivalent groups of primiparas who are at each respective point in their pregnancy. The data from each group would then be compared using statistical measures.

In contrast to the cross-sectional design, the *longitudinal design* collects data from the same group at different points in time. For instance, the investigator conducting the same maternal-fetal attachment study could elect to utilize a longitudinal design. In that case, the investigator would test the same group of primiparas at each data collection point. By collecting data from each subject at the twelfth, twenty-fourth, and thirty-sixth weeks of pregnancy, a longitudinal perspective of the attachment process is accomplished.

There are many advantages and disadvantages to both designs. When assessing the appropriateness of a cross-sectional study versus a longitudinal study, the research consumer should first assess what the goal of the researcher was in light of the theoretical framework. In the example of the maternal-fetal attachment study the researcher is looking at a developmental process; therefore a longitudinal design seems more appropriate. However, the disadvantages inherent in a longitudinal design must also be considered. Data collection may be of long duration because of the time it takes for the subjects to progress to each data collection point. In the attachment study, it would take each woman 24 weeks to complete the data collection process. It would take the investigator 6 months to complete the data collection *if* all of the subjects were obtained at one time. This does not even account for intervening variables of subject mortality such as attrition, miscarriage, or complications of pregnancy that might occur after the study has begun. These realities make a longitudinal design costly in terms of time, effort, and money. There is also a chance of confounding variables that could affect the interpretation of the results. Subjects in such a study may respond in a socially desirable way that they believe is congruent with the investigators' expectations. This is similar to the Hawthorne effect discussed in Chapter 9. However, despite the pragmatic constraints imposed by a longitudinal study, the researcher should proceed with this design if the theoretical framework supports a longitudinal developmental perspective.

The advantages of a longitudinal study are that each subject is followed separately and thereby serves as her own control, increased depth of responses can be obtained, and early trends in the data can be investigated.

In contrast, cross-sectional studies are less time-consuming, less expensive, and thus more manageable for the researcher. Since large amounts of data can be collected at one point, the results are more readily available. Additionally, the confounding variable of maturation, resulting from the elapsing of time, is not present. However, the economic accomplishments are sacrificed in terms of the investigator's lessened ability to establish an in-depth developmental assessment of the interrelationship of the phenomena being studied. Thus the researcher is unable to determine if the change that occurred is related to the change that was predicted by the hypotheses because the same subjects were not followed over a period of time. In other words, the subjects are unable to serve as their own controls (see Chapter 8).

In summary, it is important for the consumer to realize that longitudinal studies begin in the present and end in the future. On the other hand, cross-sectional studies look at a broader perspective of a cross section of the population at a specific point in time.

Retrospective and Prospective Studies

Retrospective studies are basically epidemiological in nature and are essentially the same as an ex post facto study. The term *retrospective* is mainly used by epidemiologists, whereas the term *ex post facto* is preferred by social scientists. Nevertheless, the investigator attempts to link present events to events that have occurred in the past. In example of a retrospective study conducted by Sideleau (1984), data such as sibling position, number of children in the family, and integrity of the family unit were examined in relationship to the diagnosis of mental illness in hospitalized adolescents and adults. The investigator began with a theoretical framework that was derived from a systematic retrospective search to identify the factors related to the development of mental illness. The findings of such retrospective studies can provide the basis for further investigation and require additional research information.

Prospective studies are also commonly used by epidemiologists. Prospective studies explore presumed causes and then move forward in time to the presumed effect. As such, they are much like longitudinal studies; they start in the present and end in the future. For example, a researcher might wish to test the incidence of alcohol consumption during pregnancy in relation to resulting low birth weight infants. To test this hypothesis, the investigator would draw a sample of pregnant women, some who regularly consumed alcohol during their pregnancy and others who did not. The occurrence of low birth weight infants in both groups would then be analyzed. This data would allow the investigator to assess whether regular alcohol consumption during pregnancy was related to the birth weight of the infant.

Prospective studies are less common than retrospective studies. This may be explained by the fact that it can take a long time for the phenomenon of interest to become evident in a prospective study. For example, if researchers were studing pregnant women who regularly consume alcohol, it would take 9 months for the effect of low birth weight in the subjects' infants to become evident. The problems inherent in a prospective study are therefore similar to those of a longitudinal study. However, prospective studies are considered to be stronger than retrospective studies because of the degree of control that can be imposed on extraneous variables that might confound the data.

• Causality in Nonexperimental Research

A great concern of nurses when they are conducting research is the issue of causality. Scientists are interested in explaining cause-effect relationships. Historically, researchers have said that only experimental research can support the concept of causality. For example, nurses are interested in discovering what causes anxiety in many settings. If we can find out the causes, we could develop interventions that perhaps would prevent or decrease the anxiety. Causality makes it necessary to order events chronologically. That is, if we find in a randomly assigned experiment that event one (stress) occurs before event two (anxiety), and that those in the stressed group were anxious whereas those in the unstressed group were not anxious, we can say that the hypothesis of stress causing anxiety is supported by these empirical observations. If these results were found in a nonexperimental study where some subjects underwent the stress of surgery and were anxious, and others did not have surgery and were not anxious, we would say that there is an association or relationship between stress (surgery) and anxiety. But on the basis of the results of a nonexperimental study we could not say that the stress of surgery *caused* the anxiety.

Newer methods of statistical analysis can add to what can be supported with nonexperimental data. Multiple regression techniques allow for the statistical control of many variables (Pedhazur, 1982). Recently researchers have been using sophisticated statistical techniques such as Path Analysis and LISREL, that analyze nonexperimental data in a way that either supports or does not support the concept of causality.

• Critiquing Nonexperimental Designs

Criteria for critiquing nonexperimental designs are presented in the box below. When critiquing nonexperimental research designs, the consumer should keep in mind

---

Critiquing Criteria

1. Which nonexperimental design is utilized in the study?
2. Based on the theoretical framework, is the rationale for the type of design evident?
3. Is the utilized design congruent with the purpose of the study?
4. Is the utilized design appropriate for the research problem?
5. Is the utilized design suited to the data collection methods?
6. Does the researcher present the findings in a manner that is congruent with the utilized design?
7. Does the research go beyond the relational parameters of the findings and erroneously infer cause-effect relationships between the variables?
8. Are there any reasons to believe that there are alternative explanations for the findings?
9. Where appropriate, does the researcher discuss the threats to internal and external validity?
10. How does the author deal with the limitations of the study?

that such designs offer the researcher the least amount of control. The first step in critiquing nonexperimental research is to determine which type of design was utilized in the study. Often a statement describing the design of the study appears in the abstract and in the methods section of the report. If such a statement is not present, the reader should closely examine the paper for evidence of which type of design was employed. The reader should be able to discern that either a survey or interrelationship design was used as well as the specific subtype. For example, the reader would expect an investigation of self-concept development in children from birth to 5 years of age to be an interrelationship study utilizing a longitudinal design.

Next the critiquer should evaluate the theoretical framework and underpinnings of the study to determine if a nonexperimental design was the most appropriate approach to the problem. For example, the numerous mother-infant attachment studies discussed throughout this text are all theoretically suggestive of a nonmanipulable interrelationship between attachment and any of the independent variables under consideration. As such, a nonexperimental correlational, longitudinal, or cross-sectional design is suggested by these studies. Investigators will use one of these designs to examine the relationship between the variables in naturally occurring groups. Sometimes the reader may think that it would have been more appropriate if the investigators had used an experimental or quasi-experimental design. However, the reader must recognize that pragmatic or ethical considerations may have also guided the researchers in their choice of design (see Chapters 3 and 8).

Then the evaluator should assess whether or not the problem is at a level of experimental manipulation. Many times researchers just wish to examine if relationships exist between variables. Therefore when one critiques such studies, the purpose of the study should be determined. If the purpose of the study does not include describing a cause-effect relationship, the researcher should not be criticized for not looking for one. However, the evaluator should be wary of a nonexperimental study in which the researcher suggests a cause-effect relationship in the findings.

Finally, the factor(s) that actually influence changes in the dependent variable are often ambiguous in nonexperimental designs. As with all complex phenomena, multiple factors can contribute to variability in the subjects' responses. When an experimental design is not used for controlling some of these extraneous variables that can influence results, the researcher must strive to provide as much control of them as possible within the context of a nonexperimental design. For example, when it has not been possible to randomly assign subjects to treatment groups as an approach to controlling an independent variable, the researcher may use a strategy of matching subjects for identified variables. For example, in a study of infant birth weight, pregnant women could be matched on variables such as weight, height, smoking habits, drug use, and other factors that might influence birth weight. The independent variable of interest, such as the type of prenatal care, would then be the major difference in the groups. The reader would then feel more confident that the only real difference between the two groups was the differential effect of the independent variable because the other factors in the two groups were theoretically the same. However, the consumer should also remember that there may be other influential variables that were not matched, such as income, education, and diet. Rival factors represent a major influence on the interpretation of a nonexperimental study because they impose limitations on the generalizability of the results.

• Summary

Nonexperimental research designs are used in studies that construct a picture or make an account of events as they naturally occur. The major difference between nonexperimental and experimental research is that in nonexperimental designs the independent variable is not actively manipulated by the investigator.

Nonexperimental designs can be classified as either survey studies or interrelationship studies. Survey research collects detailed descriptions of existing phenomena and uses the data either to justify current conditions and practices or to make more intelligent plans for improving them. Survey studies and interrelationship studies are both descriptive and exploratory in nature. Interrelationship studies endeavor to trace the interrelationships between variables that provide deeper insight into the phenomena of interest. Correlational, ex post facto, prediction, and developmental studies are examples of interrelationship studies. Developmental studies are further broken down into categories of cross-sectional, longitudinal, retrospective, and prospective studies. The advantages and disadvantages of each type of design must be considered by the researcher and critiquer when evaluating the merits of nonexperimental design.

Nonexperimental research designs do not enable the investigator to establish cause-effect relationships between the variables. Consumers must be wary of nonexperimental studies that make causal claims about the findings. Nonexperimental designs also offer the researcher the least amount of control. Rival factors represent a major influence on the interpretation of a nonexperimental study because they impose limitations on the generalizability of the results and as such should be fully assessed by the critical reader.

The critiquing process is directed toward evaluating the appropriateness of the selected nonexperimental design in relation to factors such as the research problem, theoretical framework, hypothesis, methodology, and the data analysis and interpretation.

• References

Bello, A., Haber, J., King, V., and King, R. (1980). *Identified factors predicting student success or failure in an associate degree nursing program.* In Teaching tomorrow's nurse: A nurse educator reader, Wakefield, Mass., Nursing Resources, Inc., pp. 174-182.

Brodie, B. (1974). Views of healthy children toward illness, *American Journal of Public Health,* **64:**1156-1159.

Campbell, D.T., and Stanley, J.C. (1963). *Experimental and quasi-experimental designs for research,* Chicago, Rand McNally College Publishing Co.

Fox, D.J. (1982). *Fundamentals of research in nursing,* 4th ed., East Norwalk, Conn., Appleton-Century-Crofts.

Littlefield-Derby, V., LoBiondo-Wood, G., and Olney-Springer, M. (1981). Changing the system to meet the needs of the patient and nurse, *The American Journal of Maternal Child Nursing,* 6(4):225-230.

Newman, M.A., and Gaudina, J.K. (1984). Depression as an explanation for decreased subjective time in the elderly, *Nursing Research,* **33**(3):137-139.

Pedhazur, E.J. (1982). *Multiple regression in behavioral research,* New York, Holt, Rinehart, & Winston, Inc.

Sideleau, B. (1984). Relationship between birth order and family size constellation and integrity to the development of mental illness in adolescence and adulthood. Unpublished doctoral dissertation, Teachers College, Columbia University, New York.

Van Dalen, D.B. (1979). *Understanding educational research: An introduction,* New York, McGraw-Hill Book Co.

• Additional Readings

Huck, S.W., and Sandler, H.M. (1979). *Rival hypotheses,* New York, Harper & Row, Publishers.

Kerlinger, F.H. (1973). *Foundations of behavioral research,* 2nd ed., New York, Holt, Rinehart & Winston, Inc.

Sherwen, L.N., and Toussie-Weingarten, C. (1983). *Analysis and application of nursing research: Parent-neonate studies,* Belmont, Calif., Wadsworth Health Sciences Division.

Waltz, C.F., and Bausell, R.B. (1981). *Nursing research: Design, statistics and computer analysis,* Philadelphia, F.A. Davis Co.

11

Additional Types of Research

Geri LoBiondo-Wood

LEARNING OBJECTIVES

After reading this chapter, the student should be able to do the following:

- Identify the historical, methodological, case study, and evaluative types of research.
- Describe each of these types of research.
- Distinguish and differentiate between each of these types of research.
- Identify the purposes of each of these types of research.
- Describe the general format of each of these types of research.
- Evaluate each of these types of research by applying the critiquing principles relevant to each type.

KEY TERMS

case study   phenomenological research
evaluative research   philosophical research
external criticism   primary source
historical research   psychometrics
internal criticism   secondary source
methodological research

The major types of experimental and nonexperimental designs have been introduced in previous chapters. Although they are very important to the development of a scientific knowledge base, experimental and nonexperimental designs are not the sum total of all research designs. Other types that complement the science of research utilize a different perspective to identify research problems or topics, form hypotheses, and collect, analyze, and interpret data. These additional types of designs are valid and useful and may be considered for special cases of nonexperimental research. They lend another means of viewing and interpreting phenomena that give further breadth and knowledge to nursing science and practice. These additional types of research are utilized to evaluate the past, study one unit in depth, develop measurement tools, evaluate programs, and study the principles of nursing as a science and an art. These types of research, though less frequently encountered in journals and as frameworks of studies, are important links to the development of nursing research. These types are historical, case study, methodological, evaluative, and philosophical. The purpose of this chapter is to present a brief description of each of these types and their respective goals. The principles for evaluating each type and its contribution to nursing within a consumer perspective are also presented.

• Historical Research

History, as we experience it in the form of written and verbal communication, is an account of past events. The reconstruction of history in writing or historiography allows us to view the occurrences of the past and to visualize the shaping of events, eras, and people. Unlike historiography, historical research is the systematic compilation of data and the critical presentation, evaluation, and interpretation of facts regarding people, events, and occurrences of the past. Its process is not the mere writing or chronicling of historical events as in a term paper, but like other research designs, it is based on the gathering of data related to either research questions or hypotheses. Unlike other previously discussed design types (see Chapters 9 and 10), in historical research data are not manipulated nor are new data generated. The data are facts from the past that are judged for authenticity. The goal of such research is to interpret the facts of the past to gain a clearer understanding of contemporary practice and issues. An example of historical research is *Hospitals, paternalism and the role of the nurse* (Ashley, 1976). In this extensive study, Ashley traced the factors that contributed to the current role of the nurse and the roots of paternalism in hospitals.

The idea has been previously stressed that when reviewing a piece of research, it should be obvious to the reader that the researcher is widely read and prepared in the specific and related topics of the study (see Chapter 5). This principle also applies in historical research because the investigation requires not only an understanding of a specific person or historical event, but also the context of the time and place of the occurrence. This broad knowledge and data base are present in Ashley's study.

The design of historical research may seem to be more flexible because statistics are not generally used, but this is not the case. Historical research must pass tests of validity and reliability in a process as carefully prescribed as those delineated for any other form of research (Christy, 1975). Hockett (1955) stated that the aim of historical research was to make use of raw statements to arrive at facts. A statement is defined as being nothing more than what someone has said. In light of the possibility of error when judging statements, it becomes the duty of the historian to doubt every statement until it is critically tested (Hockett, 1955, p.13).

PROBLEM IDENTIFICATION

One of the first steps in historical research is to identify the problem area and the purpose of the study. As with other research designs, the historical investigation should reflect the delimitations of study. The period, patterns, or population to be studied should be limited. This provides a researcher with the opportunity for in-depth research that can unfold new dimensions of an issue, relationship between events, or parallel developments or factors inherent in attitude or value formation (Krampitz, 1981). For example, Wheeler (1985) explored the editorial position and content of each issue of the first 20 years of the *American Journal of Nursing* in relation to the emergence of nursing as a profession. Even though the exploration of 20 years of one journal seems to be a vast and time-consuming project, the investigator cites the following sound reasons for the choice: (1) a period of 20 years was selected because those years represented the emergence of professional literature in the context of a large professional association, and (2) the editorial leadership remained fairly stable during that time, since the first major shift occurred in 1920. A reviewer of such a study may question the span of years or the use of one journal, but Wheeler's rationale provides definite parameters of the study.

Generally, in addition to a problem statement, a historical investigation will identify research questions. Inherent in these questions are implied and not always explicitly stated hypotheses (Best, 1970). The following are examples for the Wheeler study (1985):

- What professional issues captured the attention of nurses during this period and how were they conceptualized?
- How was the socialization of nurses into the profession presented?
- Who were the major contributors to the journal and what disciplines or occupations did they represent?
- To what extent did the journal's content attempt to define and influence "professionalism in nursing?"
- To what extent did the journal's content reflect an awareness of and influence by the major social or political movements of the time?

The specific research questions provide the investigator with a direction derived from the identified problem area. The questions provide not just for the mere chronicling of the journal's content but more importantly, set the stage for the interpretive study of the journal to investigate the emergence of professional issues.

Another example of a historical study with specific problem identification and research questions was done by Kalish, Kalish, and Clinton (1982). To answer the following questions these investigators focused on prime-time televison programs that were broadcast during the period of 1950 to 1980:

- What is the scope of nursing practice portrayed on television?
- What specific nursing actions are most commonly shown on television, and has their emphasis changed over time?
- What factors are associated with the nurses and nursing actions shown on television?
- Are certain aspects of professional nursing more highly exposed than others to the viewing public?

The studies cited are only two of a slowly growing number of interesting historical research studies. The identification of historical studies as a design and method of research has only recently become more widely accepted. Christy (1975) believed this was because of nursing's need to provide answers to immediate clinical, educational, or administrative problems, and nurses may have thought of historical research as more of a search than research. From the scope of the research questions delimited in these two studies, it becomes obvious how these studies are not only interesting, but they also show how negative portrayals of nurses and nursing may influence the public's views of the profession and its members.

DATA COLLECTION

After the research problem and questions have been delimited, the investigator needs to locate and identify data sources. This may not be easy in a historical investigation. Depending on the period of investigation and the location of the needed documents, data may be difficult to locate. It has been said that historical researchers should be free of allergies to dust because they may spend much of their time in old archives.

There are two categories of data sources: primary and secondary. Whenever possible, data should include primary sources. *Primary sources* are original documents, films, letters, diaries, records, artifacts, periodicals, tapes, or eyewitness accounts (see Chapter 5). In other words, in historical research the reviewer should be able to identify the use of firsthand information. In the Wheeler study (1985) the *American Journal of Nursing* represents a primary source. In the Kalish, Kalish, and Clinton study (1982) the films of television shows represent a primary source. An example of an eyewitness account may be found in the New York State Nurses' Association Archives. The Association is compiling videotaped oral histories of nursing leaders. The gathering and use of primary sources is necessary to confirm events or statements in a historical investigation.

Secondary sources are accounts of events written by someone other than the person involved (see Chapter 5). They are used when primary documents are missing or limited. Secondary sources represent a summation or interpretation of events by others. Secondary sources provide a view of an event by someone other than a participant in that event. It is important to remember when critiquing and assessing data sources that the further the review of an event moves from the originator, the greater the risk of error and distortion. Examples of secondary sources are verbal or written secondhand accounts, textbooks, reference books, and encyclopedias. At times, gathering primary data may be highly difficult, but the goal of the historian is to provide primary documentation. Primary documentation provides stronger reliability and validity in the study's data analysis.

DATA ANALYSIS

Historiographers have developed two processes of data evaluation: external criticism and internal criticism. The critiquer of a historical study should be able to recognize the researcher's attempts at interpretation of data based on these processes. *External criticism* establishes the validity of the data: is the document what it seems to be? External criticism is therefore the researcher's evaluation of the credibility and authenticity of the document. In the Wheeler study (1985) and the Kalish, Kalish, and Clinton study (1982) the external criticism applied by the investigators and the reviewer can be easily assessed. In the case of a primary source that is a handwritten letter or document, external criticism may be more difficult to assess. For example, Palmer (1983) conducted a study that looked at Florence Nightingale's life. In the study she used documents that were handwritten by Nightingale. To use these as primary sources, Palmer needed to establish that the handwriting was Nightingale's and that the documents were, therefore, authentic primary sources. The researcher also needed to validate the age of the paper as well. Unsigned letters or memos may present problems for historical researchers. Other aspects of external criticism are ghostwriting and time: was the document written by an assistant? Was the document dated or, if undated, has the time of writing been established?

The test of reliability for the historical researcher is internal criticism. *Internal criticism* establishes the reliability or consistency of the information within the document. In this process the researcher moves from the document itself to the content of the document. This may be the most difficult step for the historical researcher. During this process the researcher needs to determine whether or not the data regarding the event or occurrence are unbiased. The primary need of the researcher is to understand the document. This means not reading *into* the work and understanding the meaning of the words and colloquialisms of the time. Therefore the researcher needs to avoid taking statements out of context, be aware of historical nuances that may have affected the statements, compare the statements or data with other accounts of the same event, and be aware of possible biases of the document's originator. These steps for weighing and judging the data are critical to the soundness and usefulness of the investigation. The historical researcher accomplishes them as judiciously and carefully as one who is doing an empirical study.

Most historical research does not utilize statistical measures. Examples of exceptions to this are the works of Kalish, Kalish, and Clinton (1982) and Kalish, Kalish, and Young (1983). In these studies the investigators used methods of coding and content analysis to statistically review the data gathered.

SYNTHESIS AND THE RESEARCH REPORT

The historical researcher analyzes and then synthesizes the data to form a cohesive picture that addresses the research questions or hypotheses. Synthesis of the data for the final research report requires a great deal of selection based on expert judgment. The raw data are generally massive and require careful selection by the researcher to avoid bias and still portray a representative and appealing piece. The final written report therefore differs from an empirical research report. It may also seem more like a literary piece of work than a research study. The written report seen in a journal does not cite for the reader which statements or data are from primary and secondary sources. Nor do the investigators specifically relate the measures of external and internal criticism. The historical research accomplishes these steps in the analysis and presents an unbiased account of the research questions.

There is the problem of subjective analysis in historical research. Because of this, the "how" of the incident frequently takes precedence over the "why" questions (Krampitz, 1981). It is therefore the critiquer's responsibility to use her knowledge of the historical research process to infer and judge the merits of the piece, its usefulness, and generalizability. Historical research thus becomes an important link for learning about past roles, events, and occurrences. By learning from the past, we can avoid repeating its negative aspects and build on its positive aspects. Nursing needs to understand its history and scrutinize its past through historical research to build on its strengths. Understanding the purposes and format of historical research is an important goal of the research consumer.

• Methodological Research

Methodology is a general term and has many meanings. It may mean different ways of doing research for different purposes, ways of stating hypotheses, methods of data collection, measurement, and techniques of data analysis. Methodology also includes aspects of the philosophy of science as an overall critical approach to research (Kerlinger, 1979). As you will find in succeeding chapters (see Chapters 12 and 13), methodology influences research strongly. *Methodological research* is the controlled investigation of the theoretical and applied aspects of mathematics, statistics, measurement, and the means of gathering and analyzing data (Kerlinger, 1979).

The most significant and critically important aspect of methodological research that will be addressed in measurement and statistics, or their combination, is called *psychometrics*. Psychometrics deals with the theory and development of measurement instruments or measurement techniques through the research process. Psychometrics thus deals with the measurement of a concept, such as anxiety or interpersonal conflict, with reliable and valid tools (see Chapter 13 for a discussion of reliability and validity). Psychometrics is a most critical issue for nurse researchers. Many of the tools utilized by nurse researchers have been developed by other disciplines, such as psychology and sociology, and may not necessarily be totally appropriate for nursing's use. Since nurses have become more sophisticated in their investigations and knowledge of research, the need for appropriate tools to measure phenomena of interest has become recognized. Methodological research is critical to the reliability and validity of a study. For example, Klein (1983) conducted a study on the use of contraceptives in women seeking abortion and their perception of the chance and ability to conceive. While the study's purpose and problems were clear, the tool that was developed and used by the author, the consistency, chance, and ability inventory, exhibited various psychometric problems. When studies have inherent psychometric problems, they render the findings questionable or limited.

The main problem for nurse researchers is locating appropriate measurement tools. In the Klein study an important concept, risk-taking behavior, may impinge on contraceptive use and thereby clinical practice, and so it needed to be measured. The appropriate tool was lacking, so the author developed one. Many of the phenomena of interest to nursing practice and research are intangible, such as interpersonal conflict and maternal-fetal attachment. The intangible nature of various phenomena, yet the recognition of the need to measure them, places methodological research in an important position.

Methodological research differs from other designs of research. First, it does not include all of the research process steps as discussed in the introduction to Part II: The Research Process. Second, to implement its techniques, the researcher must have a sound knowledge of psychometrics or must consult with a researcher knowledgeable in psychometric techniques. The methodological researcher is not interested in the interrelationship of the independent variable and dependent variable nor in the effect of an independent variable on a dependent variable. The methodological researcher is interested in identifying an intangible construct and making it tangible with a paper-and-pencil tool or observation protocol.

Basically a methodological study includes the following steps:
1. Defining the construct
2. Formulating the item
3. Testing the tool's reliability and validity

These steps require a sound, specific, and exhaustive literature review to identify the theories underlying the construct. This literature review provides the basis of item formulation. Once the items have been developed, the researcher assesses the tool's reliability and validity (see Chapter 13). Various aspects of these procedures may differ according to the tool's use, purpose, and stage of development.

Examples of methodological research can be found in the studies done by Hoskins (1981, 1983). In these studies, Hoskins identified the construct of interpersonal conflict and defined it conceptually and operationally. The steps of the tool development process as it was applied to the interpersonal conflict scale are outlined (see Chapter 13). Many more examples of psychometric development can be found in nursing research literature (Benoliel, McCorkle, and Young, 1980; Cranley, 1981; Norbeck, Lindsey, and Carrieri, 1981, 1983; and Rees, 1980). Psychometric or methodological studies are found primarily in research reporting journals. The specific procedures of methodological research are beyond the scope of this textbook, but the reader is urged to look closely at the tools that are utilized in studies. References of psychometric or methodological research are provided in the additional readings section of this chapter.

• Case Study

The case study is a design based on an in-depth investigation of one or several samples. The *case study* is an in-depth study of an individual, a group, or an institution. Whereas other studies sample a broad number of individuals, the case study samples a narrow number in depth. Case studies investigate selected observations as they occur and use the principles of inductive reasoning (see Chapter 2). Freud used the case study method extensively. The case study may be implemented with either a descriptive or experimental approach. The purposes of a case study may be to identify principles of behavior and thereby provide a mechanism for documenting and analyzing all aspects of information from the sample unit (descriptive approach) or to investigate the sample unit's response to an experimental intervention over a period of time (experimental approach). The case study has been used only limitedly in nursing research. The argument is made that case studies are limited in scope because of the few cases researched, and therefore the conclusions are not widely applicable or generalizable to a wider population. On the positive side, because of the depth of the case study design, a wider range of information can be gathered and not lost because of design restrictions.

Even though they are limited, case studies have an important place in nursing research; some examples are the classic works of Rubin (1967a; 1967b). Based on a theoretical framework, Rubin explored the development of the maternal role during pregnancy. This and other subsequent works led to the development of a framework of the maternal role-taking process and allowed for further hypothesis-generating research. The case study allow for an in-depth exploration of newer or unexplored concepts and may provide information that would be unobtainable through other designs. Holm (1983) provides a review of the methods of the case study and an argument for its usefulness in nursing research.

Case studies have the most flexible format. Barnard (1983) noted that she had the most difficulty in critiquing case studies because of their lack of a common format. Yet the reviewer should still be able to identify a specific problem area that is substantiated by a theoretical framework. Data may be gathered by the following various methods: interviews, observations, paper-and-pencil tests, physiological measurements, and treatments, administrations, or interventions. Rubin (1967a; 1967b) utilized interviews and observations. The use of multiple methods and a flexible design does not preclude the use of scientific rigor. The user of the case study approach should employ as much depth and scientific analysis as possible to gain the level of knowledge desired to yield information that is not available through other means. This can be done by attempting to study as many aspects of a particular situation, concept, or clinical problem.

For the reviewer of a case study, the following points should be elucidated:
1. A specific problem should be identified.
2. The data gathered should reflect an in-depth study of the phenomena of interest.
3. A time period for data collection should be identified.
4. The data sources and procedures should be presented.
5. An analysis and interpretation of data should be presented.

One of the major criticisms of the case study approach is the potential for investigator bias. This may be decreased by the use of standardized procedures or protocols (see Rubin 1967a, 1967b). The case study can be a useful avenue, especially in clinical practice. Holm (1983) suggests its use by clinicians to study how a client's response to a treatment, for example, the effectiveness of breathing exercises, may be quantified by tidal volume, vital capacity, and respiratory rate. Barnard (1983) suggests using one of the 11 functional health patterns as formulated by Gordon (1982). An example would be to structure the report of the nursing management of a diabetic child's nutrition and metabolism pattern, the activity and exercise pattern, the roles and relationship pattern, or some combination of these patterns. The research goal would be to describe overall patterns of behavior and their changes after nursing intervention. For the research consumer, this could be used as a basis for a clinical conference and a learning mechanism for the nursing staff. It may also be a suggestion to the staff to use new or different approaches to care and become a hypothesis for a future study. Though not widely generalizable, the case study may be a useful learning tool for the research consumer because it provides a microscopic examination and analysis of the patterns and responses of one or a few persons.

• Evaluative Research

Recently there has been an increased emphasis placed on the evaluation of the services and methods of care. Health care consumers and their supporting agencies need and rightfully require documentation of the effectiveness of care. Therefore nursing is becoming increasingly more accountable for its practice (see Chapter 1). This emphasis requires the use of research that can help to validate the use of treatments and programs. Evaluative research provides the needed approach. *Evaluative research* is the utilization of scientific research methods and procedures to evaluate a program, treatment practice, or policy; therefore it utilizes analytic means to document the worth of an activity. Evaluative research is not a separate design, it may be implemented with either an experimental or nonexperimental approach. As a type of research, it impinges directly on practice as an applied method. Bigman (1961) further delineates the following purposes and uses of evaluative research:

1. To discover whether and how well the objectives are being fulfilled
2. To determine the reasons for specific successes and failures
3. To direct the course of the experiment with techniques for increasing effectiveness
4. To uncover the principles underlying a successful program
5. To base further research on the reasons for the relative success of alternative techniques
6. To redefine the means to be used for attaining objectives and even to redefine subgoals, in the light of the research findings

These purposes, though general, are applicable to evaluative research in nursing. Evaluative research in nursing has mainly been applied to educational program evaluation and not to clinical practices. Evaluation, therefore, involves more than judging, it also includes understanding and redefining (Suchman, 1967). Within an evaluative study, the reviewer should be able to note the following steps (U.S. Department of Health, Education, and Welfare, 1955):

1. Identify the goals to be evaluated
2. Analyze the problems that the activity must manage
3. Describe and standardize the activity
4. Measure the degree of change that takes place
5. Determine whether the observed changes are a result of the activity or some other cause
6. Indicate some of the effects

The major weakness in evaluative research is the reliability and validity of the measures of effectiveness. Evaluative studies may incorporate either an experimental or nonexperimental design depending on the purposes of the evaluation. An example of an evaluative nursing study that used random subject assignment was done by Oberst, Graham, Geller, Stearns, and Tiernan (1981). In this study the investigators compared the effectiveness of two approaches to urinary catheter management in controlling postoperative urinary function in 110 clients after an abdominoperineal resection or a low anterior bowel resection. The researchers evaluated the effectiveness of a straight gravity drainage system and a 6-day progressive catheter clamping program. Within the literature review and introduction to the study the authors analyzed the problems of postoperative urinary function. The method and procedures sections of this study clearly and specifically outlined the descriptions and standardization procedures of the activity. This study also meets the criteria of measuring the degree of change by gathering baseline data on such variables as the voiding history of each client; the presence or absence of prostatism, cystocele, or rectocele; and the type and extent of surgery. The researchers measured the differences in observed dysfunction rates with preset guidelines and through the use of statistical measures. The determination of what the observed differences were related to, and the durability of the effects, are dealt with in the results and discussions sections of the investigation. This study is an excellent example of an evaluative approach to a clinical problem because of the systematic investigative approach to the problem and the researcher's ability to present the basis for further research.

When evaluative research is applied to the functioning of a specific program, problems may arise. Polit and Hungler (1983) note that such research can be seen as threatening by individuals in the programs undergoing evaluation and may lead to a lack of cooperation. It may also be a problem when deciding how to measure a program's effectiveness, especially if the program is complex and has many broad goals. Nursing research related to program evaluation is mainly conducted on educational programs. An example of a program evaluation was done by Griggs (1977). In this study, Griggs evaluated the effectiveness of an autotutorial minicourse for nurses and hospital personnel that dealt with nosocomial infections and diseases related to the use of respiratory therapy equipment. The use of diagnosis-related groups (DRGs) and the need to document the effectiveness of care may contribute to an increase in evaluative research.

• Other Types of Research

The reviewer of research will also find attitional designs of research, but with less frequency. These are the *philosophical* and the *phenomenological* approaches. They are based on the investigation of the truths and principles of existence (ontology), knowledge (epistemology), conduct (ethics), and the description of experience as it is lived (phenomenology) (Brody, 1981). These studies focus on the philosophical reasoning of relationships. The analysis of data is accomplished through logical rather than statistical means. The mechanisms of these approaches are as specific and systematic as in other designs. The method and critique of these designs are beyond the scope of this textbook; the reader is referred to a variety of sources for the methods and their uses as a design in nursing research studies (Brody, 1981; Oiler, 1980, 1982; Paterson and Zderad, 1976; Psathas, 1973; and Stevens, 1971).

• Critiquing Other Types of Research

The criteria for critiquing the types of research presented in this chapter are given in the box on p.152. From your review of this chapter, you have found additional means of investigating phenomena related to nursing practice and theory. When critiquing these additional types of research, it is important for the consumer to first identify the type of research that was employed in the investigation. Once the type of research is identified, its specific purpose and format needs to be understood by the consumer. Understanding the format of a specific type allows the reviewer to apply the relevant principles of critiquing to the respective study. The format and methods of each type of research will vary. Knowing how they vary allows a consumer to assess if the most appropriate design was utilized, and even though the format and methods vary, it is important to remember that all research has a central goal: to answer questions scientifically. Therefore, when critiquing one of the additional types of research outlined in this chapter, it is important for the consumer to determine if the question or problem being posed is consistent with the purpose of the research. The study's format should then meet the criteria of the specific research. Finally, the merits of

Critiquing Criteria

Historical Research

1. Does the historical study overall isolate a specific event, occurrence, person, or time frame and do the following:
   a. Identify the problem area, research questions, and the purpose of the study?
   b. Discuss the occurrence within the context of its time and place?
   c. Set limitations with a rationale?
   d. Present the use of primary sources as well as secondary sources?
   e. Reflect the use of external criticism as well as internal criticism in the analysis?
   f. Critically present and evaluate the occurrence in an attempt to answer the question of how the occurrence evolved?

Methodological Research

1. Does the methodological study identify a specific construct or phenomenon that the developed tool will measure?
2. Is the construct defined?
3. Can the investigator's methods of item formulation be recognized? (Examples are client records, literature review, clinical experience, and related research and theory.)
4. Did the investigator perform reliability and validity tests and which specific types were used?
5. Did the investigator omit a specific type of reliability or validity test? If so, which one was omitted?

Case Study

1. Is the problem area or process to be research identified by a theoretical rationale?
2. Is the sampling frame identified?
3. Do the data collected reflect a depth of information?
4. Has the data collection protocol been established?
5. Has a time period for data collection been identified?
6. Are data sources and procedures presented?
7. Are the analysis and interpretation of the data presented and within the context of the originally identified problem area?
8. How has the investigator avoided bias in the interpretation of the problem area?
9. Does the study generalize beyond the boundaries of its findings?

Evaluative Research

1. Does the study identify a specific program or treatment that it will evaluate?
2. Are the goals to be evaluated identified?
3. Is the problem(s) that the activity must cope with analyzed and described?
4. Is the activity to be analyzed, described, and standardized?
5. Is measurement of the degree of change that occurs identified?
6. Is there a determination of whether the observed change is related to the activity or to some other causes?

the study should be determined by how well the investigator applied the format at each step in the study. It is within the steps and the format of a particular study that the consumer should find how well the investigator applied the research process.

• Summary

It is obvious that researchers have many types of research to choose from when addressing a research problem. The choice of one of the additional research types depends not only on the level of a problem, but also on the type of the problem. When the researcher or consumer wishes to explore relationships and facts of the past, the historical design should be utilized. When addressing the need or search for reliable and valid measurement tools, the methodological approach is the most appropriate type of research. An in-depth investigation of a single case or entity is uniquely addressed by the case study approach, whereas the evaluation of how well a program or practice functions fairly requires the use of evaluative research. Finally, if the question is related to experience, logic, and philosophy, the researcher and consumer should seek a philosophical or phenomenological approach. Each type of research can and does answer nursing questions related to the science of nursing. The research consumer should be aware of the purpose of each type when deciding the overall appropriateness, usefulness, and generalizability of the study.

• References

Ashley, J. (1976). *Hospitals, paternalism and the role of the nurse,* New York, Teachers College Press.

Barnard, K. (1983). The case study method: A research tool, *Maternal Child Nursing,* **8**:36.

Benoliel, J.Q., McCorkle, R., and Young, K. (1980). Development of a social dependency scale, *Research in Nursing and Health,* **3**:3-10.

Best, J.W. (1970). *Research in education,* Englewood Cliffs, N.J., Prentice-Hall, Inc.

Bigman, S.K. (1961). Evaluating the effectiveness of religious programs, *Review of Religious Research,* **2**:99-110.

Brody, E.B. (1981). Research design: General introduction. In Krampitz, S.D., and Pavlovich, N., eds., *Readings from nursing research,* St. Louis, The C.V. Mosby Co., pp. 40–48.

Christy, T.E. (1975). The methodology of historical research: A brief introduction, *Nursing Research,* **24**:189-192.

Cranley, M. (1981). Development of a tool for the measurement of maternal attachment during pregnancy, *Nursing Research,* **30**:281-284.

Gordon, M. (1982). *Nursing diagnosis: Process and application,* New York, McGraw-Hill Book Co.

Griggs, B.M. (1977). A systems approach to the development and evaluation of a minicourse for nurses, *Nursing Research,* **26**:34-41.

Holm, K. (1983). Single subject research, *Nursing Research,* **32**:253-255.

Hockett, H.C. (1955). *Critical method in historical research and writing,* New York, Macmillan Publishing Co., Inc.

Hoskins, C.N. (1981). Psychometrics in nursing research: Construction of an interpersonal conflict scale, *Research in Nursing and Health,* **4**:243-249.

Hoskins, C.N. (1983). Psychometrics in nursing research—further development of the interpersonal conflict scale, *Research in Nursing and Health,* **6**:75-83.

Kalish, B.J., Kalish, P.A., and Young, R.L. (1983). Television news coverage of nurse strikes: A resource management perspective, *Nursing Research,* **32**:175.

Kalish, P.A., Kalish, B.J., and Clinton, J. (1982). The world of nursing on prime time television, 1950 to 1980, *Nursing Research,* **31**:358-363.

Kerlinger, F. (1973). *The foundations of behavioral research,* New York, Holt, Rinehart, & Winston, Inc.

Kerlinger, F. (1979). *Behavioral research: A conceptual approach,* New York, Holt, Rinehart, & Winston, Inc.

Klein, P.M. (1983). Contraceptive use and perceptions of chance and ability of conceiving in women electing abortion, *Journal of Obstetrics and Gynecology*, **12**:167-171.

Krampitz, S.D. (1981). Research design: Historical. In Krampitz, S.D., and Pavlovich, N., eds., *Readings for nursing research*, St. Louis, The C.V. Mosby Co. pp. 54-58.

Norbeck, J.S., Lindsey, A.M., and Carrieri, V.L. (1981). The development of an instrument to measure social support, *Nursing Research*, **30**: 264-269.

Norbeck, J.S., Lindsey, A.M., and Carrieri, V.L. (1983). Further development of the Norbeck Social Support Questionnaire: Normative data and validity testing, *Nursing Research*, **32**:4-9.

Oiler, C. (1980). *A phenomenological perspective in nursing*, Unpublished doctoral dissertation, Teachers College, Columbia University, New York.

Oiler, C. (1982). The phenomenological approach in nursing research, *Nursing Research*, **31**:178-181.

Oberst, M.T., Graham, D, Geller, N.L., Stearns, M.W., and Tiernan, E. (1981). Catheter management programs and postoperative urinary dysfunction, *Research in Nursing and Health*, **4**:175-181.

Palmer, I.S. (1983). Nightingale revisited, *Nursing Outlook*, **31**:229-233.

Paterson, J. and Zderad, L. (1976). *Humanistic nursing*, New York, John Wiley & Sons, Inc.

Polit, D. and Hungler, B. (1983). *Nursing research: Principles and methods*, 2nd ed., Philadelphia, J.B. Lippincott Co.

Psathas, G. (1973). *Phenomenological sociology: Issues and applications*, New York, John Wiley & Sons, Inc.

Rees, B.L. (1980). Measuring identification with the mothering role, *Research in Nursing and Health*, **3**:49-56.

Rubin, R. (1967). Attainment of the maternal role. Part I: Processes, *Nursing Research*, **16**:237-245.

Rubin, R. (1967). Attainment of the maternal role. Part II: Models and referrants, *Nursing Research*, **16**:342-346.

Stevens, B. (1971). A phenomenological approach to understanding suicidal behavior, *Journal of Psychiatric Nursing*, **9**:33-35.

Suchman, E.A. (1967). *Evaluative research*, New York, Russell Sage Foundation.

U.S. Department of Health, Education and Welfare. (1955). *Evaluation in mental health*, Publication #413, Washington, Government Printing Office.

Wheeler, C.E. (1985). The American Journal of Nursing and the socialization of a profession, 1900-1920, *Advances in Nursing Science*, **7**: 20-34.

• Additional Readings

A guide to research instruments. (1981). *Image*, October, p. 92.

Barzun, J., and Reaff, H.E. (1977). The modern researcher, Chicago, Harcourt Brace Jovanovich, Inc.

Campbell, D., and Fiske, D. (1959). Covergent and discriminant validation by the multitrait-multimethod matrix, *Psychological Bulletin*, **56**: 81-105.

Fox, D.J. (1982). *Fundamentals of research in nursing*, Norwalk, Conn., Appleton-Century-Crofts.

Hersen, M., and Barlow, D.H. (1977). *Single-case experimental designs*, New York, Pergamon Press.

Kalish, B.J., and Kalish, P.A. (1976). Is history of nursing alive and well, *Nursing Outlook*, **24**: 362-366.

Kratochwill, T.R. (1978). Single subject research, New York, Academic Press.

Matejski, M.P. (1979). Humanities: The nurse and historical research, *Image*, **11**:80-85.

Newton, M.E. (1965). The case for historical research, *Nursing Research* **14**: 20-26.

Notter, L.L. (1972). A case for historical research in nursing, *Nursing Research*, **21**:483.

Norman, E.M. (1981). Who and where are nursing's historians? *Nursing Forum*, **20**:138-152.

Nunnally, J. (1978). *Psychometric theory*, New York, McGraw-Hill Book Co.

Perry, D.S. (1983). The early midwives of Missouri, *Journal of Nurse-Midwifery*, **28**:15-28.

12

Data Collection Methods

Margaret Grey

LEARNING OBJECTIVES

After reading this chapter, the student should be able to do the following:
- Define the types of data collection methods utilized in nursing research.
- List the advantages and disadvantages of each of these methods.
- Critically evaluate the data collection methods utilized in published nursing research studies.

KEY TERMS

close-ended items   operational definition
concealment   operationalization
content analysis   reactivity
intervention   scale
objective   systematic
open-ended items

Nurses use all of their senses when collecting data from the clients for whom they provide care. Nurse researchers also have available many ways to collect information about their research subjects. The major difference between the data collected when performing client care and the data collected for the purpose of research is that the data collection methods employed by researchers need to be objective and systematic. By *objective*, we mean that the data must not be influenced by anyone who collects the information; by *systematic*, we mean that the data must be collected in the same way by everyone who is involved in the collection procedure.

The methods that researchers use to collect information about subjects are the identifiable and repeatable operations that define the major variables being studied. *Operationalization* is the process of translating the concepts that are of interest to a researcher into observable and measurable phenomena. There may be a number of ways to collect the same information. For example, a researcher interested in measuring anxiety physiologically could do so by measuring sweat gland activity or by administering an anxiety scale such as the State-Trait Anxiety Scale. The researcher could also observe clients to see if they displayed anxious behavior. The method chosen by the researcher would depend on a number of decisions regarding the problem being studied, the nature of the subjects, and the relative costs and benefits of each method.

This chapter's purpose is to familiarize the student with the various ways that researchers collect information from and about subjects. The chapter will provide nursing research consumers with the tools for evaluating the selection, utilization, and practicality of the various ways of collecting data.

• Data Collection Methods

In general, data collection methods can be divided into the following five types: physiological, observational, interviews, questionnaires, and records or available data. Each of these methods has a specific purpose as well as certain pros and cons inherent in their use. We will discuss each type of data collection method and then compare their respective uses and problems.

PHYSIOLOGICAL MEASUREMENT

In everyday practice, nurses collect physiological data about clients, such as their temperature, pulse rate, and blood pressure. Such data are frequently useful to nurse researchers as well. Consider the study conducted by Lim-Levy (1982) concerning the effect of oxygen inhalation on oral temperature (see Appendix A). The researcher wanted to know whether oxygen administered by nasal cannula affected the subject's oral temperature. To study this problem, it was important to measure the temperature similarly for all subjects. Thus Lim-Levy consistently utilized a specific type of thermometer for all of the measurements of temperature.

Lim-Levy's study is an excellent example of the use of a particular type of data collection method, physiological. Physiological and physical measures may require specialized technical instruments for collecting information and frequently require specialized training. Such measurements can be physical, such as weight and temperature; chemical, such as blood sugar level; microbiological, such as cultures; or anatomical, such as x-ray examinations. What makes these measurements different from our observations of client behavior is that they require the use of special equipment to make the observation. We can say, "That client weighs a lot," but to determine how much the client weighs requires the use of a sensitive instrument, a scale.

Physiological measurement is particularly suited to the study of two types of nursing problems. Such measures may be important criteria for determining the effectiveness of certain nursing actions. This was true in the study by Wolfer and Visintainer (1975) where the researchers were interested in how a children's preoperative education program affected their postoperative recovery (see Appendix B). Another nursing problem with physiological parameters is the study of ways to improve the performance of certain nursing actions, such as the measuring and recording of clients' physiological data.

The advantages of utilizing physiological data collection methods include their objectivity, precision, and sensitivity. Such methods are generally quite objective because unless there is a technical malfunction, two readings of the same instrument taken at the same time by two different nurses are likely to yield the same result. Since such instruments are intended to measure the variable being studied, they offer the advantage of being precise and sensitive enough to pick up subtle variations in the phenomenon of interest. It is also unlikely that a subject in a study can deliberately distort physiological information.

Physiological measurements are not without inherent disadvantages, however. Some instruments, if they are not available through a hospital, may be quite expensive to obtain. In addition, such instruments often require specialized knowledge and training to be used accurately. Another problem with such measurements is that just by using them, the variable of interest may be changed. Although some researchers think of these instruments as being nonintrusive, the presence of some types of devices might change the measurement. For example, the presence of a heart rate monitoring device might make some clients anxious and increase their heart rate. In addition, nearly all types of measuring devices are affected in some way by the environment. Even a simple thermometer can be affected by the subject drinking something hot immediately before the temperature is taken. Thus it is important to consider whether the researcher controlled such environmental variables in the study. Finally, there may not be a physiological way to measure the variable of interest. Occasionally researchers try to force a physiological parameter into a study in an effort to increase the precision of measurement. However, if the device does not really measure the phenomenon of interest, the validity of its use is suspect (see Chapter 13).

OBSERVATIONAL METHODS

Sometimes nurse researchers are interested in determining how subjects behave under certain conditions. For example, a researcher might be interested in whether subjects actually comply with certain recommendations about their health, such as stopping smoking. We might ask such subjects about their behavior, but they may distort their responses to please the researcher. Therefore observing the subject may give a more accurate picture of the subject's behavior than asking.

Although observing the environment is a normal part of living, scientific observation places a great deal of emphasis on the objective and systematic nature of the operation. To be scientific, observations must fulfill the following four conditions (Seaman and Verhonick, 1982):

1. The observations are undertaken with certain objectives in mind.
2. The observations are systematically planned and recorded.
3. All of the observations are checked and controlled.
4. The observations are related to scientific concepts and theories.

Thus the researcher is not merely looking at what is happening, but rather is watching with a trained eye for certain specific events.

Observation is particularly suitable as a data collection method in complex research situations that are best viewed as total entities and that are difficult to measure in parts, such as studies dealing with the nursing process, parent-child interactions, or group processes. In addition, observational methods can be the best way to operationalize some variables of interest in nursing research studies, particularly individual characteristics and conditions, such as traits and symptoms, verbal and nonverbal communication behaviors, activities and skill attainment, and environmental characteristics.

Observational methods can also be distinguished by the role of the observer. This role is determined by the amount of interaction between the observer and those who are being observed. The following four basic types of observational roles are each distinguishable by the amount of concealment or intervention implemented by the observer:

1. Concealment without intervention
2. Concealment with intervention
3. No concealment without intervention
4. No concealment with intervention

Concealment refers to whether or not the subjects know that they are being observed, and *intervention* deals with whether or not the observer provokes actions from those who are being observed. When a researcher is concerned that the subjects will change the behavior being observed, the type of observation most commonly employed is that of concealment without intervention. In this case, the researcher watches the subjects without their knowledge of the observation, but does not provoke them into action. Often such concealed observations utilize television cameras, audio tapes, or one-way mirrors. An important ethical problem is created by this type of observation strategy, since observing subjects without their knowledge violates assumptions of informed consent (see Chapter 3).

When the observer is neither concealed nor intervening, the ethical question is not a problem. Here the observer makes no attempt to change the subjects' behavior and informs them that they are to be observed. Because the observer is present, this type of observation allows a greater depth of material to be studied than if the observer is separated from the subjects by an artificial barrier such as a one-way mirror. Participant observation is a commonly used observational technique where the researcher functions as a part of a social group to study the group in question. The problem with this type of observation is *reactivity,* or the distortion created when the subjects change their behavior because they are being observed.

The two other types of observations involve some kind of intervention by the observer. No concealment with intervention is employed when the researcher is observing the effects of some intervention introduced for scientific purposes. Since the subjects know that they are participating in a research study, there are few problems with ethical concerns, but reactivity is a problem with this type of study.

Concealed observation with intervention involves staging a situation and observing the behaviors that are evoked in the subjects as a result of the intervention. Because the subjects are unaware of their participation in a research study, this type of observation has fallen into disfavor and is rarely used in nursing research.

Observations may be structured or unstructured. Unstructured observational methods are not characterized by a total absence of structure, but usually involve collecting descriptive information about the subjects of interest. In participant observation, the observer keeps field notes that record the activities as well as the observer's interpretations of these activities. Field notes are not usually restricted to any particular type of action or behavior; rather, they intend to paint a picture of a social situation in a more general sense. Another type of unstructured observation is the use of anecdotes. Anecdotes are not necessarily funny, but usually focus on the behaviors of interest and frequently add to the richness of research reports by illustrating a particular point.

On the other hand, structured observations involve specifying in advance what behaviors or events are to be observed and preparing forms for record keeping, such as categorization systems, checklists, and rating scales. Whichever system is employed, the observer watches the subject and then marks on the recording form what was seen. In any case, the observations must be similar among the observers (see Chapter 13 for a detailed explanation of interrater reliability). Thus it is important that observers be trained to be consistent in their observations and ratings of behavior.

Scientific observation has several advantages as a data collection method, the main one being that observation may be the only way for the researcher to study the variable of interest. For example, what people say that they do is often not what they really do. Therefore if the study is designed to obtain substantive findings about human behavior, observation may be the only way to ensure the validity of the findings. In addition, no other data collection method can match the depth and variety of information that can be collected when utilizing these techniques. Such techniques are also quite flexible in that they may be used in both experimental and nonexperimental designs, and in laboratory and field studies.

As with all data collection methods, observation also has its disadvantages. We mentioned the problems of reactivity and ethical concerns when we discussed the concealment and intervention dimensions. In addition, data obtained by observational techniques are vulnerable to the bias of the observer. Emotions, prejudices, and values can all influence the way that behaviors and events are observed. In general, the more that the observer needs to make inferences and judgments about what is being observed, the more likely it is that distortions will occur. Thus it is important to consider how observational tools were constructed and how observers were trained and evaluated in judging the adequacy of observational methods.

INTERVIEWS AND QUESTIONNAIRES

Subjects in a research study often have information that is important to the study and that can be obtained only by asking the subject. Such questions may be asked orally by a researcher in person or over the telephone in an interview, or they may be asked in the form of a paper-and-pencil test. Both interviews and questionnaires have the purpose of asking subjects to report data for themselves, but each has unique advantages and disadvantages as well.

Survey research relies almost entirely on questioning subjects with either interviews or questionnaires, but these methods of data collection can also be utilized in other types of research. No matter what type of study is conducted, the purpose of questioning subjects is to seek information. This information may either be of direct interest, such as the subject's age, or it may be of indirect interest, such as when the researcher uses a combination of items to estimate to what degree the respondent has some trait or characteristic. An intelligence test is an example of how an individual item is combined with several others to develop an overall scale of intelligence. When items of indirect interest are combined to obtain an overall score, the measurement tool is called a *scale*.

The investigator determines the content of an interview or questionnaire from the literature review (see Chapter 5). When evaluating these methods, the reader should consider the content of the schedule, the individual items, and the order of the items. We will deal with the content question in the next chapter. The basic standard for evaluating the individual items in an interview or questionnaire is that the item must be clearly written, so that the intent of the question and the nature of the information sought is clear to the respondent. The only way to know if the questions are understandable to the target respondents is to pilot test them in a similar population. Items must also ask only one question, be free from suggestion, and use correct grammar. Items may also be open-ended or close-ended. *Open-ended* items are used when the researcher wants the subjects to respond in their own words, or if the researcher does not know all of the possible alternative responses. *Close-ended* items are used when there are a fixed number of alternative responses. Many scales use a fixed response format called a Likert scale. Likert scales are lists of statements on which respondents indicate whether they "strongly agree," "agree," "disagree," or "strongly disagree." Structured, fixed-response items are best utilized when the question has a fixed number of responses and the respondent is to choose the one closest to the right one. Fixed response items have the advantage of simplifying the respondent's task and the researcher's analysis, but they may miss some important information about the subject. Unstructured response formats allow such information to be included, but require a special technique to analyze the responses. This technique is called *content analysis* and is a method for the objective, systematic, and quantitative description of communications and documentary evidence.

Interviews and questionnaires are commonly utilized in nursing research. They are both strong approaches to gathering information for research because they approach the task directly. In addition, both have the ability to obtain certain kinds of information, such as the subjects' attitudes and beliefs, that would be difficult to obtain without asking the subject directly. All methods that involve verbal reports, however, share a problem with accuracy. There is often no way to know whether what we are told is indeed true. For example, people are known to respond to questions in a way that makes them look good. This response style is known as *social desirability*. Since there is no way to tell if the respondent is telling the truth or responding in a socially desirable way, the researcher usually is forced to assume that the respondent is telling the truth.

Questionnaires and interviews also have some specific purposes, advantages, and disadvantages. Questionnaires and paper-and-pencil tests are most useful when there is a finite set of questions to be asked and the researcher can be assured of the clarity and specificity of the items. Questionnaires are good when the purpose is to collect information. Face-to-face techniques or interviews are best utilized when the researcher may need to clarify the task for the respondent or is interested in obtaining more personal information from the respondent. Telephone interviews allow the researcher to reach more respondents than face-to-face interviews and allow for more clarity than questionnaires.

Researchers face difficult choices when determining whether to use interviews or questionnaires. The final decision is often based on what instruments are available and their relative costs and benefits.

Both face-to-face and telephone interviews offer some advantages over questionnaires. All things being equal, interviews are better than questionnaires because the response rate is almost always higher and this helps to eliminate bias in the sample (see Chapter 14). Respondents seem to be less likely to hang up the telephone or to close the door in a interviewer's face than to throw away a questionnaire. Another advantage of the interview is that some people, such as children, the blind, and the illiterate could not fill out a questionnaire, but they could participate in an interview.

Interviews also allow for some safeguards to be built into the interview situation. Interviewers can clarify misunderstood questions and observe the level of the respondent's understanding and cooperativeness. In addition, the researcher has strict control over the order of the questions. With questionnaires, the respondent can skip around, answering questions in any order. Sometimes changing the order of the questions can change the response.

Finally, interviews allow for richer and more complex data to be collected. This is particularly so when open-ended responses are sought. Even when close-ended response items are used, interviewers can probe to understand why a respondent answered in a particular way.

Questionnaires also have certain advantages. They are much less expensive to administer than interviews, because interviews require the hiring and training of interviewers. Thus if a researcher has a fixed amount of time and money, a larger and more diverse sample can be obtained with questionnaires. Questionnaires also allow for complete anonymity, which may be important if the study deals with sensitive issues. Finally, the fact that there is not an interviewer present assures the researcher and the reader that there will be no interviewer bias. Interviewer bias occurs when the interviewer unwittingly leads the respondent to answer in a certain way. This problem is especially pronounced in studies that are unstructured interview formats. A subtle nod of the head, for example, could lead a respondent to change an answer because the respondent thinks that this answer is what the researcher wants to hear.

RECORDS OR AVAILABLE DATA

All of the data collection methods discussed thus far concern the ways that nurse researchers gather new data to study phenomena of interest. Not all studies, though, require a researcher to acquire new information. Sometimes existing information can be examined in a way to study a problem. The use of records and available data is frequently considered to be primarily the province of historical research, but hospital records, care plans, and existing data sources, such as the census, can also be utilized for collecting information. What sets these studies apart from a literature review is that these available data are examined in a new way and are not merely summarized.

The use of available data has certain advantages. Since the data collection step of the research process is often the most difficult and time consuming, the use of available records often allows for a significant savings of time. If the records have been kept in a similar manner over time, as with the National Health and Examination Surveys, analysis of these records allows for the examination of trends over time. In addition, the use of available data decreases problems of reactivity and response bias. The researcher also does not have to ask individuals to participate in the study.

On the other hand, sometimes institutions are reluctant to allow researchers to have access to their records. If the records are kept so that an individual cannot be identified, then this is usually not a problem. However, the Privacy Act, a federal law, protects the rights of individuals who may be identified in records. Another problem that affects the quality of available data is that the researcher only has access to those records that have survived. If the records available are not representative of all of the possible records, then the researcher may have a problem with bias. Often there is no way to tell if the records have been saved in a biased manner, and the researcher has to make an intelligent guess as to their accuracy. For example, a researcher might be interested in studying socioeconomic factors associated with the suicide rate. These data are frequently underreported because of the stigma attached to suicide, and so the records would be biased.

Another problem has to do with the authenticity of the records. The distinction of primary and secondary sources is as relevant here as it was in discussing the literature review (see Chapter 5). A book, for example, may have been ghostwritten, but credit accorded to the known author. It may be difficult for the researcher to ferret out these types of subtle biases.

Nonetheless, records and available data constitute a rich source of data for study. Kalish, Kalish, and Clinton (1982) provide an excellent example of the use of available data in studying the image of American nurses on television.

• Locating Tools and Measuring Phenomena of Interest

We have said that the data collection phase of the research process is often the most difficult and time-consuming aspect. In addition, since nursing research is still relatively young, only a few good instruments exist to measure phenomena of interest. Finally, since the quality of the study's findings rest to a large extent on the quality of the data collection methods, this aspect of a research study demands painstaking efforts on the part of the researcher. Thus the process of selecting and evaluating the available tools to measure the variables of interest is of critical importance to the potential success of an investigation. In this section, we review how a researcher selects operations to measure the variables of interest, so that the consumer can make a reasonable judgment about the methods utilized in a published study.

Selection of the data collection method begins during the literature review. In chapter 5, we noted that one purpose of the review was to provide clues to instrumentation. As the literature review is conducted, the researcher begins to explore how previous investigators defined and operationalized variables similar to those of interest in the present study. The researcher uses this information to define conceptually the variables to be studied. Once a variable has been defined conceptually, the researcher returns to the literature to define the variable operationally. This *operational definition* translates the conceptual definition into behaviors or verbalizations that can be measured for the study. In this second literature review the researcher searches for measuring instruments that might be utilized as is or adapted for use in the study. If instruments are available, the researcher needs to obtain permission for their use from the author.

It is often the case that no suitable measuring device exists, so then the researcher needs to decide if the variable is important to the study and a new device should be constructed. This is often a problem in nursing research, as many variables of interest have not been studied. The construction of new instruments for data collection that have reasonable reliability and validity (see Chapter 13) is a difficult and time-consuming task. Sometimes researchers decide not to study a variable if no suitable measuring device exists; other times, the researcher may decide to invest the time and energy into tool development. Either decision is acceptable depending on the goals of the study and the goals of the researcher.

Whether the researcher chooses to use available methods or create new ones, once the variables have been operationally defined, the researcher needs to decide on how the data collection phase of the study will be implemented. This decision deals with how instructions for the data collection task will be given to the respondents. The reseacher must consider ways to minimize the participants' anxiety, maintain their motivation to complete the data collection, and make the procedures as similar as possible for all participants. All of these procedures go together to form a kind of "cookbook" for the research project that tells those who are gathering the data exactly how respondents are to be contacted and what should be said and not said.

• Critiquing Data Collection Methods

Evaluating the adequacy of data collection methods from written research reports is often problematic for new nursing research consumers. This is because the tool itself is not available for inspection and the reader may not feel comfortable about judging the adequacy of the method without seeing it. However, a number of questions can be asked as you read to judge the method chosen by the researcher. These questions are listed in the box on p.165.

All studies should have clearly identified data collection methods. The conceptual and operational definitions of each important variable should be present in the report. Sometimes it is useful for the researcher to explain why a particular method was chosen. For example, if the study dealt with young children, the researcher may explain that a questionnaire was deemed to be an unreasonable task, so an interview was chosen.

Once you have identified the method chosen to measure each variable of interest, you should decide if the method utilized was the best way to measure the variable. If a questionnaire was utilized, for example, you might wonder why the decision was made not to use an interview. In addition, consider whether the method was appropriate to the clinical situation. Does it make sense to interview clients in the recovery room, for example?

Once you have decided if all relevant variables are operationalized appropriately, you can begin to determine how well the method was carried out. For studies utilizing physiological measurement, it is important to determine if the instrument was appropriate to the problem and not forced to fit it. The rationale for selecting a particular instrument should be given. For example, it may be important to know that the study was conducted under the auspices of a manufacturing firm that provided the measuring instrument. In addition, provision should be made to evaluate the accuracy of the instrument and those who use it.

Several considerations are important when reading studies that utilize observational methods. Who were the observers and how were they trained? Is there any reason to believe that different observers saw events or behaviors differently? Remember that the more inferences the observers are required to make, the more likely

Critiquing Criteria

1. Are all of the data collection instruments clearly identified and described?
2. Is the rationale for their selection given?
3. Is the method used appropriate to the problem being studied?
4. Is the method used appropriate to the clinical situation?
5. Are the data collection procedures similar for all subjects?

Physiological Measurement

1. Is the instrument used appropriate to the research problem and not forced to fit it?
2. Is a rationale given for why a particular instrument was selected?
3. Is there a provision for evaluating the accuracy of the instrument and those who use it?

Observational Methods

1. Who did the observing?
2. Were the observers trained to minimize any bias?
3. Was there an observational guide?
4. Were the observers required to make inferences about what they saw?
5. Is there any reason to believe that the presence of the observers affected the behavior of the subjects?
6. Were the observations performed utilizing the principles of informed consent?

Interviews and Questionnaires

1. Is the schedule described adequately enough to know if it covers the subject?
2. Is there clear indication that the subjects understood the task and the questions?
3. Who were the interviewers and how were they trained?
4. Is there evidence of any interviewer bias?

Available Data and Records

1. Are the records that were utilized appropriate to the problem being studied?
2. Are the data examined in such a way as to provide new information and not summarize the records?
3. Has the author addressed questions of internal and external criticism?
4. Is there any indication of selective bias in the available records?

there will be problems with biased observations. Also consider the problem of reactivity; in any observational situation, the possibility exists that the mere presence of the observer could change the behavior in question. What is important here is not that reactivity could occur, but rather how such reactivity could affect the data. Finally, consider whether the observational procedure was ethical. The reader needs to consider whether subjects were informed that they were being observed, whether any intervention was performed, and whether subjects had agreed to be observed.

Interviews and questionnaires should be clearly described to allow the reader to decide whether the variables were adequately operationalized. Sometimes the researcher will reference the original report about the tool, and the reader may wish to read this study before deciding if the method was appropriate for the present study. The respondents' task should be clear. Thus provision should be made for the subjects to understand both their overall responsibilities and the individual items. In the interview situation, who were the interviewers? Does the researcher explain how they were trained to decrease any interviewer bias?

Available data are subject to internal and external criticism. Internal criticism deals with the evaluation of the worth of the records. Internal criticism primarily refers to the accuracy of the data. The researcher should present evidence that the records are genuine. External criticism is concerned with the authenticity of the records. Are the records really written by the first author? Finally, the reader should be aware of the problems with selective survival. The researcher may not have an unbiased sample of all of the possible records in the problem area, and this may have a profound effect on the validity of the results.

Finally, the reader should consider the data collection procedure. Is any assurance provided that all of the subjects received the same information? In addition, it is important to try to determine if all of the information was collected in the same way for all of the subjects in the study.

Once you have decided that the data collection method used was appropriate to the problem and the procedures were appropriate to the population studied, then the characteristics of the instruments themselves need to be considered. These characteristics are discussed in the next chapter.

• Summary

This chapter's purpose was to familiarize the student with the various methods that researchers utilize to collect information from and about subjects. Data collection methods are described as being both objective and systematic. The data collection methods of a study provide the operational definitions of the relevant variables.

The following five types of data collection methods were described: physiological, observational, interviews, questionnaires, and available data or records. The purposes, advantages, and disadvantages of each method were presented.

Physiological measurements are those methods that use technical instruments to collect data about clients' physical, chemical, microbiological, or anatomical status. Such instruments are particularly suited to the study of the effectiveness of nursing care and the ways to improve the provision of nursing care. Physiological measurements are objective, precise, and sensitive. However, they may be very expensive and they may distort the variable of interest.

Observational methods are frequently utilized in nursing research when the variables of interest deal with events or behaviors. Scientific observation requires preplanning, systematic recording, controlling the observations, and relationship to scientific theory. This method is best suited to research problems that are difficult to view as a part of a whole. Observers may be passive or active and concealed or obvious. Observational methods have several advantages, the most important one being the flexibility of the method to measure many types of situations. In addition, observation allows for a great deal of depth and breadth of information to be collected, depending on the problem being studied. Observation has several disadvantages, too. Reactivity, or the distortion of data as a result of the observer's presence, is a common problem in nonconcealed observations. If the observer is concealed, however, there are ethical considerations. Finally, observations may be biased by the person who is doing the observing.

Interviews and questionnaires are the most commonly utilized data collection methods in nursing research. Both have the purpose of asking subjects to report data for themselves. Items on questionnaire and interview schedules may be of direct or indirect interest and can be combined into scales. Scales provide an estimate of the degree to which the respondent possesses some trait or characteristic. Either open-ended or close-ended questions may be utilized when asking subjects questions. The form of the question should be clear to the respondent, free from suggestion, and grammatically correct.

Questionnaires, or paper-and-pencil tests, are particularly useful when there are a finite number of questions to be asked and the researcher is sure that the questions are clear and specific. Questionnaires are also much less costly in time and money to administer to a large number of subjects, particularly if the subjects are widespread. Another advantage of the questionnaire over the interview is that questionnaires have the potential to be completely anonymous. In addition, there is no possibility of interviewer bias.

Interviews, on the other hand, are best utilized when it is important to have a large response rate and an unbiased sample, because the refusal rate for interviews is much less than that for questionnaires. Interviews also allow for some portions of the population who would be precluded by the use of a questionnaire, such as children and the illiterate, to participate in the study. An interviewer can clarify the questions and maintain the order of the questions for all participants.

Records and available data are also an important source for research data. The use of available data may save the researcher considerable time and money when conducting a study. This data collection method reduces problems with reactivity and ethical concerns as well. However, records and available data are subject to problems of availability, authenticity, and accuracy.

Finally, the criteria for evaluating data collection methods utilized in published research studies were presented. A critical evaluation of this aspect of a research study should emphasize the appropriateness, objectivity, and consistency of the method employed.

• References

Fox, D.J. (1982). *Fundamentals of research in nursing,* Norwalk, Conn., Appleton-Century-Crofts.

Kalish, P.A., Kalish, B.J., and Clinton, J. (1982). The world of nursing on prime time television, 1950-1980, *Nursing Research,* **31**:358.

Lim-Levy, F. (1982). The effect of oxygen inhalation on oral temperature, *Nursing Research,* **31**:150.

Polit, D.F., and Hungler, B.P. (1983). *Nursing research: Principles and methods,* 2nd ed., Philadelphia, J.B. Lippincott.

Seaman, C.C.H., and Verhonick, P.J. (1982). *Research methods for undergraduate students in nursing,* Norwalk, Connecticut, Appleton-Century-Crofts.

Wolfer, J., and Visintainer, M.A. (1975). Pediatric surgical patients' and parents' stress responses and adjustment as a function of psychological preparation and stress-point nursing care, *Nursing Research,* **24**:244-255.

13

Measurement Principles

Carol Noll Hoskins

LEARNING OBJECTIVES

After reading this chapter, the student should be able to do the following:
- Discuss the principles of measurement.
- Summarize the common characteristics of self-report inventories.
- Compare and contrast the questionnaire, test, and scale as types of self-report inventories.
- Discuss the direct observation of behavior as a type of measurement tool.
- Summarize the criteria for data collection when using direct observation as a form of measurement.
- Define validity.
- Compare and contrast content, criterion-related, and construct validity.
- Define reliability.
- Explain the purpose of test-retest, alternate form, split-half, statistical, and interrater reliability.
- Describe the tool development process.
- Identify critiquing criteria for measurement tools.
- Use the critiquing criteria to evaluate the measurement aspects of a research report.

KEY TERMS

alternate form reliability	quantitative measurement
chance errors	questionnaire
construct validity	ratio
content validity	reliability
criterion-related validity	scale
direct observation	split-half reliability
error variance	statistical reliability
interrater reliability	systematic errors
interval	test
nominal	test-retest reliability
ordinal	validation sample
qualitative measurement	validity

The subject of measurement is a crucial part of critiquing and conducting research, and a brief review of some points that have already been made is needed. As we have observed, a large component of nursing practice is, or should be, based on scientific knowledge developed through systematic investigation. The research process poses and seeks answers to questions about nursing interventions or the theoretical bases for those interventions. As noted, a characteristic of a profession is that it claims to base its practice on science. Without research endeavors that build its theory base, a profession will have a limited body of knowledge that is often inadequate or inappropriate for improving its practice because it was developed by other disciplines.

Once identified, a research problem must be studied within a theoretical framework. As we have seen, it is preferable to phrase the problem as a question that asks whether there is a relationship between specific variables or behaviors of interest. For example, Wolfer and Visintainer (1975) (see Appendix A) were interested in whether psychological preparation and continued supportive care to parents and their hospitalized child would be related to a decrease in upset behavior and an increase in coping and adjustment. The nursing care variables and outcome behaviors that were of interest in this study were not arbitrarily linked. On the contrary, the proposed relationships were logically derived from previous research findings and composed only part of the entire set of interrelationships that made up the theoretical framework. Wolfer and Visintainer's discussion of the theoretical framework's development is a good example of a systematic explanation of some phenomena. The theoretical framework helps the researcher to identify the variables needed to explain the phenomena and suggests the nature of the relationships between them; for example, Wolfer and Visintainer hypothesized that an increase in supportive care would be related to a decrease in behavioral disturbances.

When conducting research it is usually possible to study or test only a part of the theory. For example, Wolfer and Visintainer could have examined any number of independent variables that were identified in their theory, such as parental rooming-in. The rationale for selecting the designated variables for study was discussed by the authors and appeared to be logical.

With this study and background in mind, let us consider why measurement principles are a major concern of nurses who use research findings in practice and nurse scientists who design and conduct studies in the first place. It may be readily seen that the hypothetical relationships between the variables cannot be tested unless the variables are observable or measurable. This chapter will introduce the principles of measurement, the different forms of measurement tools, and the principles of validity and reliability and discuss the availability of measurement tools.

• Principles of Measurement

Principles of measurement provide a foundation for understanding the measurement process. Both the investigator and the critiquer of a research study need to understand the principles of this process to critically evaluate their own or another's work. The following discussion illustrates the importance of applying established principles when defining the variables that are to be measured, establishing objectivity in the measurement process, and considering the levels of measurement when selecting or constructing a tool.

DEFINITION OF THE VARIABLES TO BE MEASURED

Initially, the variables must be clearly defined both conceptually and operationally (see Chapters 6 and 7). If the behavior that we wish to measure has not been defined, our confidence in the study's findings must be greatly reduced. In Wolfer and Visintainer's study the independent variables of stress-point nursing care, psychological preparation, and supportive care were defined conceptually as the "provision of information about what to expect and how to respond" before six designated events in the child's care, "along with support and reassurance during these events." The content areas of the information given to the parent and child were discussed further, as well as the methods that were used to encourage the child to express his feelings, perceptions, and understanding by means of verbalization, rehearsal, and play. The conceptual definition was clear and easily understood although it lacked specificity and had to be located by the reader in the study's text. Also, there were no indications that the degree of the subjects' participation, understanding, or response to these interventions was measured by an appropriate objective measurement device. Although the encouragement of the child's active participation served this purpose to some extent, the point here is that the evaluation of the child's response appeared to be a subjective one by the research nurse.

The dependent variable or outcome behavior, the degree of upset, was conceptually defined as "the emotional state of a child at a given point in time, primarily in terms of verbal and nonverbal expressions of fear, anxiety, or anger." It meets the criterion of telling us exactly what is meant by stress response and thus implies possibilities for observation and measurement.

Wolfer and Visintainer went on to provide a clear operational definition of upset behavior that specified exactly what had to be done to carry out the required observations or measurements. "Blind observer ratings of the child's upset behavior and cooperation with procedures at five potential stress points" were to be done with the monitoring of "pulse rates at admission and before and after the blood test and preoperative injections; resistance to induction; recovery room medications; ease of fluid intake; time to first voiding; posthospital adjustment." In addition, the "mother's rated satisfaction with various aspects of the nursing and medical care they received; and mother's rating of the adequacy of information they received" were to be measured as indicators of the dependent variable. Each of these 10 outcome behaviors was described further in terms of measurement by a rating scale or another procedure that permitted objective quantification of the variable.

This detailed description of behaviors that were observed or measured in the study by Wolfer and Visintainer emphasizes the importance of definitions that indicate exactly what it is that the researcher intended to observe or measure. Variables that are not clearly defined both conceptually and operationally cannot be measured with any satisfactory degree of accuracy or consistency. When this process is incomplete, the reader will find it difficult to interpret the findings.

OBJECTIVITY IN MEASUREMENT

Once the definitions satisfy the criteria, we may then consider some of the measurement principles or guidelines that are helpful when evaluating the instruments used in the study. As already indicated, the selected method of observation or measurement should be *objective,* meaning that anyone following a prescribed set of rules will assign the same ratings or scores to what is observed. The *interrater reliability,* or agreement among observers or research nurses, needs to be at a maximum. For example, the method used by Wolfer and Visintainer to administer the manifest upset scale maximized objectivity and interrater reliability. Their five-point scale assigned a rating of *1* to indicate little or no fear or anxiety (calm appearance, no crying, no verbal protest), a rating of *3* to indicate a moderate amount (some temporary whimpering and/or mild verbal protest), and a rating of *5* to indicate extreme distress (agitated, hard crying or screaming and/or strong verbal protest). These rules for assigning ratings to clearly defined, observed behaviors of interest were one of the means of ensuring objectivity. Two research nurses observing the behaviors of a child at the same time should have been close in their scores or ratings with such operational definitions.

In the case of tests, scales, and questionnaires that are self-administered, the instructions to the respondents must provide the same clarity. The subjects need to understand precisely how to read the items and how to use the response format. Factors such as whether there are right or wrong answers or any time limitations need to be stated. These techniques should keep the measurement as objective as possible and the level of measurement error low.

LEVELS OF MEASUREMENT

After the behavior or trait of interest has been defined and the importance of objectivity has been clarified, the researcher asks the question, "To what degree does the subject possess the behavior, trait, or attitude being studied?" The question immediately implies a primary objective of measurement, the need to differentiate between persons. To accomplish this goal, we use a dimension or a scale of items where each item has at least two response categories with ratings assigned according to whether the subject exhibits more or less of the behavior. This procedure permits the establishment of an *ordered dimension,* that is, the subjects are assessed according to the degree that they exhibit a behavior in relation to others.

The level of assessment or measurement is reflected in the response format that accompanies each item. Table 13-1 identifies levels of assessment or measurement and their characteristics and provides an example that illustrates each level. This table indicates that the researcher must identify the appropriate level of assessment for the variables under consideration before selecting a specific measurement tool. The levels of measurement are also discussed in Chapter 15. The evaluator of a research report will want to determine whether or not an appropriate level of assessment was utilized by the researcher.

• *Table 13-1* Levels of Measurement

Level of measurement	Characteristics	Example
Nominal	Simply categorizes the clients or subjects into two categories. The categories are mutually exclusive, meaning that a subject can be assigned to only one category, since there is no ambiguity or overlap of the categories. This level of measurement does not permit precise differentiation among subjects.	The subjects in the Wolfer and Visintainer study were either parents or children.
Ordinal	Systematically categorizes clients or subjects in an ordered manner. Ordinal measures also do not permit a high level of differentiation among subjects.	If Wolfer and Visintainer had been interested in the variables of socioeconomic status as a possible contributing factor to coping and adjustment, they might have used ordered categories of low, middle, and high socioeconomic status.

Continued.

• *Table 13-1*   Levels of Measurement—cont'd

Level of measurement	Characteristics	Example
Interval	Provides different levels or gradations in response, and the differences or intervals between responses are assumed to be approximately equal. This permits a finer distinction among individuals for a defined trait or behavior. There is no true zero in an interval level scale, that is, no known zero quantity of the trait or behavior.	A response format that provides such response possibilities as *strongly agree, agree, undecided, disagree,* and *strongly disagree* represents interval levels of measurement. Psychological measurements are considered interval level scales, since we can rarely, if ever, claim that a subject possesses a zero quantity of the trait that these devices measure, such as anxiety or fear.
Ratio	Permits the same fine distinction among individuals for a defined trait or behavior as the interval level of measurement. However, this level of measurement does theoretically have a true zero, that is, the trait, attribute, or parameter being measured can potentially exhibit a zero quantity.	Physiological measures such as components of blood, urine, or other parameters can conceivably be stated as having a level of zero.

• Measurement Tools

Readers of research reports will observe that many forms of tools have been devised to measure the numerous characteristics that are manifested by humans and that are of interest to the nurse investigator. They include questionnaires wherein the subject reports self-perceptions, projective techniques used to predict how a subject will associate with a specified set of symbols, and rating procedures that require an observer to judge the traits or behaviors of subjects or clients.

CHARACTERISTICS OF MEASUREMENT TOOLS

Despite their superficial differences, the evaluator of a research report needs to understand that there are identifiable commonalities among these measurement methods. Table 13-2 summarizes the common characteristics of different types of measurement tools. They are useful guidelines for researchers who are evaluating a potential measurement tool and readers who are critically assessing a measurement tool that has

• *Table 13-2*   **Common Characteristics of Different Types of Measurement Tools**

Common characteristics	Example
The well-constructed scale, test, interview schedule, or other form of index should consist of an objective standardized measure of samples of a behavior that has been clearly defined. Observations should be made on a small but carefully chosen sampling of the behavior of interest, thus permitting us to feel confident that the samples are representative.	In their study of stress response and adjustment, Wolfer and Visintainer selected 10 behaviors that were assessed as being representative of "upset behavior" as it had been defined. The basis for such a decision should be the findings from a thorough review of previous theoretical and research literature.
The tool should be *standardized,* that is, a set of uniform items and response possibilities, that are uniformly administered and scored.	In the study by Wolfer and Visintainer, the evaluation of the childrens' response to the nursing interventions consisted of an objective assessment by the research nurse in various settings. Without specific criteria and ratings for the observed behaviors, the evaluations would be based on the nurses' subjective impressions that may have varied significantly between observers and conditions.
The items of a measurement tool should be unambiguous; they should be clear-cut, concise, exact statements with only one idea per item. Negative stems or items with negatively phrased response possibilities result in a double negative and ambiguity in meaning and scoring.	In constructing a tool to measure job satisfaction, a nurse-scientist writes the following items, "I never feel that I don't have time to provide good nursing care." The response format consists of, "Agree," "Undecided," and "Disagree." It is very likely that a response of "Disagree" will not reflect the respondent's true intent because of the confusion that is created by the double negatives.
The type of items used in any one test or scale should be restricted to a limited number of variations. Subjects who are expected to shift from one kind of item to another may fail to provide a true response as a result of the distraction of making such a change.	Mixing true-or-false items with questions that require a yes-or-no response and items that provide a response format of five possible answers is conducive to a high level of measurement error.
Items should not provide irrelevant clues. Unless carefully constructed, an item may furnish an indication of the expected response or answer. Furthermore, the correct answer or expected response to one item should not be given by another item.	An item that provides a clue to the expected answer may contain value words that convey cultural expectations, such as, "A good wife enjoys caring for her home and family."

Continued.

• *Table 13-2*   Common Characteristics of Different Types of Measurement Tools—cont'd

Common characteristics	Example
The items of a measurement tool should not be made difficult by requiring unnecessarily complex or exact operations. Furthermore, the difficulty of an item should be appropriate to the level of the subjects being assessed. Limiting each item to one concept or idea helps to accomplish this objective.	A test constructed to evaluate learning in an introductory course in research methods may contain an item that is inappropriate for the designated group, such as, "A nonlinear transformation of data to linear data is a useful procedure before testing a hypothesis of curvilinearity."
The diagnostic, predictive, or measurement value of a tool depends on the degree to which it serves as an indicator of a relatively broad and significant area of behavior known as the universe of content for the behavior. As we have already emphasized, a behavior must be clearly defined before it can be measured. The definition is developed from the universe of content, for example, the information and research findings that are available for the behavior of interest. The items should reflect that definition. To what extent the test items appear to accomplish this objective is an indication of the face validity of the instrument.	Two nurse researchers, A and B, are studying the construct of client satisfaction. Each has defined this construct in a different way. Consequently, the measurement tool that each nurse devises will include different questions. The questions on each tool will reflect the universe of content for client satisfaction as defined by each researcher.
The instrument should also adequately cover the defined behavior. The primary consideration is whether the number and nature of items in the sample are adequate. If there are too few items, then the accuracy or reliability of the measure must be questioned. In general, there should be a minimum of 10 items for each independent aspect of the behavior of interest.	Very few people would be satisfied with an assessment of such traits as intelligence if the scales were limited to 3 items.
The measure must prove its worth by an empirically demonstrated correspondence between the individual's performance on the instrument and the actual behavior of the respondent. Here we are concerned with the *validity* of the tool; that is, whether it really measures what it is purported to measure.	A person who has a high score on an instrument that measures anxiety should exhibit behavioral or physiological signs of anxiety that correspond with the test score, such as pacing, diaphoresis, and palpitations.

been used in a study. As the reader can see, there are many factors to consider when assessing the merit of a measure. In fact, it is often a good practice to have a test or scale that is being considered for use submitted to a colleague or expert in psychometrics for critical analysis of the tool.

FORMS OF MEASUREMENT TOOLS

We have a notion of the characteristics that are common to all measurement tools, but we also need to be aware of some of the differences between the individual types of measures and to consider the strengths and weaknesses of each type. For the purpose of discussion, we will categorize the measures most commonly used by nurse practitioners and investigators into self-report inventories and observational methods.

Self-Report Inventories

The self-report inventories include tests, scales, and questionnaires. Although it is used less frequently than the test and scale in research, the questionnaire is still a useful direct method of obtaining information for studying relationships and testing hypotheses. The questionnaire, as opposed to the interview method of data collection, is self-administered and highly structured. When a questionnaire is used as the main instrument of a research study, the following criteria must be met:

- The questions, their sequence, and the wording are fixed.
- The instrument must be carefully constructed and pretested.
- The instrument must be subjected to the same criteria of reliability, validity, and objectivity as any other measuring instrument.

The forms of measurement used most frequently in research are self-report inventories composed of individual items that are self-perceived and self-reported, such as tests and scales. In a *test* each item has one response with a rating or score assigned by the examiner. Inferences are made from the total score as to what degree the subject possesses whatever trait, emotion, attitude, or behavior the test is supposed to measure.

An example of a test that is commonly used in the health sciences is the Minnesota Multiphasic Personality Inventory (MMPI) (Anastasi, 1976). The MMPI is a personality test designed for adults 16 years of age and older. It is made up of 550 affirmative statements to which the subject gives a response. Five sample items are shown in Fig. 13-1. The responses are treated as diagnostic or symptomatic of specific behaviors known as criterion behaviors. In the case of the MMPI, the criterion behaviors are characteristic of 10 psychiatric diagnoses and the 10 individual scales are composed of items that differentiate between a clinical group with the specific diagnosis and a normal control group.

The advantages and disadvantages of the MMPI are presented in Table 13-3. This table reinforces the point that even widely accepted and used scales have both strengths and weaknesses (Anastasi, 1976).

A *scale* differs from a test in that a scale provides a set of response symbols for each item whereas a test provides only one response possibility. For example, response

I do not tire quickly.	True	False	Cannot say
Most people will use somewhat un-fair means to gain profit or an advantage rather than lose it.	True	False	Cannot say
I am worried about sex matters.	True	False	Cannot say
When I get bored I like to stir up some excitement.	True	False	Cannot say
I believe I am being plotted against.	True	False	Cannot say

Responses consist of *True, False,* or *Cannot say.* In the individual form of the test, the statements are printed on separate cards that the respondent sorts into the three categories. In the group form, the statements are printed in a test booklet and the responses are recorded on an answer sheet.

Fig. 13-1 Illustrative items from the Minnesota Multiphasic Personality Inventory. (Reproduced from Anastasi, A. [1976]. *Psychological testing,* New York, McMillan & Co.)

• *Table 13-3* **Advantages and Disadvantages of the MMPI**

Advantages	Disadvantages
Norms are provided as standard scores that may be used in plotting profiles. The validation of the test has been carried out over time by the accumulation of empirical data about persons who show specific profile patterns. Items that serve as checks on carelessness, misunderstanding, and the presence of particular response sets are included. Response set refers to a tendency on the part of the respondent to answer items in one way, which often leads to a score that is not truly indicative of the subject's level of the behavior or trait being measured.	The use and interpretation of the scores are complex. The inventory is long. Some of the scales are "multidimensional," meaning that they measure more than one criterion behavior. There are high correlations between some of the scales, indicating that some items on both scales measure similar things, thus making their value in differential diagnosis questionable. The reliabilities of some of the scales are inadequate. Some scales of the MMPI assess behavior that is so variable over time that the claim for retest reliability or stability may not be made.

possibilities may range on a five-point scale from strongly disagree to strongly agree. The instructions for the respondents must be clear, simple, and unambiguous.

An example of a scale is the Partner Relationship Inventory (PRI) (Hoskins, 1986). It is composed of 40 items and is designed to measure the perceived degree of fulfillment of interactional and emotional needs in partners; a long form of the scale has 80 items. Five sample items are shown in Fig. 13-2. As with the test, an examiner using the PRI quantifies the response to each item by assigning a rating or score according to rules. For the PRI, a *4* is assigned to a response of "definitely feel," *3* to "feel slightly," *2* to "cannot decide," and *1* to "definitely to not feel." The

---

Each of the sentences below describes a feeling. Please use the rating scale next to each sentence to describe your feelings *at this moment*. If you circle the double check (XX) it means that you *definitely feel* this *at the moment*. If you circle the single check (X) it means that you *feel slightly* this way *at the moment*. If you circle the question mark (?) it means that this does not apply or you *cannot decide* if this is true *at the moment*. If you circle the no (no) it means that you *definitely do not feel* this way *at the moment*.

EXAMPLES:

I can share my feelings freely with my partner	(XX)	X	?	no
I can share my feelings freely with my partner	XX	(X)	?	no
I can share my feelings freely with my partner	XX	X	(?)	no
I can share my feelings freely with my partner	XX	X	?	(no)

Please mark all the items. Your first reaction is best.

1. My partner and I think alike on most things	XX	X	?	no
2. My partner has little insight into my feelings	XX	X	?	no
3. My partner and I talk very little about the day's events	XX	X	?	no
4. I long for more warmth and love from my partner	XX	X	?	no
5. My partner appreciates my efforts	XX	X	?	no

A response of definitely feel (XX) is scored as 4, feel slightly (X) as 3, cannot decide (?) as 2, and definitely do not feel (no) as 1 for items 2, 3 and 4. Items 1 and 5 are reverse scored, that is, 4 becomes 1, 3 becomes 2, 2 becomes 3, and 1 becomes 4.

Fig. 13-2   PRI illustrative items and instructions. Reproduced from Hoskins, C.N. (1985). Palo Alto Consulting Psychologists Press, Inc.

• *Table 13-4*   **Positive and Negative Features of the PRI**

Positive features	Negative features
The material for this scale is taken from an extensive review of the theoretical and research literature as well as from case records, counseling interviews, and similar sources. The review was used for content validation; that is, the validity of the content of the items was established from a large spectrum of investigators who have studied the area of interest.	With the given response format, an accurate reply to some of the negatively phrased items requires a relatively high level of cognitive appraisal
The use of a response format that actually suggests the magnitude of the problem by providing a set of response possibilities rather than one.	The inventory requires that the subject be conscious of feelings and expectations in relation to the partner and the relationship.
The scale has been found to be highly sensitive to actual and potential areas of conflict, or discrepancy in the partners' perceptions of need fulfillment.	A neutral response between positive and negative response possibilities is desirable to control for influence on the subject's response. The PRI has only a four-point response possibility format. A balance between the number of negative and positive responses with a centered neutral response is preferable.

response to each item is regarded as an index of how intensely a specific need is perceived to be met by the partner. Table 13-4 presents the positive and negative features of the PRI.

In addition to identifying the strengths and weaknesses of the MMPI and the PRI, there are other general principles that serve as guides for critiquing a test or scale, such as the following:

- The content of the items and the response process should be examined from the perspective of the intended subjects. Suitability for the "lower bounded" individuals who are more likely to have difficulty in understanding the instructions or determining their perceptions and feelings needs to be considered more than for the persons who are not likely to have such problems.
- Individuals tend to remember extremes; that is, things that they have felt particularly good or bad about; this is a problem inherent in self-report.
- It is preferable to determine a subject's interpretation or perception at the present time, rather than from the past. Since retrospective responses are not always accurate or valid, the response format should be set in the present even though the item content may be in the past. An item that is phrased in the form of, "As you remember it today, how was it then?" is preferable to, "How was it then?"
- The content of items should be as situation specific as possible, meaning that the items should be relevant to the subject's present situation and condition. When assessing marital conflict, items that pertain to actual situations where

the couple must communicate and compromise should be used, for example, responsibilities for household tasks.

- If the behavior of interest is variable over time, such as the ability of the surgical cancer client to cope with the crisis of illness (Oberst, in progress), a single observation may not be valid. Again, be sure what it is you wish to measure. A clear definition of the behavior, including whether it varies over time, must be formulated before searching for and selecting an instrument to measure it.
- There should be consistency in person and tense with no shifts from "I" to "you" in the items. Avoid double negatives, such as negatively phrased items with a no or negative response.
- Response set refers to the tendency of a subject to respond in one direction. In addition to items that detect response set, procedures may be used to identify this behavior. For example, whether most answers are "true" or "false" in the case of the MMPI may be checked by totaling the "true" items and totaling the "false" items. The causes of response set include failure of the respondent to take the testing seriously, misunderstanding of the items, and deliberate misrepresentation or nondisclosure of feelings. To reduce both types of response set, some items may be reversed. In the case of the MMPI, a response of "true" to one item should be consistent in meaning with a response of "false" to another item. In the case of the PRI, a response of "definitely feel" to the item, "I cannot please my partner" is consistent in meaning with a response of "definitely do not feel" to, "My partner is pleased with me." The scoring of the latter item is reversed from a 1 to a 4 to maintain consistency so that the total score accurately reflects the subject's intent.
- Self-report inventories have a tendency to be unstable over time, particularly in the case of the personality inventories. Some tests and scales have two forms, one where the subject is instructed to respond according to how he or she feels generally (trait) and one where the instructions are to respond according to feelings at the moment (state). The MMPI is designed to measure trait behavior, and the PRI measures state perceptions. Again, it needs to be ascertained which is of interest.

One more kind of scale of particular relevance to nursing should be mentioned, the attitude scale. Attitudes are basic to the way that a client perceives and responds to illness and therefore are a major concern of the nurse. Attitudes cannot be observed directly but are inferred from overt behavior. For example, the noncompliant behavior of a client who fails to follow nursing or medical orders is a reflection of an attitude. The *attitude* may be defined as a tendency to react favorably or unfavorably to a specific set of stimuli (Anastasi, 1976), and it is inferred from the noncompliant behavior of the client. The questions on an attitude scale are developed in this case to measure the client's reaction to specific aspects of health care. The total score is calculated from the responses to the individual questions and indicates the direction and intensity of that reaction.

Attitude scales are often developed by gathering a large number of statements relevant to the variable of interest. For example, if we are interested in developing a scale to measure clients' attitudes toward health care, we may ask several groups of people to write their opinions about an identified aspect of health care. We would select the groups on the basis of factors that may be related to the attitude of interest, such as age, sex, socioeconomic status, ethnic origin, and other demographic characteristics. The obtained list of opinions is expanded with opinions that are located in the literature review and range from very favorable to very unfavorable.

Usually the items are presented to a large group of judges for sorting into a specified number of categories. The categories are defined according to the degree of how favorable or unfavorable the statement is judged to be. The percentage of agreement among judges in placing the statements into categories provides the basis for determining the ratings that are used for scoring the statements that are selected for the final form of the scale.

However, other procedures may not involve classification of items by judges. Rather, the items are submitted directly to a large *standardization sample,* or the sample that provides the initial data for determining reliability and validity. A graded response format such as strongly agree, agree, undecided, disagree, and strongly disagree is used. The responses are scored as *5, 4, 3, 2,* and *1,* with a *5* indicating a favorable attitude and *1* an unfavorable attitude. The final selection of items is made by eliminating those that are not clearly favorable or unfavorable as well as those that cannot be categorized.

The positive features of these methods for measuring attitudes are that the items are usually relevant and unambiguous and can be distributed relatively evenly among the categories from favorable to unfavorable. If the items are submitted initially to selected judges, there is the potentially negative feature of the judges' own attitudes on the classification of the statements.

Direct Observation

A second major form of measurement is direct observation of behavior. A primary component of nursing practice is the observation of psychological and physiological behaviors in clients to evaluate any change and facilitate recovery. Here again, the nurse needs to identify the behaviors that are to be observed, whether they are a measurement of blood pressure or an assessment of attitude toward learning how to irrigate a colostomy. Furthermore, any change in such behaviors can be evaluated only within the context of previous observations of the client and the norm for that particular individual.

Nurse investigators also use the method of direct observation of behavior to test the relationships that have been stated in the hypotheses. For example, O'Brien (1980) studied the patterns of acknowledgment in parent-child communication in relation to the exploratory behavior and self-differentiation in the child. In this interesting study, O'Brien observed parent-child dyads during 30-minute periods in the home setting while they were engaged in a series of semistructured play activities. Various aspects of the mother's response to the child's assertions were observed and coded as nonevaluative recognition, positive recognition, negative recognition, direction, or nonrecognition.

Clearly, there was a basic need to define each one of the behaviors of interest in O'Brien's study so that accurate observations and measurements could be made. Parent-child communication was conceptually defined as "an interactional exchange between parent and child which includes the child's assertion and parental response to it." O'Brien operationalized parent-child communication by constructing a measurement tool, the Parent-Child Communication Schedule (PCCS). Exploratory behavior was defined as "the degree to which the child reacts to new, strange, and incongruous elements in the environment by approaching them, manipulating them or questioning them." It was measured in the nursery school setting by means of the Object Exploration Score. Self-differentiation was defined as "the sense of separate identity as manifested by the extent to which the child's experience of self and environment tends to be relatively discrete, structured, and assimilated." It was measured by the Preschool Embedded Figures Test, also in the nursery school setting. The behaviors of interest could be measured only because the conceptual and operational definitions were explicit.

Table 13-5 identifies criteria for data collection when using direct observation as a method of measurement. As with the test and scale forms of measurement, the method of direct observation of behavior has its strengths and weaknesses. In cases where the self-report inventories are not appropriate, such as gathering data from subjects who are not aware of specific feelings and behaviors or are unable to verbalize them in an interview, direct observation may be the most feasible method of mea-

• *Table 13-5*   **Criteria for Data Collection When Using a Direct Observation Method of Measurement**

Criteria	Example
The investigator must have determined the *units* of behavior that are to be observed. The larger units of behavior are known as *molar units,* meaning that a sequence of behaviors is treated as a whole. Alternatively, small *molecular units* consist of such particulate components as facial expression or tone of voice in a verbal response.	O'Brien defined the basic or molar unit of analysis as "the interactional exchange between parent and child which includes both the child's assertion and the parent's response to it." Each assertion or response constitutes a message.
The molar units are more difficult to define and have a greater tendency to be distorted by the observer's own perceptions. On the other hand, the molecular units may be so particulate that the observer forgets the larger picture of the phenomenon to be explained or understood.	In O'Brien's study, the messages constituted molecular units, "recognized as beginning when one individual begins to speak or to assert himself and as ending when another distinct thought commences, or when another person begins to speak or to assert himself, or when the speaker pauses, indicating anticipation of a response."

Continued.

• *Table 13-5*   **Criteria for Data Collection When Using a Direct Observation Method of Measurement—cont'd**

Criteria	Example
The investigator must have determined the sampling method to be used. When and how the observations are to be made must be decided. *Event sampling,* observation of a specific type of situation or interaction, can be used. Alternatively, *time sampling,* observation of a subject over a specified period of time, can be used.	O'Brien used event sampling, meaning that the parent-child dyads were observed in the home while engaged in a series of play activities. The purpose of a study by Dropkin (1978), was to determine the extent of the relationship between compliance with the care regimen and the need for social approval in the hospitalized client who had recently undergone radical head and neck surgery. Using time sampling, Dropkin completed a total of 144 observations of 50 clients from the fourth through the sixth postoperative day. The observations were made at 5-minute intervals over three 4-hour periods. The nature and frequency of social interaction was assessed to validate the need for social approval. The optimal number of self-care tasks that the client actually accomplished was noted to assess compliant behavior.
The investigator must have delineated the nature of the relationship between the observer and the subjects. There are various gradations in the extent of the subject's awareness that they are being observed. This may range from active participation with the subjects by the observer to the observer being present in the setting but not known by the subjects to be the observer. In some investigations, the investigator attempts to conceal his or her presence by using such mechanical devices as a one-way observation window. This permits an investigator to observe the subjects without the subjects being able to see the observer. In all cases, the rights of the subjects must be safeguarded by assurance of confidentiality in an informed consent.	In O'Brien's study, the investigator functioned as a nonparticipating observer after the initial introduction, explanation of the study, and instructions for the play activities were completed. In Dropkin's study, the researcher assumed a passive role, attempting to be an unobtrusive person who was natural to the setting but who observed and recorded information with little or no intervention.

• *Table 13-5*   **Criteria for Data Collection When Using a Direct Observation Method of Measurement—cont'd**

Criteria	Example
The investigator must have determined the extent of *reactivity* that the subjects will demonstrate in the presence of the observer. To what extent are the subjects likely to modify their behavior as a result of an awareness of the investigation? If reactivity is high, the generalizability of the findings will be limited.	O'Brien attempted to control for reactivity by presenting a series of semistructured tasks to the mother and child during the preobservation period that were designed to elicit their customary behavior toward each other. The tasks consisted of 10 minutes of free play with a small farm set, 10 minutes of puzzle construction, and 5 minutes of joint block construction followed by 5 minutes of continued block construction by the child while the mother completed an informational form.
The investigator must have formulated a plan for dealing with an inherent problem related to direct observation, that of having to simultaneously observe and categorize the designated units of behavior according to a predetermined set of operations. While observing the designated units of the defined behaviors, the observer is expected to assign the behaviors to predetermined categories. The categories are mutually exclusive, meaning that a behavior can be assigned to only one category.	O'Brien developed mutually exclusive categories called nonevaluative recognition, positive recognition, negative recognition, direction, and nonrecognition that were clearly defined so that there would be no ambiguity in the assignment of a behavior.
Despite procedural controls, it is difficult for the observer to perform the many cognitive operations that are involved in appraising the information derived from the observations and in categorizing the behaviors. There also may be an unmeasurable tendency to form perceptual reactions to the observations or to group subjects that may lead to a *halo effect,* that is, thinking positively or negatively about a subject.	An instructor in maternal-child nursing is responsible for both the lecture content of the course and the arrangement of clinical placements. She has evaluated each student's mastery of content based on class participation and written assignments. The instructor decides to observe the students in the clinical setting to assess mastery of clinical skills. Although student A fails to perform at an acceptable level, the instructor evaluates the student as "very good," an assessment that is actually based on the instructor's observation of excellent classroom performance.

surement. However, bias may be inadvertently introduced as a result of observer inconsistency or distractions during the data collection process.

• • •

In our presentation of measurement methods, including the self-report inventories and direct observations, we have been indirectly focusing on both qualitative and quantitative measurement. Measurement has been already defined as using a dimension or scale of items, with each item having at least two response categories and ratings that may be assigned according to whether the subject exhibits more or less of the behavior being studied. In *qualitative measurement* the items or observed behaviors are assigned to mutually exclusive categories that are representative of the kinds of behavior exhibited. On the other hand, in *quantitative measurement* the items or behaviors are assigned to categories that represent the *amount* of an exhibited characteristic (Waltz, Strickland, and Lenz, 1984). Although there is some debate over the strengths and weaknesses of each, it may be seen from the previous discussions that there are advantages and disadvantages associated with both kinds of measurement that depend on the research problem, the nature of the variables to be studied, and the design for testing the hypothesized relationships.

• Instrument Validity

When a self-report inventory or direct observation technique has been located, the investigator's task is only partially completed. Although it may appear to be appropriate for the designated use, the tool must be evaluated for the qualities of validity, reliability, and practicality. *Validity* refers to whether a measurement instrument actually measures what it is supposed to measure. There are three major kinds of validity that vary according to the kind of information provided and the purpose of the investigator. They are content validity, criterion-related validity, and construct validity.

Content validity represents the universe of content, or the domain of a given behavior. The domain provides the framework for formulating the items that should adequately represent that content. For example, the domain for the PRI (Hoskins, 1986) included the work of family theoreticians, communication theorists, investigators of interpersonal conflict in human relationships, and researchers in the areas of family conflict and patterns in conflict.

Content validity is often evaluated by submitting a tool that is being developed or considered for use to a panel of experts in the field. For example, in her study of parent-child communication and exploratory behavior, O'Brien developed the PCCS to measure patterns in interactional exchange. "The content validation of the PCCS was established by submitting the definitions of the five coding categories and specific examples of parent-child exchanges illustrative of each definition to a panel of three judges. The judges included specialists in psychiatric nursing, parent-child nursing, and community health nursing. Additionally, two of the judges were experienced family therapists. The overall agreement among the three judges was 90 percent."

In summary, content validity reflects how representative the items in a tool are of the behavioral domain. Content validity is important when its purpose is to assess the subject's performance or knowledge in that domain. A frequently cited problem with content validity is that both the subject and the behavioral domain may vary over time. With the likelihood of change in the content of a domain, as well as within persons, there is the problem of content becoming outdated and comparisons over time not being possible.

Criterion-related validity indicates to what degree the subject's performance on the measurement tool and the subject's actual behavior either in the present (concurrent) or in the future (predictive) are related. Usually an independent criterion of whatever the tool is designed to measure has been used to establish this kind of validity. For example, in the development of the MMPI, the actual psychiatric diagnoses that were based on observed behavior constituted the external criteria for establishing criterion-related validity of the tool. In norm-referenced tests, the norms established on the standardization sample are used to interpret the scores.

As noted, the criterion-related validity of a measuring tool is often established by examining the subjects' performance on the tool in relation to their performance in other settings. For example, a nurse-educator may establish the criterion-related validity of a test in medical-surgical nursing by examining the test scores in relation to performance in the clinical setting.

Criterion-related validity also indicates the effectiveness of a test that predicts an individual's behavior in specific situations. For example, if a director of a nursing service wished to predict the job performance of applicants for the position of pediatric clinical nurse specialist, a test of knowledge in this area with predictive criterion-related validity might be useful. Similarly, a tool with concurrent criterion-related validity that measures a quality, trait, or behavior actually exhibited by an individual might be used to assess selected abilities essential for implementing the highly specialized skills of a clinical nurse specialist. In some cases, such tests are useful for diagnosing deficiencies.

Approximately 50 subjects will be required for each scale or factor in the first study of the tool's validity. In the preselection of comparison groups, the range of variability in behaviors that may be related to the construct which the tool is being developed for, such as "attitude toward value of health care" in the example given earlier, often will be restricted. This fact should be considered in the interpretation of the statistical analyses.

A tool's *construct validity* is based on the extent that a test measures a theoretical construct or trait. A *construct* is an abstraction that is adapted for a scientific purpose. In research we want to observe or measure constructs to test the hypothesized relationships between them. Construct validity is established by gradually accumulating data from studies over time. The observational procedure used by O'Brien (1980) for measuring exploratory behavior was modified and tested over time for validity. Through repeated use, the relationships between the construct measured by the designated tool and other constructs are tested, and the construct's validity is either established to a greater degree or questioned further.

Construct validity may be established by a number of techniques. Developmental change is often used as a criterion, assuming that as chronological age increases, patterns in growth and development can be identified by testing and observing behavior. For example, human neurological development and its associated changes in behavioral competencies progress in a sequential manner that can be observed and documented from the prenatal stage. A second method for establishing construct validity is to demonstrate a correlation or relationship between the test being developed and an established one that measures a similar construct. A third method is factor analysis, a statistical procedure based on correlations between items. Factor analysis helps to identify clusters of correlated items that indicate a single construct or dimension. A fourth method is to use an experimental design to observe the effect of specific treatments on outcome behaviors. Physiological measures are commonly used in experimental and other designs to validate self-report inventories and direct observation techniques.

The choice of a validation method depends on the characteristics of the measurement tool and how the scores will be utilized. It is quite likely that the same inventory or observation schedule, when used for different purposes, will need to be validated in different ways.

• Instrument Reliability

Reliability refers to the proportion of accuracy to inaccuracy in measurement. In other words, if we use the same or comparable instruments on more than one occasion to measure a set of behaviors that ordinarily remain relatively constant, we would expect similar results if the tools were reliable. We would be concerned over whether the scores that were obtained for our sample of subjects were consistent, true measures of the behaviors and thus an accurate reflection of the differences between individuals. The extent of variance in test scores that is attributable to error rather than a true measure of the behaviors would be the *error variance*.

An observed score that is derived from a set of items actually consists of the true score plus error. Error may be the result of chance or it may be what is known as systematic error. *Chance errors* are errors that are difficult to control, such as a respondent's anxiety level at the time of testing. Perceptions or behaviors that occur at a specific point in time, such as anxiety in the example given, are known as state characteristics and are often beyond the awareness and control of the examiner.

Systematic errors, on the other hand, are attributable to lasting characteristics of the subject that do not tend to fluctuate from one time to another. Trait anxiety is present to some degree in most individuals on an ongoing basis and is an example of a systematic error. Both chance and systematic errors reduce the reliability and validity of a measurement tool.

Since all forms of reliability are concerned with the degree of consistency between scores that are obtained in two or more independent times of testing, they can be expressed in terms of a correlation coefficient. There are five major kinds of reliability that vary according to the nature of the tool and the data that are obtained from the standardization sample. They are known as test-retest, alternate form, split-half, statistical, and interrater reliabilities (Anastasi, 1976). Table 13-6 defines each form of reliability and indicates the limitations of each type.

• *Table 13-6*   Forms of Instrument Reliability

Type	Definition	Limitations	Example
Test-retest	Administration of the same instrument twice to the same subjects under the same conditions within a prescribed time interval and comparison of the paired scores to estimate the reliability of the instrument. The correlation between the scores should be high if the measurement tool is stable and reliable.	The experience and practice of taking a test twice may lead to different degrees of improvement among subjects. Also, if the interval between the test and retest is short, there may be a tendency for some individuals to recall their previous responses.	A newly developed reading comprehension test is given to all incoming freshmen nursing students. After 6 weeks the test is administered again to the same group of students under the same testing conditions.
Alternate form	Two or more alternate forms of a test are constructed. The forms are alike in every way except that the particular references and wording of items are different. The alternate forms of the test are administered to the same subjects at different times and then the scores of the two tests are correlated to determine the degree of relationship between them. The alternate forms of a test should be highly correlated if the measurements are to be reliable.	A major problem associated with alternate form reliability is a lack of availability of alternate forms. The development and validation of alternate forms requires a large pool of items initially. Shrinkage occurs when items are eliminated because they do not correlate well with other items. Another shortcoming of alternate form reliability is that if the behavior that the forms are designed to measure is prone to a significant practice effect, the alternate forms will reduce such an effect but will not eliminate it.	There are two alternate forms of the Partner Relationship Inventory (Hoskins, 1986) that may be used in a repeated-measures design. A second edition of the scale has six alternate forms. An item on one form, for example, "I am able to tell my partner just how I feel," is consistent with the paired item on the second form, "My partner tries to understand my feelings." A pharmacology test that requires arithmetic calculations of drug dosages is prone to a

Continued.

• *Table 13-6* **Forms of Instrument Reliability—cont'd**

Type	Definition	Limitations	Example
Alternative form—cont'd		A third consideration is that the nature of the test itself may change with repeated administrations. For example, once a problem has been solved, the solution to any problem involving the same principle is relatively easy. Similarly, once a set of items designed to elicit a specific perception has been administered over several occasions, the subjects may become weary and begin to respond in a random or nonreflective manner.	practice effect and one would expect an improvement in performance on a second test. The nursing students in a physical diagnosis class are provided with a list of observations and laboratory findings for a client with congestive heart failure. They are to determine the diagnosis. The same problem appears on the certification examination 3 months later. Asking a respondent to reply to the item, "My partner appreciates my efforts," on repeated testing occasions may become tiresome and annoying. The subject may cease to reflect on true feelings and randomly select a response.
Split-half	An index of the comparison between the scores on one half of a test with those on the other half, often performed on the basis of the odd-numbered versus the even-numbered items. It provides a measure of consistency in response to items that reflects spe-	A difficulty with the split-half method is that the correlation between halves will vary depending on how the items are divided, for example, into quarters, halves or odd-even parts, which raises some questions regarding what is the *actual* reliability.	A 30-item self-concept scale is administered to a group of subjects. The test is divided into presumably equivalent halves. The odd-numbered items represent one half and the even-numbered ones represent the other. Scores are

obtained for each half of the self-concept scale, and the two sets of scores are correlated. A high correlation, r = 0.85, between the two halves indicates a high degree of internal consistency between the items.

cific content. If the scores on the two halves are approximately equal, the test may be considered to be reliable. Split-half reliability is sometimes labeled as the coefficient of internal consistency, since only one administration of a single form of the test is required. The method is appropriate only when the test is unidimensional, that is, all of the items are designed to measure only one construct, and when the level of difficulty of the items is equally balanced between the two halves. In general, there should be a minimum of 10 items per dimension, and more are preferable. When assessing reliability by the split-half method, thus shortening the test and reducing the numbers of items, a statistical formula known as the Spearman-Brown formula is used to estimate reliability. The calculated correlation coefficient is actually the reliability for a half-test but the formula provides for doubling the length of the test.

Continued.

• *Table* 13-6   Forms of Instrument Reliability—cont'd

Type	Definition	Limitations	Example
Statistical tests	In addition to the Spearman-Brown formula, the statistical tests of reliability include the Kuder Richardson formula and Cronbach's coefficient alpha. The Kuder Richardson technique yields a correlation coefficient that is based on the internal consistency of the responses to all of the items of a single form of a test that is administered one time. Coefficients of reliability of 0.80 or higher are desirable but are not frequently found for the behavioral measures that are of particular interest to nurses.	The problems or disadvantages of the statistical tests of reliability are that the variations within respondents over time are not considered. Some tests, such as the Kuder Richardson formula, also imply that there is a single right or wrong answer. These statistical tests of reliability are not appropriate for scales that provide a response format of three or more response possibilities. In such cases the Cronbach coefficient alpha formula is applied.	A 40-item empathy scale, with a four-point response format, is administered to a group of subjects. In light of the response format, Cronbach's coefficient alpha is computed to estimate the internal consistency reliability of the scale. A correlation of r = 0.82 indicates that there is a high degree of internal consistency among the items; that is, performance on one item would be expected to correlate highly with other items on the same empathy scale.
Interrater	An index of the consistency between scorers is usually used with the direct observation method. It may also refer to the degree of agreement between judges who are evaluating the degree of congruence between newly constructed test items and the related universe of content.	A potential limitation is the effect of the observers' or scorers' own attitudes and perceptions on their evaluations.	O'Brien obtained a measure of interrater reliability when she developed the PCCS. "The reliability of coding observations with the PCCS was assessed through the use of videotaped interactions of five parent-child dyads engaged in tasks similar to those of the

An index of the consistency between scorers is the interrater reliability. It may be expressed in terms of a correlation coefficient between the observed behaviors by two or more observers or in terms of a percentage of agreement between scorers.

proposed study. Following a period of training, the investigator and two observers independently coded the videotaped interactions of the five parent-child dyads. When an identical category was recorded by each observer for the same exchange, it was scored as agreement. The percentage of agreement between the investigator and the two observers was calculated using the formula: number of agreements/(number of agreement + number of disagreement). The agreement between all ratings made by the investigator and the two observers was 84 percent and 82 percent, respectively.

In summary, the particular kind of reliability reported for an existing measurement device will depend on the tool's characteristic, the testing methodology used for the tool's initial estimation of validity and reliability, and the kind of data that were obtained from the standardization sample. Similarly, the particular technique selected for assessing the reliability of a new tool will be based on the same considerations. The different kinds of reliability vary in terms of what factors contribute to error variance. For example, a source of error variance in test-retest reliability is temporal variation; in alternate-form reliability, differences between sets of paired items; and in split-half and statistical tests of reliability, inconsistency between items. The factors that are not part of error variance are those aspects of the dimension that the tool has been designed to measure and that should be reflected in the score, as well as influential variables that can be controlled situationally or experimentally.

• Availability of Measurement Tools

For nursing research, the problems related to the search for suitable measurement devices in the past have been compounded by the fact that nursing has drawn on scientific knowledge generated by many fields of inquiry. For example, nurse-scientists have sought tools from psychology, sociology, physiology, and anthropology. It is virtually impossible for one person to be familiar with the current data-gathering devices in any one field, much less all fields.

Nevertheless, specific measures from these disciplines have proven to be extremely useful, both for measuring behaviors of interest and for learning principles of measurement. Measurement is essentially concerned with the methods used to provide quantitative and qualitative descriptions of the degree to which individuals manifest or possess specified characteristics or outcome behaviors occur. The psychological tests have been particularly valuable in this respect, for measuring both the differences between individuals and the responses of the same individual on different occasions.

A frequently cited barrier to conducting good clinical research is the lack of appropriate data-gathering instruments that meet the specifications discussed in this chapter. However, the lack is sometimes more apparent than real. For example, a suitable device may exist but the researcher was not successful in determining either its existence or the information necessary to use it. The results in this case are frustration, duplication of effort, increased costs of research, and prolongation or cessation of the research endeavor. Obviously, then, the inaccessibility of measurement tools may lead to a noteworthy waste of resources for the investigator. The consumer who reads and critiques a report of a study only evaluates the strengths and weaknesses of the tools used for a particular study and is often unaware of the difficulty involved in locating a tool that is both appropriate for the study and methodologically sound.

How can the nurse-scientist cope with these problems? Initially, it is advisable to conduct a thorough search for an instrument that is already available. Compilations of tools for the measurement of physiological and psychosocial variables that include descriptions of how the tools were developed, levels of validity and reliability, and critiques are of value (Ward and Lindeman, 1979). The appendices are also of value; they include a citation of the literature that was searched, an index of key terms for psychosocial tools, and listings of other compilations and cross references. The Mental Measurements Yearbooks (Buros, 1978) and nursing periodicals (Chinn, 1984) are also valuable sources of measurement instruments. The major nursing research journals are including an increasing number of articles that present the specific steps utilized for the development of a tool for measuring a variable relevant to nursing research and practice. The authors and reviewers are demonstrating greater knowledgeability of principles of measurement and criteria for tool construction than ever before.

Once a measurement tool is located, the principles and criteria that have been discussed in this chapter should be applied to evaluate it. In addition, the appropriateness of the tool for the intended sample may become an issue. The measurement device may need to be reevaluated in a pilot study of validity and reliability if the intended sample differs from the sample that was used for the initial validation of the tool. A basic knowledge of psychometrics is necessary to evaluate an available tool, and more advanced knowledge is required to construct an instrument. The practical aspects of a tool need to be evaluated as well. If it is relatively easy to administer in terms of explicit directions, amount of time required for completion, and training of observers or examiners, then the tool is probably acceptable. Also, the method for scoring the tool should not be excessively complex, time consuming, or expensive. Although computer scoring is efficient, it may be expensive, and the tests and scales that require highly trained personnel, such as the projective techniques, may not be practical. Finally, the interpretation of the scores should require a reasonable length of time and skill. In summary, a tool ought to be practical in terms of administration, scoring and interpretation without sacrificing the qualities of validity and reliability.

CONSTRUCTION OF NEW TOOLS

Some cases, such as testing part of a nursing theory or evaluating the effectiveness of a clinical intervention, require the development of a new instrument. Although the construction and validation of a measurement device will probably be the exception rather than the rule, there are identifiable qualifications needed for the task. Initially, a comprehensive understanding of the subject matter must be acquired. It is not possible to develop a good measurement device without adequate knowledge of the clinical or research areas of interest, whether they are sleep-wake patterns in the mother-infant dyad, outcome behaviors in stroke rehabilitation, coping strategies in cancer patients, psychological responses to a new antidepressant, or perceptions of health maintenance services in the elderly. A comprehensive knowledge of content provides the basis for a good construct definition of the behavior of interest. Next, some degree of knowledge and skill in the techniques of test and scale construction must be acquired. Many reference materials on measurement and psychometric theory are available to the nurse-scientist who intends to develop or evaluate a tool, some of which have been developed by other disciplines and some by nursing. Principles for formulating items for tests, scales, questionnaires, or rating criteria for direct observations of behavior may be found in these references (Anastasi, 1976; Nunnally, 1978; Waltz, Strickland, and Lenz, 1984). Finally, one needs to develop an ability to combine the first two qualities; that is, the application of subject matter and test construction skill to the formulation of items or rating criteria that yield an accurate measurement of the dimension of interest. In actuality, all three aspects of the measurement process are likely to become a concern of the nurse-scientist to some degree, whether it be in the context of research, practice, or education and whether a tool is to be evaluated or constructed.

For the nurse-scientist who plans to construct a tool, the procedural steps will include the following:

1. Define the construct or behavior to be measured.
2. Formulate the items.
3. Submit the final listing of the items to individuals with appropriate expertise for assessment of content validity.
4. Develop instructions for users and respondents.
5. Administer the items to a large standardization sample that is representative of the subjects for whom the test or scale is designed.
6. Analyze the data from the sample for estimation of validity and reliability.

Again, the principles that have been presented in this chapter are applicable. To define the behavior to be measured will require an exhaustive review of the literature and an examination of both published and unpublished tests and scales that have been designed to measure the same or a related construct. Attention should be focused on how the construct was defined, the item content and form, the response format, and the procedures that were used to establish validity and reliability. The theory, research findings, and other data that are identified are then synthesized, leading to the actual development of the definition of a construct or behavior that requires a measurement tool.

After the construct is defined, the investigator asks to what degree does a subject or client possess that trait or behavior, implying, of course, the use of a measurement tool composed of items. The basic principles for item formulation are followed, with attention to such factors as consistency between item content and construct definition and representation of the content area as identified from the literature. A minimum of 10 items with two response categories should be developed for each behavioral dimension to be measured. When the items are administered to a sample of representative subjects, consistency in testing conditions and uniformity in scoring procedures are basic to standardization and objectivity, thus reducing the chances of measurement error.

The analyses of the data that are collected from the standardization sample usually include determination of the variance in item responses, estimation of validity and reliability, and generation of either norm-referenced or criterion-referenced data. Criterion-referenced tools measure a subject's status in terms of well-defined performance standards. On the other hand, norm-referenced tools evaluate an individual's performance against those of others, and the individual is placed in a position relative to other subjects in a specified group. Establishing validity by criterion referencing is indicated in some cases, whereas in others norm referencing is more appropriate. For example, a nurse-educator may want to use a norm-referenced text to measure learning in an introductory course of research methods and a criterion-referenced test to evaluate the performance of clinical skills.

Clearly, the task of tool development for measuring constructs and outcome behaviors that are of interest to the nursing profession calls for a long-term effort by clinical nurse-researchers, investigators skilled in psychometrics, and practitioners. The identification of research problems ideally begins with the practitioner, the planning and conduct of research are the tasks of nurses qualified to assume these responsibilities, and the measurement of key variables in the theoretical framework is facilitated by the nurse-scientist with expertise in psychometrics. The link should be collaboration, and the outcome improved client care.

CONCLUSION

Accurate, dependable measurement is a fact of life in modern technical societies. It is indispensable in many professions such as medicine, engineering, nursing, and education. However, while recognizing the pervasiveness and usefulness of measurement in education and nursing, it must be kept in mind that measurement is a tool, a means to an end, and not an end in itself. In nursing our objective is to measure constructs so that we can test theories and enhance the existing body of nursing knowledge, or we use measurement tools to assess current practice and thereby develop nursing interventions that will positively influence health care and outcome behaviors in the client.

• Critiquing the Measurement Tool

Criteria for critiquing measurement tools are outlined in the box on p. 198.

The methods of measurement and discussion of instrumentation are usually found in the methodology section of the research report. The research consumer critically evaluates the congruence between the specific behavior of interest and the conceptual and operational definition of the variable. Other areas to be evaluated are the method of observation, the item and response format, and the scoring technique. The degree of reliability and validity that has been established is also of central importance. In cases where a new measurement tool has been developed, has the researcher utilized the appropriate procedures for accomplishing this task?

The reviewer of a research report will want to determine whether the measurement tool assesses the behavior of interest as defined by the researcher. For example, if the researcher intends to measure anxiety, a specific conceptual definition of the type of anxiety to be measured is required. The way that construct is to be measured must also be specified, that is, operationally defined. Let us say that a researcher wanted to study state anxiety and conceptually defined it as such. The researcher may contemplate using a tool such as the State-Trait Anxiety Scale (STAI) (Spielberger, Gorsuch, and Lushene, 1968) and would examine the literature pertaining to the

---

Critiquing Criteria

1. Are the instruments appropriate for the data collection method being used?
2. Have the measures been derived from an identified conceptual framework?
3. Have the variables that are to be measured been conceptually and operationally defined?
4. Is the selected method of observation or measurement procedure objective?
5. Has the appropriate level of measurement been selected for the variables of the study?
6. Is there a systematic response format and scoring procedure for the measure?
7. How has the researcher attempted to minimize any observer bias in the case of direct observation?
8. Was the issue of measurement error addressed?
9. Is there a sufficient number of questions to adequately measure the specific behavior of interest?
10. Was an appropriate method used to test the reliability of the measurement tool? Is the reliability of the instrument adequate?
11. Was an appropriate method used to determine the validity of the measurment tool? Is the validity of the instrument adequate?
12. Have the strengths and weaknesses of the measurement tool been identified?

STAI to see if the definition of state anxiety was consistent with the researcher's definition of the construct. If it was consistent and other psychometric properties of the tool were satisfactory, both the researcher and the evaluator would feel confident about using the tool in the study. If state anxiety was the only variable of interest, only the state anxiety subscale of the STAI would be used by the researcher. When direct observation is the selected method of measurement, the conceptual definition of the behavior, the specific behavioral indicators to be observed, and the procedure for observing the behavior must also be congruent. Lack of congruence in this area limits the evaluation of the findings because doubt would be cast on whether or not the researcher actually measured what he or she intended to measure.

The reviewer will also examine the directions for both the researcher and the respondents, the response format of items, the observation procedure, and the scoring system for clarity, uniformity, and consistency. It is important to evaluate the items of a measuring instrument when possible. Except for a few sample questions, the items of the instrument are seldom included in a research report, and as a result, the reviewer is rarely in a position to evaluate the majority of the items. The researcher primarily engages in the item review process in advance of selecting the measure for use. Criteria for item evaluation include the following:

- Are the questions and response possibilities uniform?
- Are the items unambiguous, clear-cut, and concise?

- Are there items that are ambiguous when a negative stem is combined with a negative response?
- Is each question limited to one idea?
- Do the items provide irrelevant clues that may influence a response?
- Is the number of questions sufficient for adequate assessment of the behavior of interest?
- Is there a limited number of variations in the type of item?
- Is the difficulty of the items appropriate to the level of subjects being assessed such as their intelligence level?

The response format for the items should be based on a level of measurement appropriate for the researcher's purposes. For example, attitude scales are representative of the interval level of measurement and thus provide a finer distinction among individuals than the nominal level of measurement.

The scoring system should be clearly delineated in the report so that the evaluator understands exactly how each instrument is scored. This is particularly important when a measure contains subscales. The reviewer needs to know whether the scores for the subscales are combined into one composite score or whether the scores of each subscale are considered individually. For example, a scale designed by Haber (1984) to measure differentiation of self uses a four-point response format. The user is instructed to score the responses as follows: strongly agree *4,* agree *3,* disagree *2,* and strongly disagree *1.* Responses to items that indicate evidence of differentiation, such as "I am capable of helping myself when I am in a crisis," are scored in this manner. However, responses to items that indicate a lack of differentiation, such as, "I will change my opinions to avoid arguments with other people," are reverse scored. The scale is composed of two subscales, Emotional Maturity and Emotional Dependency. The responses to the items in each subscale are summed separately to arrive at two total scores. Thus the higher the score on each subscale, the greater the emotional maturity or lack of emotional dependency, and so it may be inferred, the higher the level of differentiation of self.

In a study utilizing an observational form of measurement the following criteria can be applied as a standard for evaluating similar issues:

1. Has the researcher formulated conceptual definitions that are clear and operational and that spell out exactly what must be done to measure the behavior?
2. Have the molar units of behavior been defined?
3. Have the molecular units of behavior been defined?
4. Has a consistent, systematic procedure for observing the units of behavior been described?
5. Has a procedure for categorizing and scoring the observed behaviors been identified?
6. Has the interrater reliability been established?
7. How has the researcher controlled for subject reactivity?
8. Has the researcher considered methods for controlling bias and the halo effect when observing and scoring?

Reliability and validity are two crucial aspects in the critical appraisal of a measure. The reviewer evaluates an instrument's level of reliability and validity and the manner in which they were established. In a research report, the reliability and validity of the data for each measure should be presented. If these data have not been presented at all, the reviewer must seriously question the merit and use of the tool.

Appropriate reliability tests should have been performed by the developer of the measurement tool and should then be included by the current user in the research report. If the initial standardization sample and the current sample have different characteristics, the reader would expect that a pilot study for the present sample would have been conducted to determine if the reliability was maintained. For example, if the standardization sample for a tool that measures "satisfaction in intimate heterosexual relationships" was made up of undergraduate college students and an investigator plans to use the tool with married couples, it would be advisable to reexamine the reliability for the latter group.

The investigator determines which type of procedure is used in the study, depending on the nature of the measurement tool and how it will be used. For example, if the instrument is to be administered twice, the researcher might determine test-retest reliability. If alternate forms have been developed for use in a repeated measures design, evidence of alternate form reliability should be presented. If the degree of internal consistency among the items is relevant, an appropriate test of internal consistency should be presented. In some instances, more than one type of reliability will be presented, but the evaluator will want to determine whether they are both appropriate. For example, the Kuder Richardson formula implies that there is a single right or wrong answer, making it inappropriate to use with scales that provide a response format of three or more response possibilities. In such cases, another formula is applied, such as the Cronbach coefficient alpha formula. Another important consideration is the acceptable level of reliability, which varies according to the type of test. Coefficients of reliability of 0.80 or higher are desirable but are not frequently found for the behavioral measurement tools that are of particular interest to nurses. The validity of an instrument is limited by its reliability; that is, less confidence can be placed in scores from tests with low reliability coefficients.

Satisfactory evidence of validity is probably the most difficult item for the reviewer to ascertain. It is the aspect of measurement that is most likely to fall short of meeting the required criteria. Validity studies are time consuming as well as complex, and sometimes researchers will settle for presenting minimal validity data. As a result, the critiquer will want to closely examine the item content of a tool when evaluating its strengths and weaknesses and endeavor to find conclusive evidence of content validity. Ideally, a panel of experts has evaluated the tool in terms of the items' congruence with the content area and their psychometric properties. Such procedures provide the reviewer with assurance that the tool is psychometrically sound and the content of the items is consistent with the conceptual framework and construct definitions. Construct and criterion-related validity compose some of the more precise statistical tests of whether the tool measures what it is supposed to measure. Ideally, an instrument should provide evidence of content validity as well as criterion-related or construct validity before a reviewer invests a high level of confidence in the tool.

As the reader can see, the area of measurement is complex. The measurement aspects of research reports can be evaluated in varying degrees of depth. The research consumer should not feel inhibited by the complexity of this topic, but may use the guidelines presented in this chapter to systematically assess the measurement aspects of a research study. Collegial dialogue is also an approach to evaluating the merits and shortcomings of an existing as well as a newly developed instrument that is reported in the nursing literature. Such an exchange promotes the understanding of methodologies and techniques of measurement, stimulates the acquisition of a basic knowledge of psychometrics, and encourages the exploration of alternative methods of observation.

• Summary

Measurement is a crucial aspect of conducting and critiquing research. Principles of measurement include the following: defining the variable(s) to be measured both conceptually and operationally, determining the level of measurement for the specified variables, and ensuring objectivity of the measurement tool.

There are many different types of measurement tools, but despite their differences, they all have characteristics in common. The common characteristics provide a guide for determining the strengths and weaknesses of a measurement tool. One type of measurement tool is the self-report inventories, such as questionnaires, scales, and tests. Another type of measurement is the direct observation of behavior. Each type of measurement has specific characteristics as well as advantages and disadvantages.

Validity refers to whether an instrument measures what it is purported to measure. It is a crucial aspect of evaluating a tool in terms of whether it really measures what it is supposed to measure. Three types of validity are content validity, criterion-related validity, and construct validity. The choice of a validation method is important and is made by the researcher on the basis of the characteristics of the measurement device in question and its utilization.

Reliability refers to the proportion of accuracy to inaccuracy in a measurement device. The five major types of reliability are the following: test-retest, alternate form, split-half, statistical, and interrater reliability. Again, the selection of a method for establishing reliability will depend on the characteristics of the tool, the testing method that is used for collecting data from the standardization sample, and the kind of data that are obtained.

One of the problems in nursing research is locating an appropriate tool that is psychometrically satisfactory. The researcher cannot be familiar with tools from all of the disciplines, but literature reviews, measurement indexes, and yearbooks provide good sources for locating tests and scales from nursing and the behavioral sciences. Nurse researchers are increasingly developing their own measurement instruments to test part of a nursing theory or evaluate the effectiveness of a clinical intervention. Thus the procedural steps of tool development are becoming an essential aspect of nursing education. They may be applied when constructing or critiquing measurement devices. In this chapter, these steps have been presented along with the principles of measurement.

• References

Anastasi, A. (1976). *Psychological testing*, New York, Macmillan, Inc.

Buros, O.K. (1978). *Mental measurements yearbooks*, New Jersey, Gryphon Editions Ltd.

Chin, P.L. (Ed.) (1984). Research Tools, *Advances in Nursing Science*, 7:(1) entire issue.

Dropkin, M.J. (1978). Influence of social approval upon postoperative compliance in patients undergoing radical head and neck surgery: a pilot exploration. (Unpublished Master's thesis.)

Haber, J.E. (1984). An investigation of the relationship between differentiation of self, complementary psychological need patterns, and marital conflict, *Dissertation Abstracts International*, 45:7. (University Microfilms p.2102-B).

Hoskins, C.N. (1983). Psychometrics in nursing research—Further development of The Interpersonal Conflict Scale. *Research in Nursing and Health*, 6:75-83.

Hoskins, C.N. (1986). *Partner Relationship Inventory*, Palo Alto, California, Consulting Psychologists Press, Inc.

Nunnally, J.C. (1978). *Psychometric theory*, New York, McGraw-Hill, Inc.

Oberst, M.J. (1983). Postdischarge crisis in cancer patients, NCI grant CA 26767-03 (in progress).

O'Brien, R.A. (1980). Relationship of parent-child communication to child's exploratory behavior and self-differentiation, *Nursing Research*, 29: 150-156.

Spielberger, C.D., Gorsuch, R.L., Lushene, R. (1968). Self-evaluation questionnaire, Palo Alto, California, Consulting Psychologists Press, Inc.

Waltz, C., Strickland, O., Lenz, E. (1984). *Measurement in nursing research*, Philadelphia, F.A. Davis Co.

Ward, M.J., Lindeman, C.A. (eds.) (1979). *Instruments for measuring nursing practice and other health care variables I and II*. Washington, D.C.: U.S. Government Printing Office.

Wolfer, J.A., Visintainer, M.A. (1975). Pediatric surgical patients' and parents' stress responses and adjustment as a function of psychologic preparation and stress-point care, *Nursing Research*, 24:244-255.

14

Sampling

Judith Haber

LEARNING OBJECTIVES

After reading the chapter, the student should be able to do the following:
• Identify the purpose of sampling.
• Define population, sample, and sampling.
• Compare and contrast a population and a sample.
• Discuss the eligibility criteria for sample selection.
• Define nonprobability and probability sampling.
• Identify the types of nonprobability and probability sampling strategies.
• Compare the advantages and disadvantages of specific nonprobability and probability sampling strategies.
• Discuss the factors that influence determination of sample size.
• Discuss the procedure for drawing a sample.
• Formulate a sampling plan for a research study.
• Identify the criteria for critiquing a sampling plan.
• Use the critiquing criteria to evaluate the sampling section of a research report.

KEY TERMS

accidental sampling   random sampling
cluster sampling   representative sample
delimitations   sample
element   sampling
nonprobability sampling   sampling interval
population   sampling unit
probability sampling   simple random sampling
purposive sampling   stratified random sampling
quota sampling   systematic sample

Sampling is the process of selecting representative units of a population for study in a research investigation. Although sampling is a complex process, it is a familiar one. In our daily lives we gather knowledge, make decisions, and formulate predictions based on sampling procedures. For example, nursing students may make generalizations about the overall quality of nursing professors as a result of their exposure to a sample of nursing professors during their undergraduate programs. Clients may make generalizations about a hospital's food during a 1-week hospital stay. It is apparent that limited exposure to a limited portion of these phenomena forms the basis of our conclusions and so a great deal of our knowledge and decisions is based on our experience with samples.

Scientists also derive knowledge from samples. Many problems in scientific research cannot be solved without employing sampling tools. For example, when testing the effectiveness of a medication for cardiac clients, the drug is administered to a sample of the population for whom the drug is potentially appropriate. The scientist must come to some conclusions without administering the drug to every known cardiac client or every laboratory animal in the world. But because human lives are at stake, the scientist cannot afford to casually arrive at conclusions based on the first dozen cardiac clients who are available for study. The consequences of arriving at erroneous conclusions or making inaccurate generalizations from a small, nonrepresentative sample are much more severe in scientific investigations than in everyday life. Consequently, research methodologists have expended considerable effort to develop sampling theories and procedures that produce accurate and meaningful information. Essentially, researchers sample representative segments of the population because it is rarely feasible or necessary to sample the entire population of interest to obtain relevant information.

This chapter will familiarize the research consumer with the basic concepts of sampling as they pertain to the principles of research design, nonprobability and probability sampling, sample size, and the related critiquing process.

• Sampling Concepts

POPULATION

A *population* is a well-defined set that has certain specified properties. A population can be composed of people, animals, objects, or events. For example, if a researcher is studying undergraduate nursing students, the type of educational preparation of the population must be specified. In this instance the population consists of undergraduate students enrolled in a generic baccalaureate nursing program. Examples of other possible populations might be all male clients admitted for a first myocardial infarction in hospital ABC during the year 1984; all children with asthma in the state of New York; or all men and women with a diagnosis of depression in the United States. These examples illustrate that a population may be broadly defined and potentially involve millions of people, or narrowly specified to include only several hundred people.

The reader of a research report should consider whether or not the researcher has identified the population descriptors that form the basis for the *eligibility criteria* that are used to select the sample from the array of all possible units, be they people, objects, or events. Let us consider the population previously defined as undergraduate nursing students enrolled in a generic baccalaureate program. Would this population include part-time as well as full-time students? Would it include students who had previously attended another nursing program? How about foreign students? Would freshmen through seniors qualify? Insofar as it is possible, the researcher must demonstrate that the exact criteria used to decide whether an individual would or would not be classified as a member of a given population were specifically delineated. The population descriptors that provide the basis for eligibility criteria should be evident in the sample. That is, the characteristics of the population and the sample should be congruent. The degree of congruence is evaluated to assess the representativeness of the sample. For example, if a population was defined as full-time, American-born, senior nursing students enrolled in a generic baccalaureate nursing program, the sample would be expected to reflect these characteristics.

Eligibility criteria may also be viewed as *delimitations,* or those characteristics that restrict the population to a homogeneous group of subjects. Examples of delimitations include the following: sex, age, marital status, socioeconomic status, religion, ethnicity, level of education, age of children, and diagnosis. In a study investigating maternal-fetal attachment the researcher established several of the following delimitations:

- Marital status—married
- Previous pregnancy—none
- Status of current pregnancy—non-high risk pregnancy
- Age—over 18 years of age

These delimitations were selected because their potential effect on the attachment process would limit the validity of the findings as well as the ability to generalize about the findings. Let us consider the criterion of no previous pregnancy. If women who had previously been pregnant, either successfully or unsuccessfully, were grouped with women in their first pregnancy, the researcher would end up with three groups of pregnant women who had potentially experienced the attachment process in different ways because of their different pregnancy histories. The heterogeneity of this sample group would inhibit the researcher's ability to meaningfully interpret the findings and make generalizations. It is much wiser to either study only one homogeneous group or include all three groups as distinct subsets of the sample and study the attachment process comparatively. The reader should remember that delimitations are not established in a casual or meaningless way, but they are established to control for extraneous variability or bias. Each delimitation should have a rationale, presumably related to a potential contaminating effect on the dependent variable. The careful establishment of sample delimitations will increase the precision of the study and contribute to the accuracy and generalizability of the findings.

The population criteria establish the _target population,_ that is, the entire set of cases about which the researcher would like to make generalizations. A target population might include all undergraduate nursing students enrolled in generic baccalaureate programs in the United States. It is often not feasible, because of time, money, and personnel, to pursue utilizing a target population. An _accessible population,_ one that meets the population criteria and that is _available,_ is used instead. For example, an accessible population might include all full-time generic baccalaureate students attending school in Connecticut. Pragmatic factors must also be considered when identifying a potential population of interest.

The reader should know that a population is not restricted to human subjects. It may consist of hospital records; blood, urine, or other specimens taken from clients at a clinic; historical documents; or laboratory animals. It is apparent that a population can be defined in a variety of ways. The important thing to remember is that the basic unit of the population must be clearly defined, since the generalizability of the findings will be a function of the population criteria.

SAMPLES AND SAMPLING

Sampling is a process of selecting a portion of the designated population to represent the entire population. A _sample_ is a set of elements that make up the population, and an _element_ is the most basic unit about which information is collected. The most common element in nursing research is individuals, but other elements can form the basis of a sample or population. A _sampling unit_ is the element or set of elements used for selecting the sample. Sometimes the sampling unit and the element represent the same thing, and other times it is more efficient to use a unit larger than the element for sampling purposes. For example, a researcher was planning a study that compared the effectiveness of different nursing interventions on the healing rate of decubitus ulcers. Four hospitals, each using a different treatment protocol, were identified as the sampling units rather than the nurses themselves or the treatment alone.

The purpose of sampling is to increase the efficiency of a research study. The novice reviewer of research reports must realize that it would not be feasible to examine each and every element or unit in the population. When sampling is properly done, it allows the researcher to draw inferences and make generalizations about the population without examining each and every unit in the population. Sampling procedures that entail the formulation of specific criteria for selection ensure that the characteristics of the phenomena of interest will be, or are likely to be, present in all of the units being studied. The researcher's endeavors to ensure that the sample is representative of the target population put the researcher in a stronger position to draw conclusions from the sample findings that are generalizable to the population.

Evaluators of research studies will find that samples and sampling procedures vary in terms of merit. The foremost criterion in evaluating a sample is its representativeness. A *representative sample* is one whose key characteristics closely approximate those of the population. If 70% of the population in a study of childrearing practices consisted of women, and 40% were full-time employees, then a representative sample should reflect these characteristics in the same proportions.

It must be understood that there is no way to guarantee that a sample is representative without obtaining a data base about the entire population. Since it is difficult and inefficient to assess a population, the researcher must employ sampling strategies that minimize or control for sample bias. If an appropriate sampling strategy is utilized, it is almost always possible to obtain a reasonably accurate understanding of the phenomena under investigation by obtaining data from a sample.

• Types of Samples

Sampling strategies are generally grouped into two categories: nonprobability sampling and probability sampling. In *nonprobability* sampling, elements are chosen by nonrandom methods. The drawback of this strategy is that there is no way of estimating the probability that each element has of being included in the samples. Essentially, there is no way of ensuring that every element has a chance for inclusion in the nonprobability sample. *Probability sampling* utilizes some form of random selection when choosing the sample units. This type of sample enables the researcher to estimate the probability that each element of the population will be included in the sample. Probability sampling is the more rigorous type of sampling strategy because it is more likely to result in a representative sample. The remainder of this section will be devoted to a discussion of different types of nonprobability and probability sampling strategies.

NONPROBABILITY SAMPLING

The nonprobability sampling strategy is less rigorous than probability sampling strategy and it tends to produce less accurate and representative samples. However, the majority of samples, not only in nursing research but in other disciplines as well, are nonprobability samples. Although such samples are more feasible for the researcher to obtain, the use of nonprobability samples does limit the ability of the researcher to make generalizations about the findings. The three major types of nonprobability sampling are the following: accidental, quota, and purposive samples.

Accidental Sampling

Accidental sampling is the use of the most readily accessible persons or objects as subjects in a study. The subjects may include volunteers, the first 25 clients admitted to hospital X with a particular diagnosis, all people who enrolled in program Y during the month of September, or all students enrolled in course Z at a particular university during 1983. The subjects are convenient and accessible to the researcher and are sometimes called a *sample of convenience*. For example, a researcher studying marital communication patterns utilized an accidental sample of the first 200 couples meeting the sample criteria and who volunteered to participate in the study. Another researcher studying the effect of group client education on cardiac rehabilitation utilized all clients transferred from coronary care unit to the intermediate coronary care unit in hospital X between September and December 1984.

The advantage of an accidental sample is that it is easier for the researcher to obtain subjects. All the researcher may have to be concerned with is obtaining a sufficient number of subjects who meet the same criteria.

The major disadvantage of an accidental sample is that the risk of bias is greater than in any other type of sample. The problem of bias is related to the fact that accidental samples tend to be self-selecting. That is, the researcher ends up obtaining information only from the people who volunteer to participate. In this case, the following questions must be raised, "What motivated some of the people to participate and others to not participate? What kind of data would I have obtained if nonparticipants had also responded? How representative are the people who did participate in relation to the population?" For example, a researcher may stop people on a street corner to ask their opinion on some issue; place advertisements in the newspaper; or place signs in local churches, community centers, or supermarkets indicating that volunteers are needed for a particular study. A researcher may even offer to pay the participants for their time. The problem is that those who choose to participate may not be typical of the population with regard to the variables being measured. There is no way to assess the biases that may be operating. In cases where the phenomena under investigation are relatively homogeneous within the population, the risk of bias may be minimal. However, in heterogeneous populations the risk of bias is great.

The evaluator of a research report should recognize that the accidental sample is the weakest form of sampling strategies. Its use should be avoided whenever possible. When an accidental sample is utilized, caution should be exercised in analyzing and interpreting the data. When critiquing a research study that has employed this sampling strategy, the reviewer will be justifiably skeptical about the external validity of the findings.

② Quota Sampling

Quota sampling refers to a form of nonprobability sampling in which knowledge about the population of interest is utilized to build some representativeness into the sample. A quota sample identifies the strata of the population and proportionally represents the strata in the sample. For example, 40% of the 5,000 nurses in city X are diploma graduates, 40% are associate degree graduates, and 20% are baccalaureate graduates. Each stratum of the population should be proportionately represented in the sample. In this case the researcher used a proportional quota sampling strategy and decided to sample 10% of a population of 5,000, or 500 nurses. Based on the proportion of each stratum in the population, 200 diploma graduates, 200 associate degree graduates, and 100 baccalaureate graduates were the quotas established for the three strata. The researcher recruited subjects who met the eligibility criteria of the study until the quota for each stratum was filled. In other words, once the researcher obtained the necessary 200 diploma, 200 associate degree, and 100 baccalaureate graduates, the sample was complete.

The researcher systematically assures that proportional segments of the population are included in the sample. The quota sample is not randomly selected, that is, once the proportional strata have been identified, the researcher obtains subjects until the quota for each stratum has been filled, but it does increase the representativeness of the sample. This sampling strategy addresses the problem of overrepresentation or underrepresentation of certain segments of a population in a sample.

The characteristics chosen to form the strata are selected according to a researcher's judgment. The criterion for selection should be a variable that would reflect important differences in the dependent variables under investigation. Age, sex, religion, ethnicity, medical diagnosis, socioeconomic status, level of completed education, and occupational rank are among those variables that are likely to be important stratifying variables in nursing research investigations.

The critiquer of a research study seeks to determine whether or not the sample strata appropriately reflect the population under consideration and whether the stratifying variables are homogeneous enough to ensure a meaningful comparison of differences between strata. Even when the preceding factors have been addressed by the researcher, the evaluator must remember that as a nonprobability sample, the quota strategy contains an unknown source of bias that affects external validity.

③ Purposive Sampling

Purposive sampling is a strategy in which the researcher's knowledge about the population and its element is utilized to handpick the cases to be included in the sample. The researcher usually selects subjects who are considered to be *typical* of the population. A purposive sample is also used when a highly unusual group is being studied, such as a population with a rare genetic disease such as Tay-Sachs disease. In this case the researcher would describe the sample characteristics very precisely to ensure that the reader will have an accurate picture of the subjects in the sample.

The researcher who utilizes a purposive sample assumes that errors of judgment in overrepresenting or underpresenting elements of the population in the sample will tend to balance out. However, there is no objective method for determining the validity of this assumption. The evaluator must be aware of the fact that the more heterogeneous the population, the greater the chance of bias being introduced in the selection of a purposive sample. Conscious bias in the selection of subjects remains a constant danger. As such, the findings from a study utilizing a purposive sample should be regarded with caution. As with any nonprobability sample, the ability to generalize is very limited.

The following are several instances when a purposive sample may be appropriate:

1. The effective pretesting of newly developed instruments with a purposive sample of divergent types of people
2. The validation of a scale or test with a known groups technique.
3. The collection of exploratory data in relation to an unusual or highly specific population, particularly when the total target population remains an unknown to the researcher.

Even when the use of a purposive sample is appropriate, the researcher as well as the critiquer should be cognizant of the limitations of this sampling strategy.

PROBABILITY SAMPLING

The primary characteristic of probability sampling is the random selection of elements from the population. *Random selection* occurs when each element of the population has an equal and independent chance of being included in the sample. Four commonly used probability sampling strategies are simple random, stratified random, cluster, and systematic sampling.

Simple Random Sampling

Simple random sampling is a laborious and carefully controlled process. Since the more complex probability designs incorporate the principles of simple random sampling in their procedures, the principles of this strategy will be presented.

The researcher defines the population (a set), lists all of the units of the population (a sampling frame), and selects a sample of units (a subset) from which the sample will be chosen. For example, if American hospitals specializing in respiratory problems are the sampling unit, then a list of all such hospitals would be the sampling frame. If certified clinical specialists constituted the accessible population, then a list of those nurses would be the sampling frame.

Once a list of the population elements has been developed, the best method of selecting a sample is to employ a table of random numbers containing columns of digits such as the one appearing in Fig. 14-1. After assigning consecutive numbers to units of the population, the researcher starts at any point on the table of random numbers and reads consecutive numbers in any direction (horizontally, vertically, or diagonally). When a number is read that corresponds with the written unit on a card, that unit is chosen for the sample. The investigator continues to read until a sample of the desired size is drawn.

```
20 09 54 18 10  49 53 20 29 11  61 32 52 06 56  20 10 38 29 96  05 01 37 99 11 32
37 42 44 92 89  62 39 80 96 99  86 23 14 11 66  63 24 70 34 00  71 99 92 49 13 74
20 80 24 12 87  56 56 05 70 10  46 61 70 51 58  22 96 40 59 60  86 65 36 87 31 10
15 68 56 48 84  93 02 49 15 78  73 46 26 22 37  84 02 31 64 22  73 94 31 90 71 46
93 15 26 67 10  63 99 16 81 49  73 44 24 67 32  47 66 86 08 14  33 44 78 97 18 30
03 71 18 44 50  31 48 18 23 96  48 21 06 89 23  63 00 09 97 85  58 35 66 61 28 25
84 31 97 89 14  96 13 61 83 59  79 12 87 04 18  40 20 11 50 28  61 48 87 44 06 53
26 06 24 52 95  01 65 30 06 10  84 92 93 22 20  56 57 72 57 99  25 70 69 19 98 43
07 09 38 25 04  65 17 20 75 07  69 63 69 10 37  31 44 66 12 39  85 54 52 02 82 33
95 03 87 65 81  03 86 59 16 03  62 88 19 19 63  32 93 05 72 94  52 78 13 63 91 30
61 94 07 43 67  25 66 92 74 77  97 32 69 76 58  25 79 15 44 55  02 38 73 19 96 62
56 81 76 05 32  62 69 99 94 05  05 85 17 10 73  59 62 22 60 68  44 93 55 92 48 59
86 72 78 41 95  08 67 30 65 95  44 50 40 29 08  65 67 45 27 81  33 16 96 58 09 52
54 75 26 06 31  52 40 70 99 12  26 35 99 71 63  18 52 50 09 02  24 57 12 03 02 01
38 94 08 93 95  38 06 71 72 80  30 74 21 08 10  91 85 70 90 68  03 75 10 86 10 78
07 80 46 11 90  58 89 94 97 21  12 25 05 73 71  32 03 11 66 37  44 29 42 75 75 76
88 50 51 24 19  33 41 09 86 10  94 70 74 99 39  58 64 53 70 07  09 62 50 56 67 81
15 97 57 96 75  56 68 65 97 29  19 47 17 22 81  21 35 81 94 46  23 41 39 54 26 78
54 79 88 81 42  21 91 38 47 51  36 25 79 78 24  43 12 59 38 22  80 04 56 74 65 66
75 85 66 33 52  21 89 44 90 49  26 74 40 83 67  37 14 74 66 61  70 22 58 66 18 53
00 13 21 22 16  00 98 72 65 81  58 01 73 67 19  36 06 65 54 55  11 24 37 30 06 11
71 94 55 21 12  81 23 78 46 98  03 40 97 49 61  62 54 35 65 65  36 37 05 82 24 82
57 58 60 36 59  97 02 01 71 64  38 67 03 17 93  92 15 20 68 65  85 27 44 28 04 80
79 79 71 49 24  15 99 69 00 36  20 23 01 29 94  54 29 66 69 26  29 88 91 43 94 34
47 98 26 41 63  08 11 99 04 76  38 61 88 05 66  44 54 92 10 89  39 17 60 78 97 71
05 64 93 40 12  20 75 35 34 63  96 36 93 43 65  14 19 36 54 78  91 51 63 94 01 77
00 84 17 34 41  10 40 47 60 98  94 26 10 54 59  05 66 26 27 72  65 43 49 18 93 76
18 65 50 05 76  03 82 95 54 20  92 77 57 54 38  45 01 73 64 62  05 58 11 51 20 20
60 60 76 75 12  92 87 41 97 28  53 75 19 93 06  08 57 15 31 56  44 15 33 46 55 14
17 67 54 91 82  94 59 46 43 98  77 30 34 89 98  64 61 28 27 25  69 28 71 14 07 16
74 13 15 78 81  02 98 91 18 06  86 15 37 27 96  71 62 44 42 89  89 70 38 37 66 92
32 93 57 33 80  92 07 48 75 39  95 93 81 04 03  75 56 18 67 25  28 08 71 75 01 04
74 01 40 47 25  97 77 31 10 73  78 68 45 55 45  17 59 52 81 94  33 38 46 27 26 30
69 36 01 63 85  62 50 52 53 95  15 76 59 20 79  06 21 23 65 60  34 29 68 18 77 16
01 53 85 65 34  40 65 14 27 22  21 79 68 95 22  20 35 49 26 49  43 20 28 73 79 49
42 55 14 47 79  69 04 42 73 12  76 41 70 23 59  65 03 69 46 59  55 41 12 02 00 14
07 31 98 53 15  89 75 07 05 25  04 14 80 89 30  64 42 85 16 05  57 20 17 22 72 75
61 04 37 16 72  47 78 91 33 70  31 21 95 10 08  23 21 63 35 03  47 19 94 90 28 06
44 96 38 19 06  14 05 56 06 06  92 86
```

Fig. 14-1   A table of random digits. (From Wilson, E. Bright, Jr.: An introduction to scientific research, New York, copyright 1952 by McGraw-Hill, Inc. Used with permission of McGraw-Hill, Inc.)

The advantages of simple random sampling are the following:
1. The sample selection is not subject to the conscious biases of the researcher.
2. The representativeness of the sample in relation to the population characteristics is maximized.
3. The differences in the characteristics of the sample and the population are purely a function of chance.
4. The probability of choosing a nonrepresentative sample decreases as the size of the sample increases.

However, the consumer must remember that despite the utilization of a carefully controlled sampling procedure that minimizes error, there is no guarantee that the sample will be representative. Factors such as sample heterogeneity and subject drop out may jeopardize the representativeness of the sample despite the most stringent random sampling procedure.

The major disadvantage of simple random sampling is that it is a time-consuming and inefficient method for obtaining a random sample. Consider the task of listing all of the baccalaureate nursing students in the United States. In addition, it may be impossible to obtain an accurate or complete listing of every element in the population. Imagine trying to obtain a list of all completed suicides in New York City for the year 1984. It is often the case that although suicide may have been the cause of death, another cause such as cardiac failure appears on the death certificate. It would be difficult to estimate how many elements of the target population would be eliminated from consideration. The issue of bias would definitely enter the picture despite the researcher's best efforts. Thus the evaluator of a research report must exercise caution in generalizing from reported findings, even when random sampling is the stated strategy, if the target population has been difficult or impossible to list completely.

Stratified Random Sampling

Stratified random sampling requires that the population be divided into strata or subgroups. The subgroups or subsets that the population is divided into are homogeneous. An appropriate number of elements from each subset are randomly selected, based on their proportion in the population. This strategy's goal is to achieve a greater degree of representativeness. Stratified random sampling is similar to the proportional stratified quota sampling strategy discussed earlier in the chapter. The major difference is that stratified random sampling utilizes a random selection procedure for obtaining sample subjects. Fig. 14-2 provides an example that illustrates the use of stratified random sampling.

The population is stratified according to any number of attributes such as age, sex, ethnicity, religion, socioeconomic status, or level of completed education. The variable selected to make up the strata should be adaptable to homogeneous subsets with regard to the attributes being studied.

The following criteria can be used for decision making in the selection of a stratified sample:

1. Is there a critical variable or attribute that provides a logical basis for stratifying the sample?
2. Does the population list contain sufficient information about the attributes that will be used to divide the sample into subsets?
3. Is it appropriate for each subset to be equal in size, or is it more appropriate for each subset to be proportionally stratified based on the proportion of each subset in the population?
4. If proportional sampling is being utilized, is there a sufficient number of subjects in each subset for basing meaningful comparisons?
5. Once the subset composition has been determined, are random procedures used for selection of the sample?

There are several advantages to a stratified sampling strategy: (1) The representativeness of the sample is enhanced, (2) The researcher has a valid basis for making comparisons between subsets if information on the critical variables has been available. (3) The researcher is able to oversample a disproportionately small stratum to adjust for their underrepresentation, statistically weigh the data accordingly, and continue to be able to make legitimate comparisons.

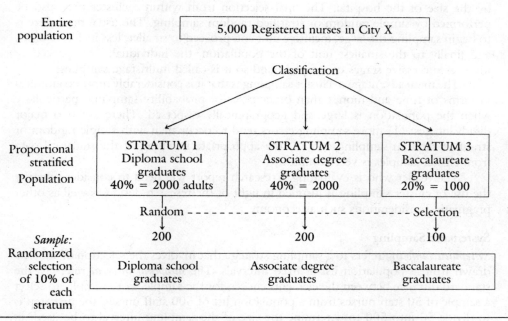

Fig. 14-2   Subject selection using a proportional stratified random sampling strategy.

The obstacles encountered by a researcher utilizing this strategy include the following: (1) The difficulty of obtaining a population list containing complete critical variable information, (2) The time-consuming effort of obtaining multiple enumerated lists, and (3) The time and money involved in carrying out a large-scale study utilizing a stratified sampling strategy. The critiquer needs to question the appropriateness of this sampling strategy to the problem under investigation. For example, if the reader refers to Fig. 14-2, it is clear that the study population consisted of diploma, associate degree, and baccalaureate degree nurses, three distinct strata. It is appropriate for the researcher to strive to proportionately represent all three strata in the study sample. This strategy would not be necessary if the researcher was studying only one of the three subsets, unless that subset was being logically divided into strata based on other attributes.

Cluster Sampling

Cluster sampling involves a successive random sampling of units that progress from large to small. The first unit consists of large units or "clusters." For example, if a sample of head nurses was desired, a random sample of hospitals might make up the cluster. A large-scale national survey would use states as the first unit and proceed to successively smaller units like counties, cities, districts, blocks, and then households.

The clusters are selected either by simple random or stratified random methods. For example, when selecting clusters of hospitals, it might be appropriate to stratify by the size of the hospital. The final selection from within a cluster may also be performed by simple random or stratified random sampling. The usual procedure is to begin sampling the large, inclusive unit and proceed to smaller, less inclusive units, and finally to the smallest unit of the population, the individual. This procedure involves successive stages of sampling and so it is called multistage sampling.

The main advantage of cluster sampling is that it is considerably more economical in terms of time and money than other types of probability sampling, particularly when the population is large and geographically dispersed. There are two major disadvantages: (1) more sampling errors tend to occur than with simple random or stratified random sampling and (2) the appropriate handling of the statistical data from cluster samples is very complex.

The reader who is evaluating a research report will need to consider whether the use of cluster sampling is justified in light of the research design as well as other pragmatic considerations such as economy.

Systematic Sampling

Systematic sampling refers to a sampling strategy that involves the selection of subjects drawn from a population list at fixed intervals. The *sampling interval* refers to the standard distance between the elements chosen for the sample. For example, to select a sample of 50 staff nurses from a population list of 500 staff nurses, the first step is to divide 50 into 500 to determine the size of the sampling interval to be used, in this case 10. Essentially every tenth element on the list would be sampled. The first element is selected randomly, using a table of random numbers. In this instance the number 51 is randomly selected from a table. The staff nurses corresponding to numbers 51, 61, 71, and so forth would be included in the sample of 50.

Systematic and simple random samplings are essentially the same type of procedure. The advantage of systematic sampling is that the results are obtained in a more convenient and efficient manner. The disadvantage of systematic sampling is that bias in the form of nonrandomness can inadvertently be introduced to the procedure. This problem may occur if the population list is arranged so that a certain type of element is listed at intervals that coincide with the sampling interval. Let us say that if every tenth nursing student on a population list of all types of nursing students in New York State were a baccalaureate student, and the sampling interval were ten, then baccalaureate students would be overrepresented in the sample. Cyclical fluctuations are also a factor. For example, if a list is kept of nursing students using the college library each day, a biased sample will probably be obtained if every seventh day is chosen as the sampling interval, for fewer and perhaps different nursing students probably study in the library on Sundays than on weekdays. Therefore caution must be exercised about departures from randomness as they affect the representativeness of the sample and as a result affect the external validity of the study.

• • •

The critiquer will want to note whether or not a satisfactory random selection procedure was carried out. If randomization was not used, the systematic sampling may have become a nonprobability quota sample. It is important to be cognizant of this issue because the implications related to interpretation and generalizability are drastically altered if the evaluator is dealing with a nonprobability sample.

• Sample Size

There is no single rule that can be applied to the determination of a sample's size. When arriving at an estimate of sample size, many factors such as the following must be considered:

1. The type of sampling procedure being utilized
2. The type of sample estimation formula being used
3. The degree of precision required
4. The heterogeneity of the attributes under investigation
5. The relative frequency of occurrence of the phenomenon of interest in the population, that is, a common versus a rare health problem
6. The projected cost of utilizing a particular sampling strategy

The sample size should be determined before the study is conducted. When probability sampling is utilized, it is possible to estimate the sample size in advance with the use of statistical procedures. This is a complex procedure beyond the scope of this text. The reader who is interested in this topic is referred to a statistical text such as that of Cohen (1977). The size of nonprobability samples can be estimated in two ways. (1) A general rule of thumb is to always use the largest sample possible. The larger the sample, the more representative of the population it is likely to be;

smaller samples produce less accurate results. (2) It is generally recommended that a sample size of 30 be selected for each subset of the data, or cell of the design. This means that if a researcher is investigating the relationship between tactile and auditory stimulation and heart rate response in premature infants, the two data subsets (independent variables) would be auditory and tactile stimulation. As such, a satisfactory sample size of 60 (2 × 30 subjects) would be required. If the researcher has an experimental and a control group and also wants to consider general differences, a minimum number of subjects in a study would be 120 (2 × 2 × 30 subjects). To precisely estimate sample size, the researcher should consult a text such as that of Cohen (1977).

The principle of "larger is better" generally holds true for both probability and nonprobability samples. Results based on small samples (under 10) tend to be unstable; that is, the values fluctuate from one sample to the next. Small samples tend to increase the probability of obtaining a markedly deviant sample. As the sample size increases, the mean more closely approximates the population values. Large samples permit the principle of randomization to work effectively, that is, to counterbalance, in the long run, atypical values.

However, the consumer should be aware that large samples do not ensure representativeness or accuracy. A large sample cannot compensate for a faulty research design. The proportion of the population that is sampled does not provide a guarantee of accurate results. It is often possible to obtain accurate results from only a small fraction of a large population. For example, a 10% probability sample of a population containing 1,500 elements will yield more precise results than a nonprobability 0.01% sample of a population with 100,000 elements.

The critiquer should evaluate the sample size in terms of whether or not it adequately represents the elements and subsets of the population. Unless representativeness is ensured, all the data in the world becomes inconsequential.

• Sampling Procedures

Criteria for drawing a sample will vary according to the sampling strategy. Regardless of which strategy is used, it is important that the procedure by systematically organized. This will eliminate the bias that occurs when sample selection is carried out inconsistently. Several general steps can be identified that will ensure a consistent approach by the researcher. Initially, the target population must be identified, that is, the entire group of people or objects about whom the researcher wants to draw conclusions or make generalizations. The target population may consist of all male clients with a first-time myocardial infarction, all children with acute leukemia, all pregnant teenagers, or all doctoral students in the United States. Next, the accessible portion of the target population must be delineated. An accessible population might consist of all clinical specialists in the state of California, or all male clients with a first-time myocardial infarction admitted to hospital X during 1983, or all pregnant teenagers in a specific prenatal clinic, or all children with acute leukemia under care at a specific hospital specializing in oncology. Then once the accessible population has been established, permission is obtained from the institution's research committee.

This permission provides free access to the desired population. Finally, a sampling plan or a protocol for actually selecting the sample from the accessible population is formulated. The researcher makes decisions about how subjects will be approached, how the study will be explained, and who will select the sample—the researcher or a research assistant. Regardless of who implements the sampling plan, consistency in how it is done is of paramount importance. The reader of a research study will want to find a description of the sample as well as the sampling procedure in the report. Based on the appropriateness of what has been reported, the critiquer is able to make judgments about the soundness of the sampling protocol that, of course, will affect the interpretations made about the findings.

When an appropriate sample size and sampling strategy have been used, the researcher can feel more confident that the sample is representative of the accessible population, but it is more difficult to feel confident that the accessible population is representative of the target population. Are clinical specialists in California representative of all clinical specialists in the United States? It is impossible to be sure about this. Researchers must exercise judgment when assessing their typicality. Unfortunately, there are no guidelines for making such judgments, and there is even less basis for the critiquer to make such decisions. The best rule of thumb to use when evaluating the representativeness of a sample and its generalizability to the target population is to be realistic and conservative about making sweeping claims relative to the findings.

• Critiquing the Sample

The criteria for critiquing the sampling technique of a study are presented in the box below. The research consumer approaches the sample section of a research report with a different perspective than does the researcher. The consumer must raise two questions. The first question asks, "If this study were to be replicated, would there be enough information presented about the nature of the population, the sample, the sampling strategy, and sample size for another investigator to carry out the study?" The second question asks, "Are the previously mentioned factors appropriate in light

---

Critiquing Criteria

1. Do the parameters of the study population specify to what population the findings may be generalized?
2. Is the sample representative of the population as defined?
3. Would it be possible to replicate the study population?
4. Is the method of sample selection appropriate? How was the sample selected?
5. What bias, if any, is introduced by this method?
6. Is the sample size appropriate? How is it substantiated?
7. Are there indications that the human rights of the subjects have been ensured?

of the particular research design, and if not, which factors require modification, especially if the study is to be replicated?"

Sampling is considered to be one important aspect of the methodology of a research study. As such, data pertaining to the sample usually appear in the methodology section of the research report. The sampling content presented should reflect the outcome of a series of decisions based on sampling criteria appropriate to the design of the study as well as the options and limitations inherent in the context of the investigation. The following discussion will highlight several sampling criteria that the research consumer will want to consider when evaluating the merit of a sampling strategy as it relates to a specific research study.

Initially the parameters or attributes of the study population should clearly specify to what population the findings may be generalized. Generally the target population of the study is not specifically identified by the researcher, but the nature of it is implied in the description of the accessible population and the sample. For example, if a researcher states that 100 subjects were randomly drawn from a population of married primiparas who vaginally delivered full-term infants at hospital L during 1985, the critiquer is able to specifically evaluate the parameters of the population. Demographic characteristics of the sample such as age, sex, diagnosis, ethnicity, religion, and marital status should also be presented as they provide further explication about the nature of the sample and enable the critiquer to evaluate the sampling procedure more accurately. For example, in a study by Krouse and Krouse (1982) titled "Cancer as a Crisis: The Critical Elements of Adjustment," the age range of the subjects were 30 to 60 years of age. Additionally, the subjects were potential mastectomy or hysterectomy candidates. The subjects were divided into three sample groups according to the diagnosis and the type of treatment. However, age was not a factor in terms of grouping subjects. The evaluator who has this demographic sample information available is able to question the validity of utilizing a sampling strategy that does not also consider the differential effect of age on an individual's adjustment to cancer. It would seem logical that there might be a difference in terms of adjustment between a 30-year-old woman and a 66-year-old woman each having a mastectomy.

It is also helpful if the researcher has presented a rationale for having elected to study one type of population versus another. For example, why did the previously cited study focus only on married primiparas who vaginally delivered full-term infants, as opposed to unmarried women or women who had had cesarean births? In a research study that utilizes a nonprobability sampling strategy, it is particularly important to fully describe the population and the sample in terms of who the study subjects are, how they were chosen, and why they were chosen. If these criteria are adhered to, the degree of heterogeneity or homogeneity of the sample can be determined. The utilization of a homogeneous sample minimizes the amount of sampling error introduced, a problem particularly common in nonprobability sampling.

Next, the defined representativeness of the population should be examined. Probability sampling is clearly the ideal sampling procedure for ensuring the representativeness of a study population. Utilization of random selection procedures such as simple random, stratified, cluster, or systematic sampling strategies minimize the occurrence of conscious and unconscious biases that, of course, would affect the researcher's ability to generalize about the findings from the sample to the population. The evaluator should be able to identify the type of probability strategy utilized and to determine whether the researcher adhered to the criteria for a particular sampling plan. In experimental and quasi-experimental studies, the evaluator must also know whether or how the subjects were assigned to groups. If the criteria have not been followed, the reader would have a valid basis for being cautious about the proposed conclusions of the study.

Although random selection is the ideal in establishing the representativeness of a study population, more often realistic barriers, such as institutional policy, inaccessibility of subjects, lack of time or money, and the current state of knowledge in the field, necessitate the utilization of nonprobability sampling strategies. Many important research problems that are of interest to nursing do not lend themselves to experimental design and probability sampling. A well-designed, carefully controlled study utilizing a nonprobability sampling strategy can yield accurate and meaningful findings that make a significant contribution to nursing's scientific body of knowledge. The critiquer needs to ask a philosophical question, "If it is not possible to conduct an experimental or quasi-experimental investigation that utilizes probability sampling, should the study be abandoned?" The answer usually suggests that it is better to carry out the investigation and be fully aware of the limitations of the methodology, than to lose the knowledge that can be gained. The researcher is always able to move on to subsequent studies that either replicate the study or utilize more stringent design and sampling strategies to refine the knowledge derived from a nonexperimental study.

The critiquer of a research study will want to apply the following criteria as a standard for evaluating the sampling plan.

1. Have the population and sample characteristics been completely described?
2. Are criteria for eligibility in the sample specifically identified?
3. Have sample delimitations been established?
4. How was the sample selected?
5. What kinds of bias are inherent in this type of selection procedure?
6. What factors influenced the researcher's choice of a sampling plan?
7. How homogeneous or heterogeneous is the sample?
8. How conservative is the researcher about the inferences and conclusions drawn from the data?
9. Does the researcher identify the limitations in generalizability of the findings from the sample to the population?
10. Does the researcher indicate how replication of the study with new samples would provide increased support for the findings?

The greatest difficulty in nonprobability sampling stems from the fact that not every element in the population has an equal chance of being represented in the sample. Therefore it is likely that some segment of the population will be systematically underrepresented. If the population is homogeneous on critical characteristics, systematic bias will not be very important. However, few of the attributes that researchers are interested in are sufficiently homogeneous to render sampling bias an irrelevant consideration.

Next, the sampling plan's suitability to the research design should be evaluated.

Experimental and quasi-experimental designs utilize some form of random selection or random assignment of subjects to groups (see Chapter 9). The critiquer evaluates whether or not the researcher adhered to the principles of random selection and assignment. Lack of adherence to such principles compromises the representativeness of the sample and the external validity of the study. The following are questions the evaluator might pose relative to this issue:

1. Has a random selection procedure been identified, such as a table of random members?
2. Has the appropriate random sampling plan been selected, that is, has a proportional stratified sampling plan been selected instead of a simple random sampling plan in a study where there are three distinct occupational levels that appear to be critical variables for stratification?
3. Has the particular random sampling plan been carried out appropriately, that is, if a cluster sampling strategy was utilized, did the sampling units logically progress from the largest to the smallest?

Random sampling should not be looked on as a cure-all. Sometimes bias is inadvertently introduced even when the principle of random selection is utilized.

Nonexperimental designs often utilize nonprobability sampling strategies. The question that can be raised by the critiquer, in this instance, is whether or not a nonexperimental design and a related nonprobability sampling plan were most appropriate for this study. It is sometimes true that if the researcher had utilized another type of design or sampling plan, she could have constructed a stronger study that would have allowed greater confidence to be placed in the findings and greater generalizability. However, the critiquer is rarely in a position to know what factors entered into the decision to plan one type of study versus another.

Then, the evaluator should determine if the sample size is appropriate and whether its size is justifiable. It is unusual for the researcher to indicate in a research article how the sample size was arrived at; this is more commonly seen in doctoral dissertations. However, the method of arriving at the sample size and the rationale should be briefly mentioned. For example, a researcher may state in a very detailed way:

> The sample size was set on the basis of a significance level of 0.05, a medium effect of 0.13, and a power of 0.95 in multiple regression analysis (Cohen, 1977). This sample size, $N = 168$, is larger than required for nine predictors with a conventional power of 0.80 ($N = 110$). The sample size was expanded to allow for the shrinkage of R^2.

The importance of this example lies not in understanding every technical word cited, but rather in understanding that this type of statement or some abbreviated form of it meets the criteria stated at the beginning of the paragraph and should be evident in the research report.

Other considerations with respect to sample size, especially where the sample size appears to be small or inadequate and there is no stated rationale for the size, are the following:

- How will the sample size affect the accuracy of the results?
- Are any subsets or cells of the sample overrepresented or underrepresented?
- Are any of the subsets so small as to limit meaningful comparisons?
- Has the researcher examined the effect of attrition or dropouts on the results?
- Has the researcher recognized and identified any limitations posed by the size of the sample?

Essentially, these criteria demand that the critiquer carefully scrutinize several important elements pertaining to sample size that have implications for the generalizability of the findings.

Finally, evidence that the rights of human subjects have been protected should appear in the sample section of the research report. The critiquer will evaluate whether permission was obtained from an Institutional Review Board that reviewed the study relative to the maintenance of ethical research standards (see Chapter 3). For example, the review board examines the research proposal to determine if the introduction of an experimental procedure may be potentially harmful and therefore undesirable. The critiquer also examines the report for evidence of informed consent on the part of subjects as well as protection of confidentiality or anonymity. It is highly unusual for research studies not to demonstrate evidence of having met these criteria. Nevertheless, the careful evaluator will want to be certain that ethical standards that protect sample subjects have been maintained.

It is evident that there are many factors to consider when critiquing the sample section of a research report. The type and appropriateness of the sampling strategy become crucial elements in the analysis and interpretation of data, in the conclusions derived from the findings, and in the generalizability of the findings from the sample to the population. As stated earlier in this chapter, the major purpose of sampling is to increase the efficiency of a research study by utilizing a sample that is representative of the particular population so that every element need not be studied, and yet generalizing the findings from the sample to the population. The critiquer needs to justify that the sampling strategy utilized provided a valid basis for feeling confident of the findings and their generalizability.

• Summary

Sampling is a process that select representative units of a population for study. Researchers sample representative segments of the population because it is rarely feasible or necessary to sample entire populations of interest to obtain accurate and meaningful information.

A *population* is a well-defined set that has certain specified properties. A population may consist of people, objects, or events. Researchers establish *eligibility criteria,* that are descriptors of the population and that provide the basis for selection into a sample. Eligibility criteria, also referred to as delimitations, include the following: age, sex, socioeconomic status, level of education, religion, and ethnicity. The researcher must identify the *target population,* that is, the entire set of cases about which the researcher would like to make generalizations. However, because of pragmatic constraints, the researcher usually utilizes an *accessible population,* one that meets the population criteria and is available.

Sampling is a process that selects a portion of the designated population to represent the entire population. A *sample* is a set of elements that comprise the population. A *sampling unit* is the element or set of elements used for selecting the sample. The foremost criterion in evaluating a sample is the *representativeness* or congruence of characteristics with the population.

Sampling strategies consist of nonprobability and probability sampling. In *nonprobability sampling* the elements are chosen by nonrandom methods. Types of non-probability sampling include accidental, quota, and purposive sampling. *Probability sampling* is characterized by the random selection of elements from the population. In *random selection* each element in the population has an equal and independent chance of being included in the sample. Types of probability sampling include simple random, stratified random, cluster, and systematic sampling.

Sample size is a function of the type of sampling procedure being used, the degree of precision required, the type of sample estimation formula being used, the heterogeneity of study attributes, the relative frequency of occurrence of the phenomena under consideration, and cost.

Criteria for drawing a sample vary according to the sampling strategy. Systematic organization of the sampling procedure minimizes bias. The target population is identified, the accessible portion of the target population is delineated, permission to conduct the research study is obtained, and a sampling plan is formulated.

The critiquer of a research report evaluates the sampling plan for its appropriateness in relation to the particular research design. Completeness of the sampling plan is examined in light of potential replicability of the study. The critiquer evaluates whether the sampling strategy is the strongest plan for the particular study under consideration.

An appropriate systematic sampling plan will maximize the efficiency of a research study. It will increase the accuracy and meaningfulness of the findings and enhance the generalizability of the findings from the sample to the population.

• References

Bright, W.E., Jr. (1952). *An introduction to scientific research,* New York, McGraw-Hill Book Co.

Brown, R.C., Jr. (1976). Research Q and A on sampling, *Nursing Research,* **25**:62.

Cohen, J. (1977). *Statistical power analysis for the behavioral sciences* (rev. ed.), New York, Academic Press.

Downs, F.S. and Newman, M.A. (1977). *A source book of nursing research,* Philadelphia, F.A. Davis Co.

Kerlinger, F.N. (1973). *Foundations of behavioral research,* New York, Holt, Rinehart & Winston, Inc.

Krouse, H.J. and Krouse, J.H. (1982). Cancer as a crisis: the critical elements of adjustment, *Nursing research,* **31**:96-100.

Levey, P.S. and Lemeshow, S. (1980). *Sampling for health professionals,* New York, Lifetime Learning.

Owens, J.F., McCann, C.S. and Hutelmyer, C.M. (1978). Cardiac rehabilitation: a patient education program, *Nursing Research,* **27**:148-150.

Polit, D.F. and Hungler, B.P. (1983). *Nursing research: Principles and methods* 2nd ed., Philadelphia, J.B. Lippincott Co.

Sudman, S. (1976). *Applied sampling,* New York, Academic Press.

Van Dalen, D.B. (1979). *Understanding educational research* (4th ed.), New York, McGraw-Hill Book Co.

15

Descriptive Data Analysis

Ann Bello

LEARNING OBJECTIVES

After reading this chapter, the student should be able to do the following:
- Define descriptive statistics.
- State the purposes of descriptive statistics.
- Identify the levels of measurement in a research study.
- Describe a frequency distribution.
- List the measures of central tendency and their use.
- List the measures of variability and their use.
- Critically analyze the descriptive statistics utilized in published research studies.

KEY TERMS

descriptive statistics	modality
frequency distribution	mode
interval measurement scales	nominal measurement scales
kurtosis	normal curve
levels of measurement	ordinal measurement scales
mean	percentile
measurement	range
measures of central tendency	ratio measurement scales
measures of variability	semiquartile range
median	standard deviation
modal percentage	

Data, no matter how carefully collected, are meaningless without organization and interpretation. Researchers would find it difficult or impossible to present the results of their studies without some method to describe the sample studied and estimate how reliably they can make predictions for the whole population.

Statistical procedures are used to give meaning to data. Procedures that allow researchers to describe and summarize data are known as *descriptive statistics*. Procedures that allow researchers to estimate how reliably they can make predictions based on data are known as *inferential statistics* (see Chapter 16). Descriptive statistical techniques reduce data to manageable proportions by summarizing them, and they also describe various characteristics of the data under study. Descriptive techniques include measures of central tendency, such as mode, median, and mean measures of variability, such as modal percentage, ranges, and standard deviation; and some correlation techniques, such as scatter plots. The research consumer does not need a detailed knowledge of how to calculate these statistics, but does need an understanding of their meaning, use, and limitations.

Measures of central tendency describe the average member of the sample, whereas measures of variability describe how much dispersion there is in the sample. If a researcher reported that the average age of students in one nursing class was 22, with the youngest member being 18 and the oldest 25, and that another nursing class' students also had an average age of 22, but the youngest member was 17 and the oldest 45, the reader would form a very different picture of the two classes. In both cases, the average member of the sample was the same but in the second class there was much greater variation or dispersion in the age of the members of the class.

This chapter and the next are designed to provide the reader of nursing research with an understanding of statistical procedures. This chapter will focus on the understanding and evaluation of descriptive statistical procedures and the next chapter will discuss inferential statistical procedures. To evaluate the appropriateness of the statistical procedures used in a study, the research consumer should have an understanding of the levels of measurement that are appropriate to each statistical technique.

• Levels of Measurement

Measurement is the assignment of numbers to objects of events according to consistently applied rules (Kerlinger, 1973). Every event that is assigned a specific number must be similar to every other event assigned that number. The level of measurement is determined by the nature of the object or event being measured. Levels of measurement in ascending order are nominal, ordinal, interval, and ratio (see Chapter 13). In chapter 13 the levels of measurement were introduced as they apply to instrumentation. The levels of measurement are important when analyzing data and are therefore being reintroduced.

The higher the level of measurement, the greater the flexibility the researcher has in choosing statistical procedures. Every attempt should be made to utilize the highest level of measurement possible so that the maximum amount of information will be obtained from the data. (see Table 15-1).

NOMINAL MEASUREMENT SCALES

Nominal measurement scales are used to classify objects or events into categories. The categories are mutually exclusive; the object or event either has the characteristic or does not have it. The numbers assigned to each category are nothing more than a label; such numbers do not indicate more or less of a characteristic. Nominal scales can be used to categorize a sample on such information as sex, hair color, marital status, or religious affiliation. In Wolfer and Visintainer's study of pediatric surgical patients (1975) (see Appendix A), there are several examples of nominal scale measurement, including the child's sex, the birth order, whether the parents roomed-in or not, and the type of surgery the child had.

• *Table 15-1*   Summary Table

Measurement	Description	Measures of central tendency	Measures of variability
Nominal	Classification	Mode	Modal percentage range
Ordinal	Relative rankings	Mode, median	Range, percentile, semiquartile range
Interval	Rank ordering with equal intervals	Mode, median, mean	Range, percentile, semiquartile range, standard deviation
Ratio	Rank ordering with equal intervals and absolute zero	Mode, median, mean	All

ORDINAL MEASUREMENT SCALES

Ordinal measurement scales are used to show relative rankings of objects or events. The numbers assigned to each category can be compared, and a member of a higher category can be said to have more of an attribute than a member of a lower category. The intervals between the numbers on the scale are not necessarily equal nor is the zero an absolute zero. For example, ordinal measurement is used to formulate class rankings where one student can be ranked higher or lower than another. However, the difference in actual grade point average between students may differ widely. Wolfer and Visintainer (1975) used ordinal scales to measure the children's emotional state. The manifest upset scale reflected the emotional state of the child at a given point in time. A low number reflected less upset than a higher number, but it is not possible to speak of a child with a score of 4 as being twice as upset as a child with a score of 2, nor as having two more upsets.

Ordinal scales are limited in the amount of mathematical manipulation possible. In addition to what is possible with nominal data, medians, percentiles, and rank order coefficients of correlation can be calculated.

INTERVAL MEASUREMENT SCALES

Interval measurement scales show rankings of events or objects on a scale with equal intervals between the numbers. The zero point remains arbitrary. For example, interval measurements are used when measuring temperature on the centigrade and fahrenheit scales. The distance between each degree is equal, but the zero point is arbitrary.

In many areas of the behavioral sciences, including nursing, there is much controversy over the classification of the level of measurement of intelligence, aptitude, and personality tests, with some regarding these measurements as ordinal and others as interval. The research consumer needs to be aware of this controversy and look at each study individually (Kerlinger, 1973). Interval scales allow more manipulation of data, including the addition and subtraction of numbers and the calculation of means. This additional degree of manipulation provides the basis for arguing the favor of classifying aptitude, intelligence, and personality tests at the interval rather than the ordinal level of measurement.

RATIO MEASUREMENT SCALES

Ratio measurement scales show rankings of events or objects on a scale with equal intervals and absolute zeros. The number represents the actual amount of the characteristic that the object possesses. This is the ideal level of measurement, but it is usually only achieved in the physical sciences and is used to measure such characteristics as height, weight, pulse, and blood pressure.

All mathematical procedures can be performed on data from ratio scales. Therefore the use of any statistical procedure is possible, as long as it is appropriate to the design of the study (see Chapters 8 and 16).

• Frequency Distribution

One of the most basic ways of organizing data is in a frequency distribution. In a *frequency distribution* the number of times each event occurs is counted, or the data are grouped and the frequency of each group is reported. An instructor reporting the results of an exam could report the number of students receiving each grade or could group the grades and report the number in each group. Table 15-2 shows the results of an exam given to a class of 51 students. The results of the exam are reported in

• *Table 15-2*   Frequency Distribution

		Frequency	
Score	Tally	Individual	Group score
90	|	1	>89 = 1
88	|	1	
86	|	1	
84	|||| |	6	80-89 = 15
82	||	2	
80	||||	5	
78	||||	5	
76	|	1	
74	|||| ||	7	70-79 = 23
72	|||| ||||	9	
70	|	1	
68	|||	3	
66	||	2	
64	||||	4	60-69 = 10
62	|	1	
60		0	
58	|	1	
56		0	
54	|	1	<59 = 2
52		0	
50		0	
TOTAL		51	51

Mean 73.1   S.D. ±12.1
Median 74   Mode 72
Range 36 (54 to 90)

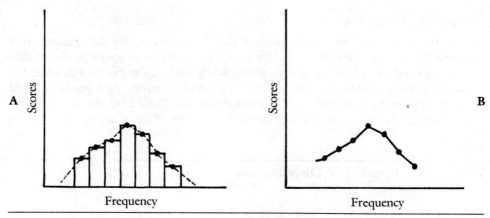

Fig. 15-1   A, Histogram and **B,** frequency polygon.

several ways. The column labeled *tally* gives the raw data for each grade, while the *frequency* column gives the results both for individual scores and for grouped scores.

When data are grouped, it is necessary to define the size of the group or the interval width so that no score will fall into two groups. The grouping of the data in Table 15-2 prevents overlap, since each score falls into only one group. If the grouping had been 70 to 80 and 80 to 90, scores of 80 would have fallen into two categories. The grouping should allow for a precise presentation of the data without any serious loss of information. Very large interval widths lead to a loss of data information and may obscure patterns in the data. If the test scores in Table 15-2 had been grouped as 40 to 69 and 70 to 99, the pattern of the scores would have been obscured.

Information about frequency distributions may be presented in the form of a table such as Table 15-2 or in graphic form. Fig. 15-1 illustrates the most common graphic forms: the histogram and the frequency polygon. The two graphic methods are similar in that they both plot scores or percents of occurrence against frequency. The greater the number of points plotted, the smoother the resulting graph will be. The shape of the resulting graph allows the observations that will further describe the data.

• Shape of Distribution

The shape of a distribution may be described in terms of symmetry, modality, and kurtosis. Each of these descriptors is independent of the others and contributes its own information about the distribution of data.

SYMMETRY

When the two halves of a distribution are folded over and they can be superimposed on each other the distribution is said to be *symmetrical*. In other words, the two halves

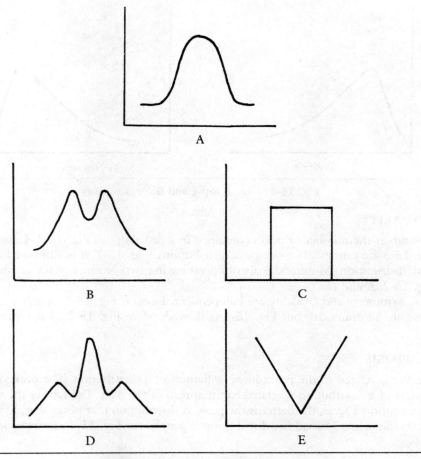

Fig. 15-2   Symmetrical shapes.

of the distribution are mirror images of each other. The overall shape of the distribution does not affect symmetry. Although the shapes in Fig. 15-2 are different, they are all symmetrical.

A distribution is *nonsymmetrical* when the peak is off-center. If one tail is longer than the other, the distribution is described in terms of *skew*. In a positive skew, the bulk of the data is at the low end of the range and there is a longer tail to the right. Worldwide individual income has a positive skew with most individuals in the low to moderate range and very few in the upper range. In a negative skew, the bulk of the data is in the high range and there is a longer tail to the left. Age at death in the United States has a negative skew, since most deaths occur at older ages. Fig. 15-3 illustrates positive and negative skews. In each diagram, the peak if off-center and one tail is longer.

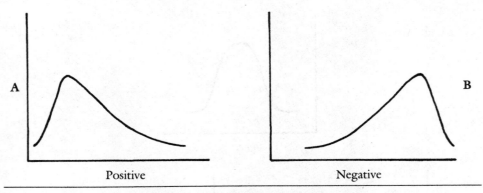

Fig. 15-3   **A,** Positive and **B,** negative skew.

MODALITY

Modality is the number of peaks contained in a distribution. Fig. 15-2 *A* and *E* and Fig. 15-3 are unimodal or one-peak distributions. Fig. 15-2, *B* is a bimodal or two-peak distribution. Multimodal distributions having two or more peaks are shown in Fig. 15-2, *B* and *D*.

Symmetry and modality are independent. Look at Fig. 15-2, *A* and Fig. 15-3; these are all unimodal, but Fig. 15-3 is skewed, while Fig. 15-2, *A* is symmetrical.

KURTOSIS

Kurtosis is related to the peakedness or flatness of a distribution. The peakedness or flatness of a distribution is related to the spread of the data. The farther the data are spead out on a scale, the flatter is the peak. A distribution that peaks sharply is called *leptokurtic,* while a broad flat distribution is *platykurtic.* Fig. 15-4 illustrates kurtosis.

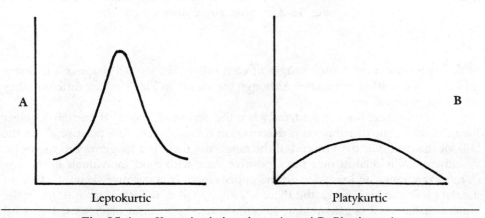

Fig. 15-4   Kurtosis: **A,** leptokurtosis, and **B,** Platykurtosis.

• **Measures of Central Tendency**

Measures of central tendency answer questions such as, "What does the average nurse think?" and, "What is the average temperature of clients on a unit?" They yield a single number that describes the middle of the group. They summarize the members of a sample. Therefore, they are known as summary statistics and are sample specific. Since they are sample specific, they will change with each sample.

The characteristics of a sample in a study are described in terms of summary statistics. The mean test score reported in Table 15-1 is an example of such a statistic. If a different group of students was given the same test, it is likely that the mean would be different.

The term *average* is really a nonspecific, general term. In statistics, there are three kinds of averages: the mode, the median, and the mean. Depending on the distribution, these may not all give the same answer to the question, "What is the average . . . ?" Each type of average has a specific use and is most appropriate to a specific kind of measurement and type of distributions.

MODE

The *mode* is the most frequent score or result and it can be obtained by inspection of the frequency distribution table or graph. A distribution can have more than one mode. The mode is most appropriately used with nominal data. It cannot be used for any subsequent calculations, and it is unstable. By unstable, we mean that the mode can fluctuate widely from sample to sample from the same population. A change in just one score in Table 15-1 would change the mode from 72. Fig. 15-2, *B* illustrates a distribution that would have two modes.

MEDIAN

The *median* is the middle score or the score where 50% of the scores are above it and 50% of the scores are below it. The median is not sensitive to extremes in high and low scores, for example, in the series of scores in Table 15-1, the 26th score will always be the median, regardless of how high or low the scores may range. The median is best used when the data are skewed and the researcher is interested in the typical score. This statistic is easy to find, either by inspection or calculation.

MEAN

The *mean* is the arithemetic average of all the scores. It is what is usually thought of when the term *average* is used in general conversation and is the most widely used measure of central tendency. Most tests of significance use the mean (see Chapter 16). The mean is affected by every score, but is more stable than the median or mode, and of the three measures of central tendency, it is the most constant, or least affected by chance. The larger the sample size, the less affected the mean will be by a single extreme score. The mean is generally considered the single best point for summarizing data.

• • •

When comparing the measures of central tendency, the mean is the most stable and the median the most typical of these statistics. If the distribution is symmetrical and unimodal, the mean, median, and mode will coincide. If the distribution is skewed, the mean will be pulled in the direction of the long tail of the distribution. With a skewed distribution, all three statistic should be reported. The mean and the median always exist in a sample and are unique; however, there may not be a single mode. The mode is the easiest to calculate, but the mean is the most useful for additional calculations.

• Measures of Variability

Variability or dispersion is concerned with the data spread. Samples with the same mean could differ in both distribution (kurtosis) and skew. Variability measures answer the following questions: is the sample homogenous or heterogenous? similar or different? If a researcher measured oral temperatures in two samples, one sample drawn from a healthy population and one sample from a hospitalized population, it is possible that the two samples will have the same mean. However, it is likely that there will be a wider range of temperatures in the hospitalized sample than in the healthy sample. Measures of variability are used to describe these differences in the dispersion of data.

As with measures of central tendency, the various measures of variability are appropriate to specific kinds of measurement and types of distribution.

Modal percentage is used with nominal data and is the percentage of cases in the mode. A high modal percentage is indicative of decreased variability.

RANGE

The *range* is the simplest but most unstable measure of variability. The range is the difference between the highest and the lowest scores. A change in either of these two scores would change the range. The range should always be reported with other measures of variability. The range in Table 15-1 is 36, but this could easily change with an increase or decrease in the high score of 90 or the low score of 54.

SEMIQUARTILE RANGE

The *semiquartile range* (semiinterquartile range) indicates the range of the middle 50% of the scores. It is more stable than the range, since it is less likely to be changed by a single extreme score. It lies between the upper and lower quartiles. The upper quartile is the point below which 75% of the scores fall, and the lower quartile is the point below which 25% of the cases fall.

PERCENTILE

A *percentile* represents the percent of cases a given score exceeds. The median is the 50% percentile. A score in the 90th percentile is exceeded by only 10% of the scores. The zero percentile and the 100th percentile are usually dropped (McNemar, 1969).

STANDARD DEVIATION

The *standard deviation* (S.D.) is the most frequently used measure of variability. It is a measure of average deviation of the scores from the mean and, as such, should always be reported with the mean. It takes all scores into account and can be used to interpret individual scores.

The standard deviation is based on the concept of the normal curve. The *normal curve* is a distribution that is symmetrical about the mean and unimodal. The mean, median, and mode are equal. The normal curve, illustrated in Fig. 15-5, is derived from the observation that repetitive measures of interval and ratio level data group themselves about the midpoint in a distribution that closely approximates the curve shown. In addition, if the means of a large number of samples of the same interval or ratio data are calculated and plotted on a graph, that curve also approximates the normal curve. This tendency of the means to approximate the normal curve is termed the *sampling distribution of the means*. The mean of the sampling distribution of the means is the mean of the population (see Chapter 16).

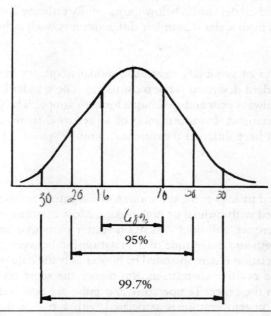

Fig. 15-5   Standard deviation.

An additional characteristic of the normal curve is that a fixed percentage of the scores fall within a given distance of the mean. As shown in Fig. 15-5, about 68% of the scores or means will fall within ±1 standard deviation of the mean, 95% within ±2 standard deviations of the mean, and 99.7% within ±3 standard deviations of the mean.

Since the mean $(\overline{X})$ and standard deviation (S.D.) for the exam in Table 15-1 was 73.1 ± 12.1, a student should know that 68% of the grades were between 85.1 and 61. If the student received a grade of 88, he would know he did better than most the class, while a grade of 58 would indicate he did not do as well as most the class.

The standard deviation is used in the calculation of many inferential statistics (see Chapter 16). One limitation of the standard deviation is that it is expressed in terms of the units used in the measurement and cannot be used to compare means that have different units of measurement. If researchers were interested in the relationship between height measured in inches and weight measured in pounds, it would be necessary for them to convert the height and weight measurements to standard units or Z scores.

Z Scores

The Z *score* is used to compare measurements in standard units. Each of the scores are converted to a Z score, and then the Z scores are used to examine the relative distance of the scores from the mean. A Z score of +1.5 means that the observation is 1½ standard deviations above the mean, while a score of −2 means that the observation is 2 standard deviations below the mean. By utilizing Z scores, a researcher can compare results from scales that utilize different units, such as height and weight.

• • •

Many measures of variability exist. The modal frequency is the easiest to calculate, but the standard deviation is the most useful. The standard deviation and the interquartile range always exist and are unique for each sample. The standard deviation is the most stable statistic. Transformation of scores to Z scores allow comparison between scores that have different measurement units.

• Correlation

Correlations are used to answer the question: to what extent are the variables related? Correlations are used with ordinal or higher data. Most correlations are discussed in Chapter 16, but here we will briefly mention scatter plots that are visual representations of the strength and magnitude of the relationship between two variables. The strength of the correlation is demonstrated by how closely the data points approximate a straight line. In a positive correlation, the higher the score on one variable, the higher the score on the other. Temperature and pulse are positively correlated; that is, generally a rise in temperature is associated with a rise in the pulse rate. In a negative correlation, the higher the score on one measure, the lower the score on the other measure. A decrease in blood volume is generally associated with a rise in the pulse rate. Fig. 15-6 illustrates a perfect positive correlation, a perfect negative cor-

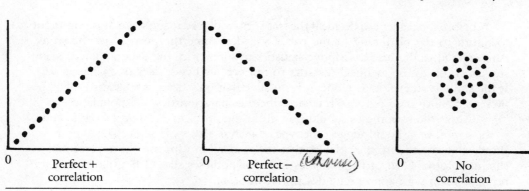

Closer this to one ⇒ positive correlation

0   Perfect +
     correlation

0   Perfect − *(inverse)*
     correlation

0   No
     correlation

Fig. 15-6   Scatter plots.

relation, and no correlation. In most research, correlation results lie between these extremes.

• Critiquing Descriptive Statistics

Many students who have not had a course in statistics feel that they cannot critique descriptive statistics. However, the student should be able to critically analyze the use of statistics, even if the student does not understand the derivation of the numbers presented. What is most important in critiquing this aspect of a research study is that the procedures for summarizing the data make sense in light of the purpose of the study. The criteria for critiquing descriptive statistics are presented in the box below.

●

Critiquing Criteria

1. Does the purpose of the study suggest the use of descriptive statistics?
2. What major variables are mentioned in the hypotheses?
3. What level of measurement is used to measure each of the major variables?
4. Is the sample size large enough to prevent one extreme score from affecting the summary statistics utilized?
5. What descriptive statistics are reported?
6. Were these descriptive statistics appropriate to the level of measurement for each variable?
7. Are there summary statistics for each major variable?
8. Is there enough information presented to judge the results?
9. Are the results clearly and completely stated?
10. If tables and graphs are used, do they agree with the text and extend it, or do they merely repeat it?

Before the reader can decide if the statistics employed made sense, it is important to return to the beginning of the paper and determine the purpose of the study. Although all studies use descriptive statistics to summarize the data obtained, many studies go on to use identical statistics to test specific hypotheses (see Chapter 16). If the study is an exploratory one, it is possible that only descriptive statistics will be presented, since their purpose is to describe the characteristics of a population.

Just as the hypotheses should flow from the problem and purpose of a study, so the hypotheses should suggest the type of analysis that will follow. The hypotheses should indicate the major variables that the reader can expect to have presented in summary form. Each of the variables in the hypotheses should be followed in the results section with appropriate descriptive information.

After studying the hypotheses, the reader should proceed to the methods section. Using the operational definition provided, the reader identifies the level of measurement employed to measure each of the variables that were listed in the hypotheses. From this information, the reader should be able to determine the measures of central tendency and variability that should be employed to summarize the data. For example, you would not expect to see a mean used as a summary statistic for the nominal variable of sex. In all likelihood, sex would be reported as a frequency distribution. The reader should expect that the means and standard deviations will be provided for measurements performed at the interval level. The sample size is another aspect of the methods section that is important when evaluating the researcher's use of descriptive statistics. The larger the sample, the less the chance that one outlying score will affect the summary statistics.

Only after these aspects of the study have been examined should the reader begin to consider the results presented by the researcher. Each important variable should have an appropriate measure of central tendency and variability presented. If tables or graphs are used, they should agree with the information presented in the text of the paper. Tables and graphs should be clearly and completely labeled. If the researcher presents grouped frequency data, the groups should be logical and mutually exclusive. The size of the interval in grouped data should not obscure the overall pattern of the data, nor should it create an artificial pattern. Each table and chart should be referred to in the text, but should add to the text and not merely repeat it. Each table or graph should have an obvious connection to the study being reported. For example, there may be one table that describes the sample and another that presents data relevant to the hypotheses being studied.

The results should be written so that they are understandable to the intended audience. The audience for nursing research is the average practicing nurse. Thus the descriptive information presented should be clear enough that the reader at that level can determine the usefulness of the study in the individual practice situation.

Descriptive statistics cannot be critiqued apart from the study as a whole. Each part of the research paper must make sense in relation to the entire paper. Therefore the reader should evaluate each portion of the paper in relation to what has preceded it. As such, the evaluation of the descriptive statistics must precede the evaluation of any inferential statistic.

• Summary

This chapter has introduced the student to the use of descriptive statistics as a means of describing and organizing data gathered in research. The focus has been on understanding the techniques rather than on their calculation.

Basic to the discussion has been an understanding of the levels of measurement utilized in a study. Each level of measurement, such as nominal, ordinal, interval, and ratio, has appropriate descriptive techniques associated with it.

Three ways of describing and summarizing data have been presented. The frequency distribution presents data in tabular or graphic form and allows for the calculation or observation of the data's characteristics, including symmetry, modality, and kurtosis. In nonsymmetrical distributions the degree and direction of the pull of the peak off-center are described in terms of skew. In modality the number of peaks is described as unimodal, biomodal, or multimodal. The relative spread of the data is described by kurtosis. Each characteristic of the frequency distribution is independent.

Measures of central tendency describe the average member of a sample. The mode is the most frequent score, the median the middle score, and the mean the arithmetic average of the scores. The mean is the most stable and useful of the measures of central tendency and with the standard deviation forms the basis for many inferential statistics as described in Chapter 16.

Measures of variability reflect the spread of the data. The modal percentage is the percent of the cases in the mode. The ranges reflect differences between high and low scores. The standard deviation is the most stable and useful measure of variability.

The standard deviation is derived from the concept of the normal curve. In the normal curve, sample scores and the means of large numbers of samples group themselves around the midpoint in the distribution, with a fixed percentage of the scores falling within given distances of the mean. This tendency of means to approximate the normal curve is called the sampling distribution of the means. A Z score is the standard deviation converted to standard units.

Finally, the concept of correlation was introduced. The scatter plot was discussed as a measure of correlation.

The principles of descriptive statistics were then applied to the critical analysis of published research reports. Special emphasis was given to the relationship of levels of measurement and appropriate descriptive techniques.

• References

Fox, D.J. (1982). *Fundamentals of research in nursing,* Norwalk, Connecticut, Appleton-Century-Crofts.

Kerlinger, F.N. (1973). *Foundations of behavioral research,* New York, Holt, Rinehart & Winston.

McNemar, Q. (1969). *Psychological statistics,* New York, John Wiley & Sons, Inc.

Polit, D.F., and Hungler, B.P. (1983). *Nursing research, Principles and methods,* 2nd ed., Philadelphia, J.B. Lippincott Co.

Shelley, S.I. (1984). *Research methods in nursing and health,* Boston, Little, Brown, & Co.

Wolfer, J.A., Visintainer, M.A. (1975). Pediatric surgical patients' and parents' stress responses and adjustment, *Nursing Research* **24:244**.

16

Inferential Data Analysis

Margaret Grey

LEARNING OBJECTIVES

After reading this chapter, the student should be able to do the following:
- Identify the purpose of inferential statistics.
- Distinguish between a parameter and a statistic.
- Explain the concept of probability as it applies to the analysis of sample data.
- Distinguish between type I and type II errors.
- Distinguish between parametric and nonparametric tests.
- List the commonly utilized statistical tests and their purposes.
- Critically analyze the statistics utilized in published research studies.

KEY TERMS

correlation

degrees of freedom

inferential statistics

level of significance (alpha level)

nonparametric statistics

null hypothesis

parameter

parametric statistics

probability

sampling error

scientific hypothesis

standard error of the mean

type I error

type II error

Inferential statistics are used to analyze the data collected in a research study. The research consumer needs to understand the purpose and application of inferential statistics, rather than how to carry out statistical procedures. Therefore the purpose of this chapter is to demonstrate how researchers use inferential statistics to draw conclusions about populations from sample data. For the reader to begin to make sense of the numbers presented in research papers that utilize inferential statistics, basic concepts and terminology will be presented in the sections that follow. Those readers who desire a more advanced discussion should refer to the Additional Readings section at the end of the chapter.

In the previous chapter we discussed *descriptive statistics*, the statistics that are utilized when the researcher needs to summarize the data. In this chapter we turn our attention to the use of inferential statistics. *Inferential statistics* combines mathematical processes and logic to allow researchers to test hypotheses about a population utilizing data obtained from random samples. Statistical inference is generally used for two purposes: to estimate the probability that statistics found in the sample accurately reflect the population parameter, and to test hypotheses about a population. In the first purpose, a *parameter* is a characteristic of a population, whereas a *statistic* is a characteristic of a sample. We use statistics to estimate population parameters. Suppose we randomly sample 100 people with chronic lung disease and use an interval scale to study their knowledge of the disease. If the mean score for these clients is 65, the mean represents the *sample statistic*. If we are able to study every client with chronic lung disease, we could also calculate an average knowledge score, and that score would be the *parameter for the population*. As you know, a researcher is rarely able to study an entire population, so inferential statistics allow the researcher to make statements about the larger population from studying the sample.

The example given alludes to two important qualifications of how a study must be conducted so that inferential statistics may be used. First, it was stated that the sample was randomly selected (see Chapter 14). Since you are already familiar with the advantages of random sampling, it should be clear that if we wish to make statements about a population from a sample, that sample must be representative. All procedures for inferential statistics are based on the assumption that the sample was drawn randomly. Second, it was stated that the scale had to reach the interval level of measurement. This is because the mathematical operations involved in doing inferential statistics require this level of measurement.

The second purpose of inferential statistics is hypothesis testing. This decision-making process helps researchers answer questions such as, "How much of this effect is the result of the change?" or, "How much of this effect is a result of chance?" Statistical hypothesis testing helps researchers to make objective decisions about the outcome of their study. The procedures utilized when making statistical inferences are based on principles of negative inference. In other words, if a researcher studied the effect of a new educational program for clients with chronic lung disease, the statistical test would actually assume there is *no* difference between the experimental group and the control group. Inferential statistics utilize a null hypothesis for testing a scientific hypothesis. The *null hypothesis* states that there is no actual relationship between the variables and that any observed relationship is merely a function of chance or sampling fluctuations.

The null hypothesis is often confusing for research students. An example may help to clarify this concept. Suppose a researcher had an innovative way to teach newly diagnosed diabetic clients about their disease. An experimental study is designed to evaluate the effect of the new program on client knowledge and metabolic control. Clients are randomly assigned to either the experimental group or the control group, the intervention is implemented, and the groups are compared at some later date. The researcher finds that the experimental group does indeed do better than the control group. There are two possible explanations for this outcome: (1) the teaching program was successful, or (2) the differences were the result of chance. The first explanation is the researcher's *scientific hypothesis,* the expectation of the researcher as to the outcome of the study. The second hypothesis is the null hypothesis. The null hypothesis stems from the fact that statistical hypothesis testing is a process of disproof or rejection. It is impossible to prove that the scientific hypothesis is true, but it is possible to show that the null hypothesis has a high probability of being incorrect. To reject the null hypothesis, then, is considered to show support for the scientific hypothesis and is the desired end of most studies that utilize inferential statistics. (see Chapter 7).

• Probability

We have shown that the researcher can never prove the scientific hypothesis, but can show support for it by rejecting the null hypothesis, that is show that the null hypothesis has a high probability of being incorrect. We have now introduced the theory underlying all of the procedures to be discussed in this chapter—probability theory. Probability is a concept that we talk about all the time, such as the chance of rain today, but we have a difficult time defining it. The *probability* of an event is the event's long-run relative frequency in repeated trials under similar conditions (Colton, 1974). In other words, the statistician does not think of the probability of obtaining a single result from a single study, but rather of the chances of obtaining the same result from an idealized study that can be carried out a large number of times under identical conditions. It is the notion of repeated trials that allows researchers to use probability to test hypotheses.

Statistical probability is based on the concept of sampling error. Remember that the use of inferential statistics is based on random sampling. However, even when samples are randomly selected, there is always the possibility of some errors in sampling. Therefore the characteristics of any given sample may be different from those of the entire population. Suppose a group of researchers has at their disposal a large group of clients with decubitus ulcers and they wish to study the average length of time ulcers take to heal with the usual nursing care. If the researchers studied the entire population, they might obtain an average healing time of 50 days, with a standard deviation of 10 days. Now suppose that the researchers did not have the money necessary to study all of the clients, but wished instead to do several consecutive studies of these clients. For this study, they first draw a sample of 25 clients, calculate the mean and standard deviation, and replace the subjects in the population before drawing the next sample. The researchers repeat this process many times, so that they might end up with 50 different means. If the researchers then placed the means in a frequency distribution, it might appear as in Fig. 16-1. This frequency distribution is a sampling distribution of the means. It illustrates that the researchers might find that one sample's mean might be 50.5, the next 47.5, the next 62.5, and so on. The tendency for statistics to fluctuate from one sample to another is known as *sampling error*.

Sampling distributions are theoretical. In practice, researchers do not routinely draw consecutive samples from the same population, but usually they compute statistics and make inferences based on one sample. However, the knowledge of the properties of the sampling distribution—*if* these repeated samples are hypothetically obtained—permits the researcher to draw a conclusion based on one sample. This is possible because the sampling distribution of the means has certain known properties.

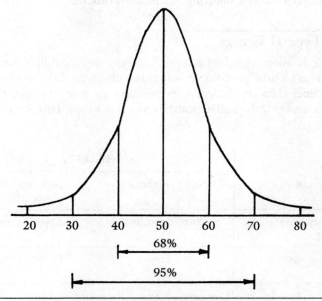

Fig. 16-1   Sampling distribution of the means.

The sampling distribution of the means follows a normal curve, and the mean of the sampling distribution will be the mean of the population. As was discussed in the previous chapter, the fact that the sampling distribution of the means is normal tells us several other important things. When scores are normally distributed, we know that 68% of the cases will fall between $+1$ S.D. and -1 S.D. or that the probability is 68 out of 100 that any one randomly drawn sample mean will lie within the range of values between plus and minus one standard deviation. In our example, if we only drew one sample, we would have a 68% chance of finding a sample mean that fell between 40 and 60. The standard deviation of a theoretical distribution of sample means is called the standard error of the mean. The word *error* is used because the various means that make up the distribution contain some error in their estimates of the population mean. The error is considered to be standard because it implies the magnitude of the average error, just as a standard deviation implies the average variation from one mean. The smaller the standard error, the less variable are the sample means and the more accurate are those means as estimates of the population value.

Although researchers rarely construct sampling distributions, standard error can be estimated because it bears a systematic relationship to the sample standard deviation and the size of the sample. This is important because it tells us that increasing the size of the sample will increase the accuracy of our estimates of population parameters. It should make intuitive sense that to increase the size of a sample will decrease the likelihood that one outlying score will dramatically affect the sample mean (see Chapter 15). The other reason that the sampling distribution is so important is that there are sampling distributions for all statistics. Researchers consult these distributions when making determinations about rejecting the null hypothesis.

• Type I and Type II Errors

The researcher's decision regarding accepting or rejecting the null hypothesis is based on a consideration of how probable it is that the observed differences are a result of chance alone. Since data on the entire population are not available, the researcher can never flatly assert that the null hypothesis is or is not true. Thus statistical inference

Conclusion of test of significance	REALITY	
	Null hypothesis is true	Null hypotheses is not true
Not statistically significant	Correct conclusion	Type II error
Statistically significant	Type I error	Correct conclusion

Fig. 16-2   Outcome of statistical decision making.

is always based on incomplete information about a population, and it is possible for errors to occur when making this decision. There are two types of error in statistical inference: type I and type II.

Type I error is the researcher's rejection of a null hypothesis that is actually true. *Type II error* is the researcher's acceptance of a null hypothesis that is actually false. The relationship of the two types is demonstrated in Fig. 16-2.

LEVEL OF SIGNIFICANCE

The researcher does not know when an error in statistical decision making has occurred. It is only possible to know that the null hypothesis is indeed true or false if data from the total population are available. However, the researcher can control the risk of making type I errors by setting the level of significance before the study begins. The *level of significance* is the probability of making a type I error, or the probability of rejecting a true null hypothesis. The minimum level of significance acceptable for nursing research is .05. If the researcher sets *alpha,* or the level of significance, at .05, the researcher is willing to accept the fact that if the study were done 100 times, the decision to reject the null hypothesis would be wrong 5 times out of those 100 trials. If, as is sometimes done, the researcher wants to have a smaller risk of rejecting a true null hypothesis, the level of significance may be set at .01. In this case the researcher is willing to be wrong only once in 100 trials. The decision as to how strictly the alpha level should be set depends on how important it is to not make an error. For example, if the results of a study are to be used to determine whether a great deal of money should be spent in some area of nursing care, the researcher may decide that the accuracy of the results is so important that an alpha level of .01 is chosen. In most studies, however, alpha is set at .05.

Perhaps you are thinking that researchers should always use the lowest alpha level possible, because it makes sense that researchers would like to keep the risk of both types of errors at a minimum. Unfortunately, decreasing the risk of making a type I error increases the risk of making a type II error. What this means is that the stricter the researcher is in preventing the rejection of a true null hypothesis, the more likely is the possibility that a false null hypothesis will be accepted. Therefore the researcher always has to accept more of a risk of one type of error when setting the alpha level.

A distinction should be made between statistical significance, as we are discussing it, and practical significance. When a researcher tests a hypothesis and finds that it is statistically significant, this means that the finding is unlikely to have happened by chance. In other words, if the level of significance has been set at .05, the odds are 19 to 1 that the conclusion the researcher makes on the basis of the statistical test performed on sample data is correct. The researcher would be wrong only 5 times out of 100. Yet such a finding may or may not have practical importance. Senator Proxmire's annual "Golden Fleece" award points out this important distinction. Senator Proxmire gives this award to researchers who have spent government monies to study unimportant topics. The results of these studies may be statistically significant, but they may have no practical value or significance. Although researchers should consider the practicality of a problem in the beginning stages of a research project (see Chapter 4), a distinction should also be made when discussing the results of a study between the statistical and the practical significance of the findings.

• Tests of Statistical Significance

Tests of significance may be *parametric* or *nonparametric*. Most of the studies in nursing research literature utilize parameteric tests, which have the following three attributes: (1) they involve the estimation of at least one parameter, (2) they require measurement on at least an interval scale, and (3) they involve certain assumptions about the variables being studied. These assumptions usually include that the variable is normally distributed in the overall population. In contrast to parametric tests, nonparametric tests of significance are not based on the estimation of population parameters, so they involve less restrictive assumptions about the underlying distribution. Nonparametric tests are usually applied when the variables have been measured on a nominal or ordinal scale.

There has been some debate about the relative merits of the two types of statistical tests. The moderate position taken by most researchers and statisticians is that nonparametric statistics are best utilized when the data cannot be assumed to be at the interval level of measurement or when the sample is small and the normality of the underlying distribution cannot be inferred. However, if these assumptions can be made, most researchers prefer to use parametric statistics because they are more powerful and more flexible than nonparametric statistics.

There are many different statistical tests of significance that researchers utilize to test hypotheses. The procedure and the rationale for their use are similar from test to test. Once the researcher has chosen a significance level and collected the data, the data are utilized to compute the appropriate test statistic. For each test, there is a related theoretical distribution that shows the probable and improbable values for that statistic. On the basis of the statistical result and the values in the distribution, the researcher either accepts or rejects the null hypothesis and then reports both the statistical result and its probability. Thus a researcher may perform a statistical test called a t-test, obtain a value of 8.98, and report that it is statistically significant at the $p.05$ level. This means that the researcher had 5 chances out of 100 to be wrong in concluding that this result could not have been obtained by chance. In addition, the likelihood of finding a statistic that is high enough to be statistically significant is increased as the sample size increases. This likelihood is indicated by the *degrees of freedom* that are often reported with the statistic and the probability value. Degrees of freedom are usually abbreviated as *df.*

Table 16-1 shows the most commonly used inferential statistics. The test that is utilized depends on the level of the measurement of the variables in question and the type of hypothesis being studied. Basically, these statistics test two types of hypotheses: (1) that there is a difference between groups, or (2) that there is a relationship between two variables.

• *Table 16-1*   Tests of Difference or Association

Level of measurement	One sample	Two samples Related	Two samples Independent	More than two samples	Correlation indexes
Nonparametric					
Nominal	Chi-square		Chi-square Fisher exact probability test	Chi-square	Phi-coefficient
Ordinal	Kolmogorov-Smirnov	Sign test Wilcoxon matched-pairs, signed rank test	Chi-square Median test Mann-Witney U	Chi-square	Spearman rank correlations Kendall rank correlations
Parametric					
Interval or Ratio	With before-after measures: Correlated *t*-test Repeated measures Analysis of variance	With matched pairs: Correlated *t*-test	Independent *t*-test Analysis of variance	Analysis of variance	Pearson product moment correlation Multiple correlation Factor analysis

TEST OF DIFFERENCE

Suppose a researcher has done an experimental study utilizing an after-only design (see Chapter 9). What the researcher hopes to determine is that the two groups are different after the introduction of the experimental treatment. If the two groups are randomly assigned and the level of measurement was at the interval level, the researcher would utilize the student's *t*-test to analyze the data. If the *t* statistic was found to be high enough as to not have occurred by chance, the researcher would reject the null hypothesis and conclude that the two groups were indeed more different than would have been expected on the basis of chance. In other words, the researcher would conclude that the experimental treatment produced the desired effect.

The *t* statistic is commonly used in nursing research, especially when the researcher wishes to test whether two group means are more different than would be expected on the basis of chance. To use this test, the variables must have been measured at the interval or ratio level, and the two groups must be independent. If the groups are related, such as in a test-retest situation, and the researcher wants to know if the subjects' scores have changed significantly, a paired or correlated *t*-test would be used.

Sometimes a researcher has either more than two groups or wants to examine the difference between before and after scores of two groups. This would be the case in a true experiment or a Solomon four-group design. Then the researcher utilizes a test called the analysis of variance. Like the *t*-test, the *analysis of variance,* often abbreviated ANOVA, searches for differences in the means of scores of variables measured at the interval level.

Researchers can also evaluate differences between groups when the data do not reach the interval level. If the level of measurement is nominal, the chi-square (χ^2) test is used. Chi-square is a nonparametric statistic that determines whether the frequency found in each category is different from what would be expected by chance. As with the *t*-test, if the calculated chi-square is high enough, the researcher would conclude that the frequencies found would not be expected on the basis of chance alone, and the null hypothesis would be rejected. The chi-square test can also be used with ordinal level data and with more than two groups. It is a commonly utilized test in nursing research.

When the data are at the ordinal level, researchers have several other nonparametric tests at their disposal. These include the sign test and the Wilcoxon matched-pairs, signed ranks test for related groups, and the median test and the Mann-Whitney U test for independent groups. Explanation of these tests is beyond the scope of this discussion, but those readers who desire further information are referred to the additional readings section at the end of this chapter.

TESTS OF RELATIONSHIPS

Researchers are often interested in exploring the relationships between two or more variables. Such studies utilize statistics that determine the *correlation,* or the degree of association, between two or more variables. Tests of the relationships between variables are sometimes considered to be descriptive statistics when they are utilized to describe the magnitude and direction of a relationship of two variables in a sample and the researcher does not wish to make statements about the larger population. Such statistics can also be inferential when they are utilized to test hypotheses about the correlations that exist in the target population.

Null hypothesis tests of the relationships between variables assume that there is no relationship between the variables. Thus when a researcher rejects this type of null hypothesis, the conclusion is that the variables are, in fact, related. Suppose a researcher is interested in the relationship between the age of clients and the length of time it takes them to recover from surgery. As with other statistics discussed, the researcher would design a study to collect the appropriate data and then analyze it utilizing measures of association. In our example, age and length of time to recovery can be considered to be interval level measurements, so the researcher would use a test called the Pearson *r,* or the Pearson product moment correlation coefficient. Once the Pearson *r* is calculated, the researcher consults the distribution for this test to determine whether the value obtained is likely to have occurred by chance. Again, the researcher reports both the value of the corrrelation and its probability of occurring by chance.

The interpretation of correlation coefficients is often problematic for students learning statistics. Correlation coefficients can range in value from $+1.0$ to -1.0 and can also be zero. A zero coefficient means that there is no relationship between the variables. A perfect positive correlation is indicated by a $+1.0$ coefficient, and a perfect negative correlation by a -1.0 coefficient. We can illustrate the meaning of these coefficients by utilizing the example from the previous paragraph. If there were no relationship between the age of the client and the length of time the client required to recover from surgery, the researcher would find a correlation of zero. However, if the correlation were $+1.0$, this would mean that the older the client, the longer it took him to recover. A negative coefficient would imply that the younger the client, the longer it would take him to recover. Of course, relationships are rarely perfect. The magnitude of the relationship is indicated by how close the correlation comes to the absolute value of 1. Thus a correlation of -0.76 is just as strong as a correlation of $+0.76$, but the direction of the relationship is opposite. In addition, a correlation of 0.76 is stronger than a correlation of 0.32. When a researcher tests hypotheses about the relationships between two variables, the test considers whether the magnitude of the correlation is large enough to not have occurred by chance. This is the meaning of the probability value or the p value reported with correlation coefficients. As with other statistical tests of significance, the larger the sample, the greater the likelihood of finding a significant correlation. Therefore researchers also report the degrees of freedom associated with the test performed.

Nominal and ordinal data can also be tested for relationships utilizing nonparametric statistics. The chi-square test can be used to study the relationships between variables measured at the nominal level, and the phi coefficient (ϕ) expresses the relationship found. Spearman rank order correlations and Kendall's tau express the correlation between variables measured at the ordinal level. All of these correlation coefficients may range in value from $+1.0$ to -1.0.

ADVANCED STATISTICS

Sometimes researchers are interested in studying more complex problems that examine more than two variables at a time. Most of these are variations on two of the tests that we have discussed—analysis of variance and multiple regression.

The analysis of variance is a powerful statistical test that can be utilized in a large number of situations. It can be expanded to encompass multiple data collection points as with time series studies, where it is called time series analysis of variance. It can also be used when a researcher believes that the results of the study will depend on some antecedent variable. This procedure is called the analysis of covariance. The *analysis of covariance test,* often abbreviated ANCOVA, is used when the analysis of variance would be used, but the researcher needs to control for another important variable that may influence the dependent variable. For example, suppose a researcher is interested in the effect of a teaching program on surgical recovery rate, but the researcher knows that the recovery rates will vary depending on the clients' age. The researcher could limit the study to just one age group, or the researcher could control for age in the analysis utilizing the analysis of covariance. If a positive result were obtained, the result would indicate that regardless of the client's age, the experimental program was effective in reducing recovery time.

Nursing problems are rarely so simple that they can be explained by only two variables. When researchers are interested in understanding more about a problem than just the relationships between two variables involved, they may use a procedure called multiple regression. *Multiple regression* is the expansion of correlation to include more than two variables, and it is utilized when the researcher wants to determine what variables contribute to the explanation of the dependent variable. For example, a researcher may be interested in determining what factors help women decide to breastfeed their infants. A number of variables, such as the mother's age, previous experience with breastfeeding, number of other children, and knowledge of the advantages of breastfeeding, might be measured and then analyzed to see if they, separately and together, predict the likelihood of breastfeeding. Such a study would require the use of multiple regression. The results of a study might help nurses to know that a younger mother who had only one other child might be more likely to benefit from a teaching program about breastfeeding than an older mother with several other children.

There are many other statistical tests of significance. Consult one of the statistics resources listed in the additional readings section at the end of the chapter if further information is desired or if a test not discussed is included in a study of interest to you.

• Example of the Use of Inferential Statistics

We have referred several times in this book to Wolfer and Visintainer's study (1975) that investigated the impact of a preoperative preparation program on children's responses and adjustment to surgery (see Appendix A). Wolfer and Visintainer utilized many of the statistics we have been discussing to test their hypotheses that the children who received the special nursing care would do better after surgery than those children who did not receive such care. Since the hypotheses being studied examined whether two groups of children would be different, the statistical tests of significance utilized were the chi-square, the *t*-test, and the analysis of variance. To use these tests, the researchers needed to assume that their variables were measured at the interval level, the variables were normally distributed, and the sample was large enough. In addition, they were not interested in just describing the sample of children studied, but rather in saying whether their findings might be similar if the total population of similar children had been studied. Thus they utilized inferential statistics.

Wolfer and Visintainer used the analysis of variance to test their hypothesis. This test was appropriate because they had four groups of children divided by age and treatment group, and they wished to determine if the mean scores on the dependent variables were significantly different. The *p* values given demonstrate that for most of the dependent variables, the treatment and the child's age were significant.

The authors also used the *t*-test and the chi-square test. Both of these were utilized to determine if the groups were similar before the introduction of the experimental program. These tests are often used in experimental studies like this one to help rule out threats to the internal validity of the findings (see Chapter 8). Characteristics of the subjects that were measured at the nominal level, such as child's sex, birth order, parental rooming-in, and type of surgery, were included in the chi-square tests. These tests determined if the experimental group and control group were equivalent. Variables that were measured at the interval level and provided pretest data for comparing the two groups were tested with the *t*-test. These variables included the children's and parents' upset behavior and the children's and parents' cooperation. As these variables might influence the ratings on the dependent variables, it was important and appropriate that they be measured at the outset of the study. This measurement and statistical analysis helped the researchers and the reader to rule out alternative hypotheses that might explain the findings of the study. Again, the researchers were able to demonstrate that the groups studied were equivalent at the initiation of the study with $p < .05$.

• Critiquing Inferential Statistical Results

Many students find that critiquing inferential statistics is difficult or even impossible, if they have not taken a course in statistics. Although there is some merit to this feeling, there are aspects of the statistical analysis that should be possible to critique without the benefit of years of statistics course work. Important questions to consider when critiquing the use of inferential statistics are listed in the boxed area below.

The first place to begin critiquing the statistical analysis of a research report is

---

Critiquing Criteria

1. Does the hypothesis indicate that the researcher is interested in testing for differences between groups or in testing for relationships?
2. What is the level of measurement chosen for the important variables?
3. Does the level of measurement permit the use of parametric statistics?
4. Is the size of the sample large enough to permit the use of parametric statistics?
5. Has the researcher provided enough information to decide whether the appropriate statistics were utilized?
6. Are the statistics utilized appropriate to the problem, the hypotheses, the method, and the sample?
7. Are the results for each of the hypotheses presented?
8. Do the tables and the text agree?
9. Are the results understandable?
10. Is a distinction made between practical significance and statistical significance? How?
11. What is the level of significance set for the study? Is it applied throughout the paper?

with the hypotheses. The hypotheses should indicate to you what type of statistics will be utilized. If the hypothesis indicates that a relationship will be found, you should expect to find indexes of correlation. If the study is experimental or quasi-experimental, the hypotheses would indicate that the author is looking for differences between the groups studied, and you would expect to find statistical tests of differences between means.

Then as you read the methods section of the paper, consider what level of measurement the author has utilized to measure the important variables. If the level of measurement is interval or ratio, the statistics will most likely be parametric statistics. On the other hand, if the variables are measured at the nominal or ordinal level, then the statistics utilized should be nonparametric. Also consider the size of the sample, and remember that samples have to be large enough to permit the assumption of normality. If the sample is quite small, for example, 5 to 10 subjects, the researcher may have violated the assumptions necessary for inferential statistics to be utilized. Thus the important question is whether the researcher has provided enough justification to utilize the statistics presented.

Finally, consider the results as they are presented. There should be enough data presented for each hypothesis studied to determine if the researcher actually examined each hypothesis. The tables should accurately reflect the procedure performed and be in harmony with the text. For example, the text should not indicate that a test reached statistical significance, when the tables indicate that the probability value of the test was above .05. If the researcher has utilized analyses that are not discussed in this text, you may want to refer to a statistics text to decide if the analysis was appropriate to the hypothesis and the level of measurement.

There are two other aspects of the data analysis section that the reader should critique. The paper should not read as if it were a statistical textbook. The results of the study in the text of the paper should be clear enough to the average reader so that the reader can determine what was done and what were the results. In addition, the author should attempt to make a distinction between practical and statistical significance. Some results may be statistically significant, but their practical importance may be doubtful. If this is so, the author should note it. Alternatively, you may find yourself reading a research report that is elegantly presented, but you come away with a "so what?" feeling. Such a feeling may indicate that the practical significance of the study and its findings have not been adequately explained in the report.

Note that the critical analysis of a research paper's statistical analysis is not done in a vacuum. It is possible to judge the adequacy of the analysis only in relationship to the other important aspects of the paper: the problem, the hypotheses, the design, the data collection methods, and the sample. Without consideration of these aspects of the research process, the statistics themselves have very little meaning. Statistics can lie; thus it is most important that the researcher use the appropriate statistic for the problem. For example, a researcher may sometimes use a nonparametric statistic when it appears that a parametric statistic is appropriate. Since parametric statistics are more powerful than nonparametric, the result of the parametric analysis may have not been what the researcher expected. However, the nonparametric result might be in the expected direction, so the researcher reports only that result.

• Summary

The purpose of this chapter was to introduce the student to the use of inferential statistics as a tool to test hypotheses about populations from sample data. The emphasis was on the appropriate use of statistical tests of hypotheses in nursing research studies.

To understand how probability is utilized by researchers when making decisions about the acceptance or rejection of a hypothesis, we discussed the theoretical distribution called the sampling distribution of the means. Because the sampling distribution of the means follows a normal curve, researchers are able to estimate the probability that a certain random sample will have the same properties as the total population of interest. Sampling distributions provide the basis for all inferential statistics.

Inferential statistics allow researchers to estimate population parameters and to test hypotheses. Since little nursing research focuses on estimation of parameters as an objective for the study, the chapter concentrated on the testing of hypotheses. The use of these statistics allows researchers to make objective decisions about the outcome of the study. Such decisions are based on the rejection or acceptance of the null hypothesis, which states there is no relationship between the variables. If the null hypothesis is accepted, this result indicates that the findings are likely to have occurred by chance. If the null hypothesis is rejected, the researcher accepts the scientific hypothesis of a relationship being present between the variables, and that this relationship is unlikely to have been found by chance.

Statistical hypothesis testing is subject to two types of error: type I and type II. Type I error occurs when the researcher rejects a null hypothesis that is actually true. Type II error occurs when the researcher accepts a null hypothesis that is actually false. The researcher controls the risk of making a type I error by setting the alpha level, or level of significance. Unfortunately, reducing the risk of a type I error by reducing the level of significance increases the risk of making a type II error.

The results of statistical tests are reported to be significant or nonsignificant. Statistically significant results are those whose probability of occurring is less than .05 or .01, depending on the level of significance set by the researcher.

Finally, a number of commonly used parametric and nonparametric statistical tests were discussed. These tests included those that test for differences between means, such as the t-test and the analysis of variance, and those that test for differences in proportions, such as the chi-square test. Tests that examine data for the presence of relationships included the Pearson r, the sign test, the Wilcoxon matched-pairs, signed ranks test, and several others. The reader was also introduced to several advanced statistical procedures such as the analysis of covariance and multiple regression.

These principles of statistical inference were then applied to the critical analysis of published research papers. The most important aspect of critiquing statistical analyses is the relationship of the statistics employed to the problem, design, and method used in the study. Clues to the appropriate statistical test to be utilized by the researcher should stem from the researcher's hypotheses. The reader should also determine if all of the hypotheses have been presented in the paper.

• References

Colton, T. (1975). *Statistics in medicine,* Boston, Little, Brown & Co.

Fox, D.J. (1982). *Fundamentals of research in nursing,* Norwalk, Connecticut, Appleton-Century-Crofts.

Polit, D., and Hungler, B. (1983). *Nursing research: Principles and methods,* 2nd ed., Philadelphia, J.B. Lippincott Co.

Wolfer, J., and Visintainer, M.A. (1975). Pediatric surgical patients' and parents' stress responses and adjustment as a function of psychologic preparation and stress-point nursing care, *Nursing Research* 24:244-255.

• Additional Readings

Bennett, S., and Bowers, D. (1976). *An introduction to multivariate techniques for the social and behavioral sciences,* New York, John Wiley & Sons, Inc.

Blalock, H.M. (1972). *Causal inferences in nonexperimental research,* New York, W.W. Norton.

Blalock, H.M. (1979). *Social statistics,* New York, McGraw-Hill Book Co.

Kerlinger, F.N., and Pedhazur, E.J. (1973). *Foundations of behavioral research,* New York, Holt, Rinehart & Winston, Inc.

Knapp, R. (1984). *Basic statistics for nurses,* Norwalk, Connecticut, Appleton-Century-Crofts.

Pedhazur, E.J. (1982). *Multiple regression in behavioral research,* 2nd ed., New York, Holt, Rinehart & Winston, Inc.

17

Computers in Research

Christine Tassone Kovner

LEARNING OBJECTIVES

After studying this chapter, the student should be able to do the following:
- Describe in general terms how a computer works.
- Compare and contrast the uses of mainframe computers and microcomputers in nursing research.
- Describe how a computer can be used in the various steps of the research process.
- Identify the steps of the research process that a computer cannot be used for and explain why.

KEY TERMS

data base	random access memory (RAM)
hardware	read only memory (ROM)
memory	software
modem	terminals
programs	time-sharing

Computer use has vastly facilitated many steps in the research process. For example, statistical tests that were infrequently performed 10 years ago because of the lengthy calculations involved are now commonly performed. It would be unusual for anyone today to analyze data from a research study without at least using a calculator, and in virtually all published quantitative research, a computer has been used. This chapter will discuss how the computer aids in carrying out the research process. This chapter includes an overview of computers and specifically identifies those steps in the research process that can be enhanced by using a computer.

• Overview of Computers

Computers are electronic devices that store and manipulate pieces of data. In simple terms, a computer is a series of electronic *on* and *off* switches.

Generally when people talk about computers, they are talking about the hardware. *Computer hardware* is the electronic equipment and includes the following four main components:
1. An input device, such as a keyboard
2. An output device, such as a monitor or a printer
3. A central processing unit (CPU)
4. The memory (RAM/ROM)

The input device is much like a typewriter, and the user simply types the information that goes into the CPU. After the instructions are entered they are stored in the computer's memory. Memory can be visualized as a series of boxes and each box has room for one message, either *on* or *off*. Memory is usually available in two types—RAM and ROM. *RAM,* or random access memory means that the user can read it, change it, or write over it. *ROM,* or read only memory as its name implies, means that the computer can read it but it cannot be changed. ROM is used for the computer's operating system and it tells the CPU what it should be doing. From the memory, the instructions go to the CPU for processing. After the information has been processed, it is sent to one or more output devices. Sometimes instructions are entered on paper cards with holes punched in them to represent the letters or numbers or on a magnetic tape directly to the CPU. Magnetic tape is similar to the tape used in audio taperecorders.

Computers can also store information. These instructions or data are stored in the memory, on floppy disks, on magnetic tape, or on cards. Information that is stored in the memory is lost when the computer is turned off. To avoid losing data, information can be stored on floppy disks that are similar to soft phonograph records or on magnetic tape. These media can be kept for long periods of time and physically transported from one computer to another. Information that is stored on cards can also be transported, but this is rarely used anymore because the cards are very bulky. Instructions that are put on disks or tapes to program the computer to do something, such as word processing or statistics, are called *software*.

• Types of Computers

The three types of computers are mainframes, minicomputers, and microcomputers. Since most researchers use mainframes or microcomputers, only those will be discussed. A mainframe is a large computer, capable of great speed, and can be used by many people at the same time. When several people are working on one mainframe at the same time it is called *time-sharing*. The mainframe is wired to many terminals. A *terminal* is an input device consisting of a keyboard and a monitor. Each person using a terminal works independently, but the people are all sharing the same mainframe. Mainframes are generally quite expensive and are owned by universities and large businesses. On the other hand, microcomputers or personal computers (PCs) are smaller and much slower than mainframes. Usually they are used by only one person at a time, are owned by individuals or small businesses, and are relatively inexpensive.

Use of either a mainframe or a microcomputer requires knowledge of the computer's operating system. The operating system directs the computer to perform the desired tasks and is the language that the computer understands. For mainframes, it is also necessary to know one of the editing systems, that is, the set of instructions used to direct the computer. The editing system is a series of short commands that will move letters and numbers around on the screen. For example, if the computer is directed to get a data file, "get file" might be typed in; however, if "het file" was typed by mistake, the spelling would need to be corrected from "het" to "get." The editing system is used to make the spelling correction. Both operating systems and editing systems vary from computer to computer. Each time the user works with a new mainframe, the operating and editing systems for that computer must be learned.

Microcomputers also have operating and editing systems. The most common disk operating systems are Microsoft Disk Operating System (MS-DOS) and Control Program for Microcomputers (CP/M). The editing systems on microcomputers serve the same purposes as those on the mainframes and the user must know its operating system before using it. If computer programs written by someone else are being used, it may not be necessary to learn the editing system.

REMOTE TERMINALS

To use a mainframe, the user communicates to the mainframe from a remote terminal. In most large universities and businesses, these terminals are "hard wired," that is, the terminals are hooked up directly by wires much like telephone cables to the computer. It is also possible to connect to a mainframe computer via the telephone. One can purchase a terminal and a *modem* (the device needed to communicate from terminal to mainframe), and then by calling the mainframe's telephone number, the user can connect to it. In this way, computer files can be accessed from any telephone in the world, including your own home telephone.

Microcomputers can also be used as terminals to communicate with a mainframe. Commercially available software tells the microcomputer to act as if it were a terminal. Access to the mainframe via telephone line and modem is then possible. The obvious advantage of using a remote terminal is the ability to use the mainframe from remote locations. Thereby making it no longer necessary to go to a computer center to use a mainframe. It is easy to enter the data, process them, and see the results from where you and your terminal are located. It is even possible to print those data wherever you are if you have a printer. The major disadvantage of using a modem and telephone connection is that it costs money to use the telephone line. Occasionally, data that are transmitted over telephone lines have errors, although there are computer programs to ensure that this does not happen.

• Software

A complicated set of directions for the computer to execute is called a *program*. Programs are called software and are written in a computer language. The computer language takes the directions and turns them into *on* and *off* switches that the CPU can manipulate. Both microcomputers and mainframes can accept sets of directions

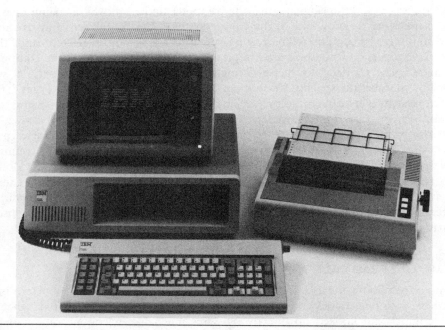

Fig. 17-1   IBM Personal Computer with keyboard, monochrome display, and 80 CPS matrix printer.

written in a computer language. Commonly used languages are FORTRAN, PASCAL, COBOL, BASIC, and LOGO. Not every computer can understand and use or compile all of these languages. It is necessary to know what languages your computer can understand.

Some software can be used by many different people. This software is sold by the person who wrote it or a company representing that person. Examples include programs that do word processing, handle statistics, set up data bases, and contain games. Thousands of these programs are available. Programs written for use on a mainframe cannot automatically run on a microcomputer becuase their operating systems differ. For example, an Apple computer's software will not work on an IBM PC. Many of the large manufacturers prepare versions of their software for a variety of computers. The word processing program Wordstar is available for the IBM PC and other computers (see Fig. 17-1). From the user's point of view, the program operates the same way on any microcomputer. From the computer's point of view, the directions it receives to process information are different and written in a language the computer can understand. Therefore, if you are able to use Wordstar on any computer, you will also be able to use it on the IBM PC. However, it will always be necessary to learn the basics of the different operating systems for each computer so you will know how to turn the machine on and ask it for the desired program.

• An Example of Data Processing in Nursing Research

Table 17-1 briefly summarizes the steps a researcher must utilize to process data on a mainframe and a microcomputer. When using a terminal to process statistical data on a mainframe such as the Cyber CDC, the researcher must "write" a program. A software program such as the Statistical Package for the Social Sciences (SPSS) (Nie et al., 1975) using an editing system called Xedit is an example of a packaged computer program. SPSS commands are similar to a series of FORTRAN programs and can be compared to baking a cake with a mix rather than from scratch. Once the program

• *Table 17-1*   Comparison of Mainframe Computers and Microcomputers for Data Processing

Mainframe computer (Cyber, CDC)	Microcomputer (IBM PC)
Network operating system: initial start-up response is the character "/". This affirms that the computer is operational.	Disk operating system: response given by the computer is "A>"
Editing system: Xedit, response is "?" or "??"	Editing system: Edlin
Software (SPSS): a statistics program	Software: EPISTAT, a statistics program
Languages: FORTRAN, PASCAL, COBOL	Languages: BASIC, and with special software can also run FORTRAN or PASCAL

is "written" (commands have to be given in the appropriate order), the researcher processes the program using the network operating system. If the researcher wants to process the same statistical data on an IBM PC, the floppy disk containing the program EPISTAT (Gustafson, 1983) is put in the disk drive and the user follows the directions that appear on the screen. Since EPISTAT is already written in BASIC, it is not necessary to use the IBM PC editing system. EPISTAT is much more user friendly or easy to use than SPSS. Processing data with SPSS on a mainframe is significantly faster than processing similar information with EPISTAT. SPSS can also perform many more statistical tests than any statistical software currently available commercially for the IBM PC. SPSS can be used on any mainframe; however, the network operating system and line editors vary from computer to computer. A simple version of SPSS is now available for the IBM PC; it is more complex than EPISTAT, both to use and in the computations it can do.

• Using the Computer in the Research Process

Many students new to the research process think that the computer is only utilized for the statistical analysis of data collected for a research study. However, this is not true. Researchers use computers to help accomplish many of the steps in the research process. This section reviews the phases of the research process in which computers can be helpful.

PROBLEM IDENTIFICATION (see Chapter 4)

The computer can be used to identify problems that can be studied. As computers are being increasingly used in clinical settings, data can be accessed from these computers to identify trends in client problems, nursing care, and delivery of nursing services. For example, the computer at a large medical center can be programmed to note all cases of infections. This can be done from laboratory records or client records. With this information, the nurse researcher can observe trends over time and decide if this problem is important enough to pursue. Another example of computer use in problem identification is in a rural hospital that might program its computer to note the incidence of decubiti. Again, the nurse researcher could monitor the incidence and decide if this were a problem to study. It should be noted that the computer is only an adjunct; real problem development occurs when the nurse thinks about clients, nurses, and care provided. In addition, reading literature about nursing research studies can set the problem identification process in motion.

LITERATURE REVIEW (see Chapter 5)

A major step in the development of a research project is the literature review. It is imperative that one knows what other work has been done on a subject of interest before designing a research project. The computer is a valuable tool for reviewing the literature. The process can be conducted from home using a microcomputer, or at most major university libraries.

The literature is listed in a data base. A *data base* is a compilation of information about something and is organized in a systematic way. Information from the data base can be presented in different ways, for example, by date, alphabetically, or by subject. Data bases exist that index everything from advertisements to health care articles to zoological literature. The most commonly used bibliographic health care data base is MEDLINE; it is produced by the United States National Library of Medicine. All articles indexed in the *Index Medicus, Index to Dental Literature,* and *International Nursing Index* since 1966 to the present are computerized in MEDLINE. MEDLINE indexes over 3,000 journals and has been including abstracts for more than a third of the citations since 1975.

To gain entry into this computer file, one needs to have an account number with either a commercial organization such as Dialog* or use the services of a library that has access to the files. The data bases are organized by key word codes. MEDLINE uses Medical Subject Headings developed by the National Library of Medicine. The specifics of the procedure vary, depending on the computer being used, but are basically as follows:

> From home, once the user has turned on the computer, the computer dials the phone number of the commercial service. An individual charge account is then entered and the actual search procedure begins. MEDLINE'S procedure is quite complicated but, in essence, the data base program requests from the user a series of key words. After the key words are entered, the MEDLINE computer will transmit, via telephone wire, the list of articles associated with the key words. They will appear on the screen or they may be printed to produce a permanent copy.

If the literature search is done at a library, the procedure is similar with either the researcher or a librarian doing the actual communicating with MEDLINE's computer. Depending on the library, the information is either printed immediately or is available at a later date. Costs for a computer search vary widely. The costs for MEDLINE include a combination of telephone charges and user time with MEDLINE. If you have an account with a commercial firm, you are usually billed monthly. Libraries generally charge on a per job basis. A typical search listing 40 articles would cost about $35. In addition, MEDLINE has completed searches for commonly requested topics. These are much less expensive and can be ordered by mail directly from MEDLINE. Specific information can be found from any major library or in the *International Nursing Index.*

Accuracy of Literature Research

The major question that arises when using a computer search concerns the accuracy of the information. Has the researcher missed any important articles? In an effort to explore this area, Fox and Ventura (1984) found that a computer search of articles about nurse practitioners did not identify a high proportion of critical studies identified from other sources. This suggests that traditional methods of reviewing literature should be used in addition to computer searches.

---

*Dialog, 3460 Hillview Avenue, Palo Alto, Calif. 94304.

Additional Uses in the Literature Search

Additional uses of the computer for literature review include abstracting services and individual reference list development. In some fields, there are commercially available abstracting services that produce references on a monthly basis using key words described by the researcher. These references are then sent to the researcher on a disk that can be accessed at will. At present, this service is not available for nursing articles, but it is expected in the near future.

The researcher can also create and store personal reference lists and abstracts. Many software programs exist that can help the researcher organize references by key words, dates, author, or any system preferred. When the researcher then wants a list of all articles with a reference to pain, for example, only that list needs to be called up from the data base.

Theoretical Rationale Development (see Chapter 6), Formulating the Hypothesis (see Chapter 7), and Selecting the Design (see Chapters 8 to 11)

At this time, computers cannot perform high level thinking skills. Therefore, computers are not helpful in these steps of the research process.

DATA COLLECTION (see Chapter 12)

Data collection can be aided by the computer in several ways. First, it is possible that the data that the researcher is interested in already exist as part of records collected for other reasons. One example is the National Health Survey, an ongoing national study about the use of health care services. Computer tapes of the surveys exist, and these tapes can either be rented and put on a mainframe or accessed from the federal government via a modem over the telephone line. Another example is the data that hospitals keep about the length of stay that are reported to various insurers and government agencies. These data can be accessed directly from the hospital.

Second, the computer can be used as a word processor to generate form letters and mailing labels that could be used in a mailed survey. The computer can be programmed so that each recipient receives a "personal" letter rather than a "Dear Colleague" letter. Survey research experts say that the response rate is higher when potential respondents receive a personalized letter.

Third, questionnaires can be prepared to use computer-readable answer sheets, like the ones we have all used to take standardized tests. These sheets are then "read" by the computer and the data are held in a file until they are analyzed.

OPERATIONALIZATION AND VARIABLE MEASUREMENT (see Chapter 13)

Operationalizing and measuring variables can be greatly enhanced by the use of the computer. Though definitions derive from theory, the researcher must choose a reliable and valid tool for measuring the variable. Many of the variables used in nursing studies are complex constructs such as pain, anxiety, or the quality of nursing care. Researchers try to measure these constructs using scales consistent with the theoretical

ITEM-TOTAL STATISTICS:

	SCALE MEAN IF ITEM DELETED	SCALE VARIANCE IF ITEM DELETED	CORRECTED ITEM-TOTAL CORRELATION	SQUARED MULTIPLE CORRELATION	ALPHA IF ITEM DELETED
IOSP1	83.00000	93.52381	.35780	.89954	.87891
IOSP2	82.50000	91.11905	.50816	.90126	.87268
IOSP3	82.22727	93.51732	.41955	.85944	.87587
IOSP4	82.09091	92.37229	.52874	.92790	.87204
IOSP5	82.90909	87.80087	.80320	.98755	.86233
IOSP6	83.13636	90.79004	.55799	.94360	.87077
IOSP7	82.72727	92.11255	.55849	.90522	.87110
IOSP8	82.54545	92.73593	.53039	.88448	.87209
IOSP9	82.18182	94.34632	.45590	.95932	.87456
IOSP10	82.36364	92.62338	.37948	.96606	.87841
IOSP11	82.63636	90.24242	.55019	.84280	.87101
IOSP12	82.40909	93.58658	.49342	.85553	.87335
IOSP13	82.90909	89.32468	.47939	.88921	.87481
IOSP14	82.63636	92.62338	.47798	.95064	.87375
IOSP15	82.81818	90.15584	.55740	.75832	.87072
IOSP16	82.68182	93.65584	.38776	.93671	.87723
IOSP17	82.45455	90.83117	.64683	.97358	.86820
IOSP18	82.50000	93.69048	.48679	.98472	.87356

A VALUE OF 99.0 IS PRINTED IF A COEFFICIENT CANNOT BE COMPUTED

Fig. 17-2   An example of reliability using SPSS.

rationale applied in the study. However, it is sometimes necessary for the researcher to develop a new scale. In either case, the reliability and validity of the tool must be assured. This is usually done by the various statistical tests discussed in Chapter 13 that can all be done quite rapidly using a computer. Thus the reliability and validity of instruments used in research studies should be available to the reader.

The following is an example. When using Hinshaw and Atwood's revision of the Risser Patient Satisfaction instrument (1982), a scale to measure the client's satisfaction with nursing care, it is necessary to know both the reliability and the validity of the scale. A common reliability test of internal consistency is the Cronbach Alpha. An example of some data and the printout describing the reliability taken from the SPSS is shown in Fig. 17-2.

For a study with 100 subjects calculating the alpha with a calculator would take several hours, but a mainframe computer can do it in less than a second.

SAMPLE SELECTION (see Chapter 14)

The selection of the sample is one of the most important aspects of the research process. As described in Chapter 14, if a volunteer sample is used, the results can be generalized only to that volunteer group. Researchers try to choose samples that will reflect the population of interest in the study. The computer can assist in several ways. There are computer programs, such as EPISTAT, that will identify the number of people in the sample necessary to achieve a stated level of significance for specific statistical tests. In addition, the computer can generate random numbers, so if the researcher wants a random sample of clients admitted to the hospital during a certain time period, random numbers can be chosen to identify chart numbers to be included in the study.

If the researcher was using a stratified sample and was interested in including the study subjects who met certain criteria, for example, clients who live in a specific part of the city, the computer could be used to choose those clients whose addresses have a specified zip code. The computer can be programmed to choose subjects along any parameters that the researcher sets. However, it should be kept in mind that the final sample is only as good as the original population list. That is, if the plan is to choose clients who live in zip code 10012, and the researcher uses as a population list those clients who go to one hospital, all those clients who live in zip code 10012 but who go to other hospitals will not be in the final sample. However, if the researcher uses a broader list of clients for the population list, the sample chosen will be more reflective of the population being studied.

ORGANIZING THE DATA FOR ANALYSIS AND ANALYZING THE DATA (see Chapter 15)

Historically, the computer has been used primarily to manipulate numbers, and this continues to be the function it best serves. When organizing the data, the computer can be used to sort the data, perhaps by generating lists of all those subjects with a particular diagnosis. When analyzing the data, the computer is an invaluable aid. Both applications require the computer to manipulate numbers.

Analyzing data is the real forte of the computer. It should always be remembered that the computer is only as good as the information put in, so if the data are inaccurate, the analysis will be inadequate. In computer lingo, this is known as the *GIGO* axiom— *Garbage In, Garbage Out*. For example if the data are best explained using multiple regression and the researcher used a *t*-test, the results will be incorrectly interpreted. It is the researcher's responsibility to analyze the data appropriately. Whether the tests requested are appropriate or not, the computer will quickly perform the statistical calculation and print the result. The researcher, not the computer, must decide if the result makes sense.

Most researchers use commercially available software packages that are already prepared to perform the most commonly required statistical programs. Of course the energetic computer user could write a program to do any statistical test required. Mainframes at most major universities have one or more general statistics programs. Two examples are SPSS and Biomedical Computer Programs (BMD). These programs are continually updated by the manufacturers to make them easier to use, more accurate, and inclusive of new statistical tests. The program used usually depends on what is available to the researcher and how familiar the faculty are with the various programs. The pros and cons of each system are not a subject for this book. The

researcher should have a record of which program (including the version, such as
SPSS version 8.3) was used, should questions about data analysis occur at a later
date.

Fig. 17-3 shows an example of data generated using an SPSS, version 8.3. This
example shows the complexity of the output generated by a multiple regression
procedure.

```
* * * * * * * M U L T I P L E   R E G R E S S I O N * * * * * * * *

DEPENDENT VARIABLE . .   PSIS

VARIABLE(S) ENTERED ON STEP NUMBER   3 . .    AGREE


MULTIPLE R           .34500    ANALYSIS OF VARIANCE    DF
R SQUARE             .11903    REGRESSION              3.
ADJUSTED R SQUARE        0     RESIDUAL               18.
STD DEVIATION        .99899    COEFF OF VARIABILITY   27.5 PCT


     SUM OF SQUARES      MEAN SQUARE        F       SIGNIFICANCE
        2.42704            .80901        .81065        .504
       17.96368            .99798


- - - - - - - - - VARIABLES IN THE EQUATION  - - - - - - - - - - -

VARIABLE        B           STD ERROR B         F           BETA
                                            _____   _____
                                           SIGNIFICANCE  ELASTICITY

AGE       -.98851754E-02  .15446952E-01  .40952759     -.1503651
                                             .530        -.13896
SEX        .32228462       .53736946     .35969401      .1490897
                                             .556         .02423
AGREE     -.41382850E-02  .34526808E-02  1.4365738     -.3079610
                                             .246        -.13667
(CONSTANT) 4.5401202       .78578315     33.383301
                                             .000


- - - - - - - - - VARIABLES NOT IN THE EQUATION  - - - - - - - - -

VARIABLE       PARTIAL      TOLERANCE              F
                                               _____
                                              SIGNIFICANCE

ALL VARIABLES ARE IN THE EQUATION.
```

Fig. 17-3   An example of multiple regression data generated by SPSS.

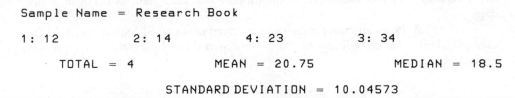

Fig. 17-4   An example of statistical data produced by the EPISTAT software package.

Statistical packages are also available for use on microcomputers. These programs are much slower than those used on the mainframe, because of the limited hardware of microcomputers. These packages also tend to be much less comprehensive than those on mainframes and include fewer statistical tests. SPSS is now available for use on some microcomputers, but the package is not identical to that used on the mainframes and includes far fewer statistics. EPISTAT is an example of a statistical program that is available to do simple statistics. This program includes only 25 tests. An example of data produced by Epistat on an IBM PC is shown in Fig. 17-4.

ANALYZING THE RESULTS (see Chapter 18)

Perhaps the most difficult part of the research process is interpreting the results. If the hypothesis is not supported, does that mean that the hypothesis is not an accurate description of events in the world, or does it mean that flaws in the design affected the results? If the hypothesis is supported, is it because the hypothesis does reflect the way events occur in the world or that the support fell in the support category on the basis of the 5% error? The answers to these and other questions raised in Chapter 18 are judgments. The computer cannot make judgments, and so the task of interpreting the result is left to the researcher and others who may read the final research report.

COMMUNICATION OF THE FINDINGS

The communication step in the research process is one of the most important. If results are not communicated to other researchers and practitioners, the nursing profession cannot advance. Results cannot and will not be used in practice. The computer, especially the microcomputer, is an aid for this step in the research process, because in addition to processing numbers, it can also process words. Using a commercially prepared software package, the researcher types on a keyboard and words appear on the monitor screen. If the researcher does not like the looks of what is written on the screen, the words are simple to change. When the researcher is happy with the final version, the report can be saved on a disk and then a printer can be used to make copies for colleagues or to submit to a journal for eventual publication. Some journals, such as *Computers in Nursing,* will accept articles directly from the disk rather than on paper. This saves both printing time and mailing costs. A copy of the article can also be transmitted over the telephone line to the disk or screen of someone else's computer for virtually instant viewing.

• Guidelines for Analyzing the Use of Computers in Published Research Studies

Almost all researchers use computers. The task for the critiquer of research reports is to decide if a computer has been used and whether it was used judiciously.

In some papers, the researcher may say, "Data were analyzed using SPSS," or, "A MEDLINE search revealed. . . ." Such statements would be presumptive evidence that the researcher utilized a computer when doing the research. If no such statement appears, the reader can make an intelligent assumption that computers were used if the sample is large, for example, greater than 20, or if inferential statistics are presented. Unless it is explicitly stated, the reader will not be able to determine if the researcher has utilized the computer for other steps of the research process.

There are no unique aspects to critiquing the written research reports that have utilized computers. The guides for critiquing the sections of a research report that can be aided by the use of a computer are presented throughout this book and should be consulted. The quality of the finished work should not be affected, either positively or negatively, by the use of a computer. The computer merely serves to facilitate the researcher's work.

• Summary

The purpose of this chapter was to discuss the use of the computer in the research process. Computers are composed of hardware and software. A computer's hardware includes an input device, output devices, central processing unit, and memory. Computers are available in the following three sizes: mainframes, minicomputers, and microcomputers, but most researchers in nursing use mainframes via terminals or microcomputers. Computer software provides the hardware with instructions to carry out procedures, such as statistical analysis or word processing.

The computer is a useful tool for researchers in many aspects of the research process. Computers can be helpful in problem identification, literature review, data collection procedures, measuring variables of interest, sample selection, data analysis, and communicating research findings. Because the computer is not capable of abstract thinking, it is not helpful for developing the theoretical rationale, formulating the hypothesis, selecting the design, and interpreting the results.

When analyzing published research reports, the reader should consider the steps in the research process where computers might be used and then consider whether appropriate steps to safeguard the quality of the work have been taken.

• References

Computers in Nursing, a bi-monthly journal published by J.B. Lippincott, East Washington Square, Philadelphia.

Fox, R.N., and Ventura, M.R. (1984). Efficiency of automated literature search mechanisms, *Nursing Research* **33**:174-177.

Gustafson, T.L. EPISTAT, available via mail at 1705 Gattis School Road, Round Rock, Texas 78664.

Nie, N., Hadlaihull, C., Jenkins, J., Steinbrenner, K., and Bent, D. (1975). *SPSS,* 2nd ed., New York, McGraw-Hill Book Co.

18

Analysis of the Findings

Geri LoBiondo-Wood

LEARNING OBJECTIVES

After studying this chapter, the student should be able to do the following:

- Discuss the difference between the results section of a study and the discussion of the results.
- Identify the format of the results section.
- Determine if both statistically supported and statistically nonsupported findings are discussed.
- Determine whether the investigator objectively reported the results.
- Describe how tables and figures were used in a research report.
- List the criteria of a meaningful table.
- Identify the format and components of the discussion of the results.
- Determine the purpose of the discussion section.
- Discuss the importance of interpreting both supported and nonsupported hypotheses.
- Discuss the importance of including generalizations and limitations of a study in the report.
- Determine the purpose of including recommendations in the study report.

KEY TERMS
findings
generalizations
limitations
recommendations

The ultimate goals of nursing research are to develop nursing theory and knowledge, to substantiate and improve nursing practice, thereby widening the scientific basis of the nursing profession. Nursing research not only serves nurses but also serves those individuals, families, and groups with whom we as nurses interact in a multitude of health care settings. From the viewpoint of the research consumer, the analysis of the results, interpretations, and generalizations that a researcher generates from a study become a highly important piece of the research project. The final sections of a research report are generally entitled results and discussion, and it is here that the researcher puts the final pieces of the jigsaw puzzle together to view the total picture with a critical eye. This process is analogous to evaluation, the last step in the nursing process. The reader of a research report may view these last sections as an easier step for the investigator, but it is here that a most critical and creative process comes into use. It is in these final sections of the report, after the statistical procedures have been applied, that the researcher will interrelate the statistical or numerical findings to the theoretical framework, literature, methods, hypotheses, and problem statements.

The final sections of published research reports are generally titled results and discussion, but other topics such as limitations of findings, implications for future research, recommendations, and conclusions may be separately addressed or subsumed within these sections. The presentational format of these areas is a function of the author's and the journal's stylistic considerations. The function of these final sections is then to interrelate all aspects of the research process and to discuss, interpret, and identify the limitations and generalizations relevant to the investigation and further nursing research. The goal of this chapter is to introduce the student to the purpose and content of the final sections of a research investigation where data are presented, interpreted, discussed, and generalized. An understanding of what an investigator presents in these sections will assist the research consumer to critically analyze an investigator's findings.

• Findings

The findings of a study are the results, interpretations, recommendations, generalizations, implications for future research, and conclusions and will be addressed by separating the presentation into two major areas. These two areas are the results and the discussion of the results. The results section will focus on the results or statistical findings of the study and the discussion of the results section will focus on the remaining topics. For both sections the rule applies, as it does to all other sections of a report, that the content needs to be presented clearly, concisely, and logically.

RESULTS

The results section of a research report is considered to be the data-bound section of the report. It is here that the researcher presents the data or numbers generated by the descriptive and inferential statistical tests and then sets the stage for the interpretations or discussion section that follows the results. The results section should then reflect the problem and hypothesis tested. The information from each hypothesis should be sequentially presented. The tests used to analyze the data should be mentioned. If the exact test that was used is not explicitly mentioned, then the values obtained should be noted. This is done by providing the numerical values of the statistics and stating the specific correlation and probability level, or *t*-value (see Chapters 15 and 16). Examples of these can be found in Table 18-1. These numbers and their signs should not frighten the novice away. These numbers are very important, but there is much more to the research process than the numbers. They are one piece of the whole. Chapters 15 and 16 conceptually present the meanings of the numbers found in studies for the novice consumer. Whether the consumer only superficially understands statistics or has an in-depth knowledge of statistics, it should be obvious that the results are clearly stated, and the presence or lack of statistically significant results should be noted. The Additional Reading section at the end of this chapter also provides further detail for those interested in the application of statistics.

The researcher is bound to present the data for all of the hypotheses posed, such as whether the hypotheses were accepted, rejected, supported, or not supported. If the data supported the hypotheses, it may be assumed that the hypotheses were proven, but this is not true. It does not necessarily mean that the hypotheses were *proven,* it only means that the hypotheses were supported and that the results suggest that the relationship as posed in the hypotheses, which were derived from the theoretical framework, were probably logical. The beginning research consumer may think that if a researcher's results were not supported statistically or only partially supported, then the study is irrelevant or possibly should not have been published, but this is also not true. If the data are not supported, the critiquer should not expect the researcher to bury the work in a file. It is as important for a critiquer of research to review and understand nonsupported studies as it is for the researcher. Information obtained from nonsupported studies can often be as useful as data obtained from supported studies. Nonsupported studies can be used to suggest limitations of particular aspects of a study's design and procedures. Data from nonsupported studies

• *Table 18-1*   **Examples of Reported Statistical Results**

Statistical test	Means of reporting results
Pearson correlation	$r = -0.39, p < .01$
Analysis of variance	$F = 3.59, df = 2, 48, p < .05$
t-test	$t = 2.65, p < .01$

may suggest that current modes of practice or current theory in an area may not be supported by research and therefore need to be reexamined and researched further. Data then assist a profession to generate new knowledge, as well as prevent static knowledge.

Generally it has been noted that an investigator will interpret the results in a separate section of the report. At times, the reader may find that the results section contains the results and the researcher's interpretations that generally fall into the discussion section. Integrating the results with the discussion in a report becomes the decision of the author. Integration of both sections may be utilized when a study contains several segments that may be viewed as fairly separate subproblems of a major overall problem.

An example of this type of integration is found in a study by Ventura, Young, Feldman, Pastore, Pikala, and Yates (1985). In this study, the investigators' purpose was to provide cost-related data from an intervention study in the care of patients with peripheral vascular disease (PVD). The study looked at various aspects of cost and hospitalization such as costs that were vascular related, and outpatient usage. Instead of two sections titled results and discussion, the investigators integrated both of these areas and discussed these areas as subproblems of the overall problem. The encompassing title that addressed results and discussion in this study was labeled *hospitalization and costs*. Subproblems or related areas tested and discussed were titled as: costs—PVD, costs—vascular related, costs—nonvascular, costs—combined total, outpatient hospital usage and time allocation, and costs for intervention. The investigators thus made use of conceptually discrete portions that flowed back to the overall problem. If integration is done in this manner, it should be consistent. That is, if one hypothesis or question is integrated, then all should. The presentation should not take on a haphazard use of integration. In the Ventura study, a consistent approach was used. Overall, the reader will generally find the data results in a separate section from the interpretation or discussion of the results.

The investigator should also demonstrate objectivity in the presentation of the results. Phrases like "analysis of variance showed that high psychosocial care resulted in significantly greater intent to adhere to a health care regimen" (Chang, Uman, Linn, Ware, and Kane, 1985) are the appropriate means to express a result. The investigators would be accused of lacking objectivity if they had stated the results in the following manner "analysis of variance showed surprisingly that high psychosocial care resulted in significantly greater intent to adhere. . . ." Opinions or reactionary statements to the data in the results section therefore are inappropriate. The box at the top of p. 271 depicts examples of objectively stated results. It is the investigator's responsibility to objectively respond to the results. This is accomplished in the last section titled discussion of results. The investigator then uses the discussion of the results section to respond to and interpret the results with a careful reflection on all aspects of the study that preceded the results.

The reader of a research report should bear in mind that the data presented are considerably reduced. A great deal more data or numbers have been generated in a study, but only the critical numbers of each test need to be presented in a report. An

Examples of Results Sections

A Pearson product moment correlation statistic, applied to depression scores in relation to the subjective time estimates, resulted in a coefficient of 0.35 ($p < .002$). Higher levels of depression were related to longer production estimates, which indicated underestimation of the interval, or decreased subjective time. Therefore, the hypothesis was supported.

(Newman and Gaudiano, 1984, p.138)

No subjects displayed significant 24-hour rhythms during the home interval from which mesors or amplitudes could be determined. The postsurgical hospitalization sodium/potassium excretion ratio was significantly higher and had an increased amplitude when compared with the home and the control groups.
(Farr, Keene, Samson, and Michael, 1984, p.142)

Hypothesis I was tested by an analysis of variance for the number of exercise steps common to both booklets . . . A two-way analysis of variance of the total number of steps available in the booklets (specific = 34, nonspecific = 20) performed correctly showed the same pattern (instruction group F [1,100] = 4.70, $p = .05$; type of surgery F [1,100] = 1.69).
Rice and Johnson, 1984, p.150)

To determine relative importance of the 35 concerns for each group, mean rankings for each concern were computed and used to create summative rank orderings.
(Broom, 1984, p.226)

example of summarized descriptive data is seen where only the means and standard deviations of age, education, income, and years married are presented rather than all of the subject information listed. Including all of the data in a published report would be too cumbersome. Individual data may be presented when a case study design is used. The condensation of data is done both in the written text and through the use of tables and figures. The use of tables and figures can facilitate the presentation of large amounts of data generated by the study. In a study on the "Impact of Arthritis on Quality of Life" (Burckhardt, 1985), the investigator presented the results in tabular form and developed figures to provide a more thorough explanation and discussion of the results. The results section then can be viewed as a summation section. Both the results of the descriptive and inferential statistics are presented for each hypothesis posed. No data should be omitted that would preclude the critiquer from gaining a full picture of the results. If tables and figures are used, they need to be concise. While the text is the major mode of communicating the results, the tables and figures serve a supplementary but independent role. The role of tables and figures is to report results with some detail that the investigator does not enter into the text. This does not mean that tables and figures should not be mentioned in the text. The amount of detail that the author uses in the text to describe the specific tabled data varies with the needs of the researcher. Fox (1982) notes that if the text includes everything that is found in the table, the table should not appear. Good tables are those that meet the following criteria:

1. They supplement and economize the text.
2. They have precise titles and headings.
3. They are not repetitious of the text.

The research consumer will find a well-written results section is systematic, logical, concise, and drawn from all of the analyzed data. All that is written in the results section should be geared to letting the data reflect the testing of the problems and hypotheses. The length of this section therefore depends on the scope and breadth of the analysis.

DISCUSSION OF THE RESULTS

In the final section of the report, the investigator interpretively discusses the results of the study. It is in this section that a skilled researcher makes the data come alive. The researcher takes the numbers and gives them meaning and interpretation. The reviewer may ask where the investigator extracted the meaning that is applied in this section. If the researcher does the job properly, you will find a return to the beginning of the study. The researcher returns to the earlier points in the study where a problem statement was identified and an independent and dependent variable were related based on a sound theoretical framework and literature review. It is in this section that the researcher discusses both the supported and nonsupported data. In this final section the limitations or weaknesses of a study are discussed in light of the design and the sample or data collection procedures. When the data are supported with a statistical significance, the discussion and interpretation are seen as a relatively easy task. The critiquer should find a discussion of how the theoretical framework was supported. In addition, the reviewer should also see the investigator's attempt to look at the data for additional or previously unrealized relationships.

Even if the data are supported, the reviewer should not believe it to be the final word. Downs (1984) cautions that the research critiquer should not be overwhelmed by small p-values, since they are not indicative of research breakthroughs. Therefore researchers and reviewers should accept statistical significance with prudence. Statistically significant findings are not the sole means of establishing the study's merit. Other considerations such as theory, sample, instrumentation, and methods should also be considered.

When the results are not statistically supported, the researcher also returns to the theoretical framework and analyzes the earlier thinking process. Results of non-supported hypotheses do not require the investigator to go on a fault-finding tour of each piece of the project. This can then become an overdone process. All research has weaknesses. This analysis is an attempt to identify the weaknesses and to suggest what the possible problem or problems were in the study. At times, the theoretical thinking is correct, but the researcher finds problems or limitations that could be attributed to the tools (see Chapters 12 and 13), the sampling methods (see Chapter

14), the design (see Chapters 8 through 11), or the analysis (see Chapters 15 and 16). Therefore when results are not supported, the investigator attempts to go on a *fact*-finding tour rather than a *fault*-finding one. The discussion is then not done to show humility or one's technical competence, but rather to enable the reviewer to judge the validity of the interpretations drawn from the data and the general worth of the study (Kerlinger, 1973).

It is in this last section of the report that the researcher ties together all the loose ends of the study. It is from here that reviewers of research can begin to think about clinical relevance, the need for replication, or the germination of a new idea for a prospective researcher. The reviewer of a research project should finally find this last section either in separate sections or subsumed within the discussion section and it should include generalizations and recommendations for future research, as well as a summary or a conclusion.

Generalizations or generalizability are inferences that the data are representative of similar phenomena beyond the study's sample to a population. Reviewers of research are cautioned not to generalize beyond the population on which a study is based. Beware of research studies that may overgeneralize. Generalizations that draw conclusions and make inferences within a particular situation and at a particular point in time are appropriate. An example of such a generalization is drawn from a study conducted by Broom (1984). This investigation was designed to identify anticipated and actual postpartum concerns about the marriage relationship during the period of transition to parenthood. Broom, when discussing the sample in light of the results, appropriately stated:

> The couples in the sample were well-educated and all had attended childbirth classes which focused on many of the relationship issues involved in transition to parenthood. . . . A replication of the study with a sample less educationally advantaged and more representative of the childbearing population might reveal even greater discrepencies in the consensus measures.

This type of statement is important for reviewers of research. It helps to guide thinking in terms of a study's clinical relevance, and it also suggests areas for further research. One study does not provide all of the answers, nor should it. It has been said that a good study is one that raises more questions than it answers. So the research consumer should not view an investigator's review of limitations, generalizations, and implications of the findings for practice as lack of research skill. These final steps of evaluation are critical links to the refinement of practice and the generation of future research. Evaluation of research, like evaluation of the nursing process, is not the last link in the chain, but a connection between findings that may serve to improve nursing theory and nursing practice.

The final area that the investigator integrates into the discussion section is the recommendations. The *recommendations* are the investigator's suggestions for the study's application to practice, theory, and further research. This requires the investigator to reflect on the question of what contribution to nursing does this study make? For examples of recommendations see Wolfer and Visintainer's study (Appendix A, page 322) and Lim-Levy's study (Appendix B, page 347). This evaluation places the study into the realm of what is known and what needs to be further known before being utilized. Fawcett (1982) noted, "It is through future exploration of the dissemination and utilization of research in nursing practice that the science of nursing will become an entity with which to be reckoned."

• Critiquing the Results and Discussion

Criteria for critiquing the results and the discussion of the results sections are found in the box below.

The results and the discussion of the results are the researcher's opportunity to examine the logic of the hypotheses posed, the theoretical framework, the methods, and the analysis. This final section requires as much logic, conciseness, and specificity as was employed in the preceding steps of the research process. The consumer should be able to identify statements of the type of analysis that was utilized and whether or not the data statistically supported the hypotheses. These statements should be straightforward and not reflect bias (see box, p. 271). Auxiliary data or serendipitous findings may also be presented. If such auxiliary findings are presented, they should be as dispassionately presented as was the hypothesis data. The statistical tests used should also be noted. The numerical value of the obtained data should also be presented (see Table 18-1). The presentation of the tests, the numerical values found, and the statements of support or nonsupport should be clear, concise, and systematically reported. For illustrative purposes, the researcher should present extensive findings in tables for the reader's consumption.

Critiquing Criteria

1. Are all of the results of each hypothesis presented?
2. Is the information regarding the results concisely and sequentially presented?
3. Are the tests that were used to analyze the data or the numerical values presented?
4. Are the results presented objectively?
5. If tables or figures are used, do they meet the following standards:
   a. They supplement and economize the text.
   b. They have precise titles and headings.
   c. They are not repetitious of the text.
6. Are the results interpreted in light of the hypotheses and theoretical framework and all of the other sections that preceded the results?
7. If the data are supported, does the investigator provide a discussion of how the theoretical framework was supported?
8. If the data are not supported, does the investigator attempt to identify the weaknesses and suggest what the possible problems were in the study?
9. Does the investigator discuss the study's clinical relevance?
10. Are any generalizations made?
11. Are the generalizations within the scope of the findings or beyond the findings?
12. Are any recommendations for future research stated or implied?

be as dispassionately presented as was the hypothesis data. The statistical tests used should also be noted. The numerical value of the obtained data should also be presented (see Table 18-1). The presentation of the tests, the numerical values found, and the statements of support or nonsupport should be clear, concise, and systematically reported. For illustrative purposes, the researcher should present extensive findings in tables for the reader's consumption.

The discussion section should interpret the data, the gaps, the limitations of the study, the conclusions, as well as the recommendations for further research. Drawing these aspects into the study should give the consumer a sense of the relationship of the findings to the theoretical framework. Statements reflecting the underlying theory are necessary, whether or not the hypotheses were supported.

If the findings were not supported, the consumer should, as the researcher did, attempt to identify without fault-finding possible methodological problems. Finally, a concise presentation of the study's generalizability and implications of the findings for practice and research should be evident. The last presentation can help the research consumer to begin to rethink clinical practice, provoke discussion in clinical settings (see Chapter 20), and find similar studies that may support or refute the phenomena being studied to more fully understand the problem.

• Summary

It is obvious that the analysis of the findings is the final step of a research investigation. It is in this section that the consumer will find the results printed in a straightforward manner. All results should be reported, whether or not they support the hypothesis. Tables and figures may be used to illustrate and condense data for presentation. Once the results are reported, the researcher interprets the results. In this presentation, usually titled discussion, the consumer should be able to identify the key topics being discussed. The key topics, which include an interpretation of the results, are the limitations, generalizations, implications, and recommendations for future research.

The interpretation of the results is the section where the researcher draws together the theoretical framework and makes interpretations based on the findings and theory. Again, both statistically supported and nonsupported results should be interpreted. If the results are not supported, the researcher should discuss the results reflecting on the theory, as well as possible problems with the methods, procedures, design, and analysis.

In this final process, research should present limitations or weaknesses of the study. This presentation is important because it affects the study's generalizability. The generalizations or inferences about similar findings in other samples are also presented in light of the findings. The research consumer should be alert for sweeping claims or overgeneralizations that a researcher may state. An overextension of the data can alert one to possible researcher bias.

Finally, the recommendations provide the consumer with suggestions regarding the study's application to practice, theory, and future research. These recommendations furnish the critiquer with a final perspective of the researcher on the utility of the investigation.

• References

Broom, B.L. (1984). Consensus about the marital relationship during transition to parenthood, *Nursing Research,* **33:**223-228.

Chang, B.L., Uman, G.C., Linn, L.S., Ware, J.E., and Kane, R.L. (1985). Adherence to health care regimens among elderly women, *Nursing Research,* **34:**27-31, (January/February).

Downs, F.S. (1984). *A sourcebook of nursing research,* 3rd ed., Philadelphia, F.A. Davis Co.

Farr, L., Keene, A., Samson, D., and Michael, A. (1984). Alterations in circadian excretion of urinary variables and physiological indicators of stress following surgery, *Nursing Research,* **33:** 140-146.

Fawcett, J. (1982). Utilization of nursing research findings, *Image,* **14:**57-59.

Fox, D.J. (1982). *Fundamentals of research in nursing,* 4th ed., Norwalk, Conn., Appleton-Century-Crofts.

Newman, M.A., and Gaudiano, J.K. (1984). Depression as an explanation for decreased subjective time in the elderly, *Nursing Research,* **33:**137-139.

Rice, V.H., and Johnson, J.E. (1984). Preadmission self-instruction booklets, postadmission exercise performance, and teaching time, *Nursing Research,* **33:**147-151.

Ventura, M.R., Young, D.E., Feldman, M.J., Pastore, P., Pikula, S., and Yates, M.A. (1985). Cost savings as an indicator of successful nursing intervention, *Nursing Research,* **34:**50-53.

• Additional Readings

Hack, S.W., Cormier, W.H., and Bounds, W.G., Jr. (1974). *Reading statistics and research,* New York, Harper & Row Publishing Co.

Kerlinger, F.N. (1973). *Foundations of behavioral research,* 2nd ed., New York, Holt, Rinehart, & Winston, Inc.

Knapp, R.G. (1985). *Basic statistics for nurses,* 2nd ed., New York, John Wiley & Sons, Inc.

Pedhazer, E.J. (1982). *Multiple regression in behavioral research,* 2nd ed., New York, Holt, Rinehart, & Winston, Inc.

Polit, D., and Hungler, B. (1983). *Nursing research: Principles and methods,* 2nd ed., Philadelphia, J.B. Lippincott Co.

Volicer, B.J. (1984). *Multivarate statistics for nursing research,* New York, Grune & Stratton, Inc.

Waltz, C., and Bausell, R.B. (1981). *Nursing research: design, statistics, and computer analysis,* Philadelphia, F.A. Davis Co.

Weinberg, S.L., and Goldberg, K.P. (1979). *Basic statistics for education and the behavioral sciences,* Boston, Houghton-Mifflin Co.

19

Evaluating the Research Project

Geri LoBiondo-Wood
Judith Haber

LEARNING OBJECTIVES

After reading this chapter, the student should be able to:
- Identify the stylistic considerations when preparing the manuscript of a research report.
- Identify the purpose of the critiquing process.
- List the steps of the critiquing process.
- Describe the criteria of each step of the critiquing process.
- Evaluate the strengths and weaknesses of a research report.
- Discuss the implications of the findings of a research report for nursing practice.
- Construct a critique of a research report.

KEY TERMS

construct replication
replication
research base
scientific merit

The preceding chapters in this book have provided the building blocks and tools for this chapter on the evaluation of a total research report. Each component of a research report raises questions that relate to criteria for evaluating the merit of a research study. In this chapter the evaluation criteria that have been presented in previous chapters will be utilized to critique a research report in a step-by-step sequence. This will serve to integrate both the research and critiquing processes.

• Stylistic Considerations

Before beginning to critique research studies, the evaluator should realize several important aspects related to the world of publishing. First, different journals have different publication goals. The market that a group of journals appeals to varies, and so the focus of the content and style of articles accepted for publication also varies. For example, *Nursing Research* is a journal that publishes articles on the conduct or results of research in nursing. The *Journal of Obstetric, Gynecologic, and Neonatal Nursing* also publishes research articles, but it also reflects articles related to the knowledge, experience, trends, and policies in obstetric, gynecological, and neonatal nursing. The emphasis in this latter journal is broader in that it contains topical as well as research articles. Consequently, the style and content of the manuscript will vary according to the type of journal to which it is being submitted.

Second, the author of a research article prepares the manuscript using both personal judgment and specific guidelines. *Personal judgment* refers to the researcher's expertise that has developed in the course of designing, executing, and analyzing the study. As a result of this expertise, the researcher is in the position to make judgments about the content that is decided to be the most important to communicate to the profession. The decision is a function of the following:

- The level of the study: experimental or nonexperimental
- The focus of the study: basic, applied, or clinical
- The audience to which the results will be most appropriately communicated

Specific guidelines refer to the umbrella protocol for preparing research manuscripts. Whenever a researcher is writing an article for publication, certain content areas must be addressed in the manuscript. The following major headings are essential sections in a research report:

- Introduction
- Methodology
- Results
- Discussion

Within each of these major sections, certain decisions can be made regarding other content to be subsumed under the major headings. Table 19-1 indentifies the

laxation training in addition to their exercise therapy; a control group of 19 patients was not taught the technique. Pretesting used two instruments to measure stress levels—the Spielberger State-Anxiety Scale and selected dimensions of the Symptom Checklist-90-Revised. At the completion of the relaxation training program, both groups of patients were retested on stress-level measures.

An analysis of covariance was used to test for the effects of the relaxation training program. The findings were: (1) posttreatment mean anxiety scores for the treatment group were significantly lower (p .05) than that of the control group; and (2) the posttest scores for the treatment group were significantly lower for the dimensions of (p .01) somatization and interpersonal sensitivity and (p .05) anxiety and depression than that of the control group. No systematic changes were induced in either the obsessive-compulsive or hostility dimension scores by the relaxation program.

The principle of enhancing the physical fitness of the cardiac patient has received increased attention in the last decade. The psychologic effects of a training program on the cardiac patient are of equal importance. Investigators report that patients who have suffered myocardial infarction tend to be more depressed and anxious than the general population. Following participation in an exercise training program, these patients showed less depression and anxiety (Hellerstein and Horsten, 1966). Another technique that shows promise as a useful treatment for psychologic distress is progressive relaxation training. Since cardiac patients are apt to experience psychologic distress, provision of various modes for managing this distress is important to insure full rehabilitative efforts.

Review of the Literature

Evidence That Cardiac Patients Are Prone to Psychologic Distress: Various psychologic responses have been observed in patients with angina pectoris and myocardial infarction. Evidence from a number of studies suggests that these psychologic characteristics may represent emotional sequelae of coronary heart disease. Rime and Bonami (1973), in a study of matched samples (30 cases and 30 controls), found significantly higher scores on the anx-

iety, obsessive-compulsive, and social introversion scales of the Minnesota Multiphasic Personality Inventory (MMPI) among patients with coronary heart disease than patients with orthopedic problems. Thiel, Parker, and Bruce (1973), in studying 50 patients with myocardial infarction, reported that these men score higher on anxiety and depression scales and display some somatization than age-matched healthy controls. Wardwell and Bahnson (1973) also observed significantly greater somatization in myocardial infarction patients than healthy community and hospitalized control groups.

Several studies suggest that emotional distress may be a precursor of coronary heart disease. Bengtsson, Hallstrom, and Tibblin (1973) found patients with angina pectoris or myocardial infarction were more likely to report a history of sustained stress, including anxiety and interpersonal conflicts, than healthy subjects. Eastwood and Trevelyan (1971) studied 124 subjects with complaints of chronic anxiety and depression and a control group without these complains. Electrocardiographic abnormalities indicative of coronary disease were more frequently found in the anxious-depressed group than in the control group. Since 90% of the subjects with abnormal electrocardiograms were previously unaware of the abnormality, the possibility of

☐ Accepted for publication December 7, 1982. Patricia Bohachick, Ph.D., R.N., is an associate professor in the graduate program for Medical-Surgical Nursing at the University of Pittsburgh.

anxiety and depression as reaction to a cardiac diagnosis seemed unlikely. Medalie, Snyder, Groen, Neufeld, Goldbourt, and Riss (1973) observed high scores on anxiety scales to be associated with the later development of angina pectoris. Friedman, Ury, Klatsky, and Siegelaub (1974) reported high scores indicative of somatization to be associated with later development of myocardial infarction. In a longitudinal study of patients with coronary heart disease, Bruhn, Paredes, Adsett, and Wolf (1974) discovered depression to be associated with an increased risk of reinfarction and sudden death.

Whether emotional distress represents a risk factor for the development of coronary atherosclerosis or a reaction to the diagnosis and physical problems of cardiac pathology remains debatable. However, evidence clearly indicates that cardiac patients are inclined to experience psychologic distress.

Effect of Progressive Relaxation on Psychologic Distress: One promising stress-reducing technique is progressive relaxation training. Improvement in subjective and behavioral measures of tension and anxiety and measures of performance and well-being have been reported to occur as a result of relaxation training (Peters, Benson, and Porter, 1977). Investigators report a significant decrease in anxiety in response to relaxation training as measured by Husek and Alexander's Anxiety Differential (Borkovec, Grayson, and Cooper, 1978), the Zukerman Multiple Affect Adjective Checklist, the Spielberger State Anxiety Scale, and empirical of state anxiety, such as heart rate and systolic blood pressure (Stoudenmire, 1975).

Paul (1969) compared progressive relaxation with hypnotic relaxation and with self-relaxation in which subjects were asked to relax to the best of their ability. In general, progressive relaxation and hypnotic relaxation produced decreases in reports of anxiety and indices of physiologic arousal that were significantly different from self-relaxation, and progressive relaxation resulted in significantly greater effects than hypnotic relaxation. Since

progressive relaxation training may have a beneficial effect on psychologic distress, relaxation training may be a useful modality for promoting cardiac rehabilitation.

Hypothesis
The posttest mean of selected psychologic variables for the experimental group will be lower than that of the control group.

Method
Sample: Volunteers for the study were recruited from a cardiac exercise program that uses exercises as a therapeutic modality for promoting cardiac rehabilitation. Data on background, variables and pretreatment psychologic measures were collected on all study subjects. After pretreatment testing and in addition to their exercise therapy, 18 patients received 3 weeks of progressive relaxation training using the technique presented by Goldfried and Davison (1976). Basically, progressive relaxation training consisted of learning to systematically tense and then relax various muscle groups while at the same time learning to attend to the feelings associated with tension and relaxation. The ultimate goal was to increase the patient's ability to identify even mild tension and to effectively eliminate that tension. Control group patients (n = 19) were not taught the technique. Criterion measures to assess achievement of the relaxation response were taken on experimental group subjects during training. At the completion of the relaxation training program, both groups of patients were retested on psychologic measures.

Psychologic Distress Measures: The first measure of psychologic distress was the Anxiety State Scale of the State-Trait Anxiety Inventory (Spielberger, Gorsuch, and Lushene, 1970). This scale attempts to measure anxiety, which is defined as a transitory emotional state characterized by perceived feelings of tension, nervousness, worry, and apprehension. The scale consists of 20 statements that require people to indicate how they feel at the moment of answering the questionnaire. Respondents indicate their answers on a 4-point rating scale ranging from Not At All to Very Much. The total score is the weighed sum of all 20 responses, and ranges from a minimum score of 20 (low anxiety) to a maximum score of 80 (high anxiety).

Alpha reliability coefficients for the Anxiety State Scale range from .83 to .92. Administration of the scale under stressful and nonstressful conditions provides evidence of the construct validity of the scale. Mean scores are reported to be considerably higher under stress conditions than under normal conditions (Spielberger et al., 1970).

The Symptom Checklist-90-Revised (SCL-90-R) is a self-report scale designed to measure psychologic symptoms. The earliest form of the instrument, The Discomfort Scale, was derived from symptoms taken from the Cornell Medical Index (Parloff, Kelman, and Frank, 1954). A major revision of the scale, termed The Hopkins Symptom Checklist, was introduced by Derogatis and his associates (1974). Based on clinical experiences and psychometric analyses, the scale was subsequently revised and validated to its present form. Designed for use primarily with psychiatric patients, the scale has been shown to be sensitive to the emotional state of nonpsychiatric patients as well (Edwards, Yarvis, Mueller, Zingale, and Wagman, 1978).

In its complete form, the instrument consists of 90 items that are clustered into scores in 9 underlying symptom dimensions: somatization, anxiety, depression, interpersonal sensitivity, hostility, obsessive-compulsiveness, phobic anxiety, paranoid ideation, and psychotism. Since normative and reliability data have been established for each dimension, selected dimensions may be used with confidence. Summary definitions of the scales used in this study and the items that comprise these are presented in Table 1.

Items of the SCL-90-R are described as a list of problems and complaints that people sometimes have. The respondent is asked to indicate how much discomfort each item has caused during the past week, including the day of answering the questionnaire. Each complaint is rated on a 5-point scale of discomfort ranging from 0 (Not At All) to 4 (Extremely). The items are then clustered into scores in the underlying symptom dimensions. Scores for the subsets are computed by calculating the mean score of the questions with the subset and each has a potential range of 0 to 4.

Two forms of reliability—internal consistency and test-retest reliability—for the SCL-90-R Symptom Dimensions are reported. The consistency with which items actually represent each symptom dimension was determined from the data of 219 symptomatic volunteers. Coefficients alpha from each of the dimensions are uniformly high, ranging from .84 to .90. Test-retest reliability coefficients for the dimensions were satisfactory, ranging between a low of .78 for hostility to a high of .86 for somatization (Derogatis, 1977).

Concurrent validity of the SCL-90-R was provided by contrasting it with other established multidimensional measures of psychopathology, the MMPI, and Middlesex Hospital Questionnaire. Each symptom dimension was shown to have its highest correlation with a like symptom construct in each of these instruments (Derogatis, 1977).

Results

To insure comparability of the experimental and control group at the outset of treatment, tests for significant differences in the pretreatment psychologic distress measures of patients in the experimental and control groups were done using an independent t test. Table 2 presents the means, standard deviations and t-test results. The t scores indicated that the two groups did not differ significantly on the various pretreatment distress level scores. Any changes on the posttreatment measures could be interpreted more confidently because of the similarity of the groups.

After establishing that there were no significant differences in the pretreatment scores of the two groups, each psychologic variable was subjected to analysis of covariance. This analysis enabled a comparison of posttreatment psychologic distress scores in both groups by statistically controlling for any differences in the pretreatment scores that were present but not significant.

The Spielberger State-Anxiety Inventory: Mean scores for this scale administered before and after the relaxation program to experimental and control groups and adjusted posttreatment mean scores are presented in Table 3. Table 4 shows the adjusted means between and within groups and the results of the F

• *Table 1*   **Summary Definitions of the Six SCL-90-R Symptom Dimensions—cont'd**

Symptom dimension	Dimension definition

I. Somatization: The *Somatization* dimension reflects distress arising from perceptions of bodily dysfunction. Complaints focused on cardiovascular, gastrointestinal, respiratory, and other systems with strong autonomic mediation are included. Headaches, pain, and discomfort of the gross musculature and additional somatic equivalents of anxiety are components of the definition. These symptoms and signs have all been demonstrated to have high prevalence in disorders demonstrated to have a functional etiology, although all may be reflections of true physical disease.

II. Depression: The symptoms of the *Depression* dimension reflect a broad range of the manifestations of clinical depression. Symptoms of dysphoric mood and affect are represented as are signs of withdrawal of life interest, lack of motivation, and loss of vital energy. In addition, feelings of hopelessness, thoughts of suicide, and other cognitive and somatic correlates of depression are included.

III. Anxiety: The *Anxiety* dimension is composed of a set of symptoms and signs that are associated clinically with high levels of manifest anxiety. General signs such as nervousness, tension, and trembling are included in definition, as are panic attacks and feelings of terror. Cognitive components involving feelings of apprehension and dread, and some of the somatic correlates of anxiety are also included as dimensional components.

IV. Interpersonal Sensitivity: The *Interpersonal Sensitivity* dimension focuses on feelings of personal inadequacy and inferiority, particularly in comparison with others. Self-depreciation, feelings of uneasiness, and marked discomfort during interpersonal interactions are characteristic manifestations of this syndrome. In addition, individuals with high scores on INT report acute self-consciousness and negative expectancies concerning the communications and interpersonal behaviors with others.

V. Obsessive-Compulsive: The *Obsessive-Compulsive* dimension reflects symptoms that are highly identified with the same name. This measure focuses on thoughts, impulses and actions that are experienced as unremitting and irresistible by the individual but are of an ego-alien or unwanted nature. Behaviors and experiences of a more general cognitive performance attenuation are also included in this measure.

VI. Hostility: The *Hostility* dimension reflects the thoughts, feelings or actions that are characteristic of the negative affect state of anger. The selection of items includes all three modes of manifestation and reflects qualities such as aggression, irritability, rage and resentment.

(Derogatis, 1977, pp.7-10)

test. The F test results for the adjusted mean changes in State-Anxiety scores were statistically significant ($p > .05$)

The Symptom Checklist-90-Revised: Pretreatment mean scores for the various dimensions of the SCL-90-R were slightly higher for the experimental group than those of the control group (Table 5). Posttreatment mean scores for each dimension were lower than pretreatment scores in both groups. The results of the analysis of covariance for the SCL-90-R dimension scores are presented in Table 6. Posttreatment mean scores for the experimental group were significantly lower for the symptom dimensions of ($p < .01$) somatization and interpersonal sensitivity and ($p < .05$) anxiety and depression than that of the control group. No systematic changes were induced in either the obsessive-compulsive or hostility dimension scores by the relaxation program.

Discussion

At the initial measurement session, the experimental group reported slightly more distress as measured by the selected dimensions of the SCL-90-R and the Spielberger State Anxiety Inventory than did the control group. While the differences in the mean scores between the two groups were not statistically significant,

the scores may have reflected a true difference between experimental and control group subjects. In an effort to insure honesty in answering the self-report items, confidentiality was assured and participants were reminded that the validity of the results depended on their answering as truthfully as possible. However, in anticipation of an intervention strategy, experimental subjects may have been more careful in recalling and/or reporting their symptoms.

The relaxation program produced a decrease in state anxiety in the trained group, which was significantly lower than that of a comparable group of untrained patients. These results are consistent with those of other investigators who report a reliable drop on the Spielberger State Anxiety Scale in response to relaxation procedures (Edelman, 1970, Stoudenmire, 1975).

There was strong support to indicate that the relaxation training programs improved self-report psychologic distress levels of the patients in the study group. Patients trained in relaxation techniques reported significantly less anxiety, interpersonal sensitivity, depression, and somatization than control group patients. These results may be contrasted with those of a study on the effects of relaxation response breaks in a working population that

• *Table 2* **Means, Standard Deviations and t Tests on Pretreatment Stress Measures for the Experimental and Control Group**

Variable	Experimental (N = 18)		Control (N = 19)		
	mean	SD	mean	SD	t Value
State anxiety	33.17	8.47	30.37	8.06	1.03
Somatization	5.67	3.91	4.84	3.91	.64
Depression	6.72	3.75	5.89	3.96	.65
Anxiety	4.33	3.36	2.95	2.82	1.36
Interpersonal sensitivity	4.11	3.07	3.95	2.53	.18
Obsessive compulsive	8.06	4.98	6.58	5.10	.89
Hostility	3.11	2.30	2.53	1.95	.84

• *Table 3* **Pretest, Posttest, and Adjusted Posttest Means for Anxiety State Scores**

Group	Pretest	Posttest	Adjusted posttest
Experimental	33.17	29.06	28.17
Control	30.37	31.58	32.42

• *Table 4* **Summary of ANCOVAS for Anxiety State Scale**

Adjusted MS between	Adjusted MS within	F (1, 34)
162.11	21.97	7.38*

$*p < .05$

used comparable measures of well-being. Peters, Benson, and Porter (1977) compared a group of subjects taught relaxation techniques with a group that received no instructions on four indices of well-being; a symptom index, illness index, performance index, and sociability-satisfaction index. The symptom index, which included a list of 51 symptoms, was comparable to the somatization scale used in this study. Additionally, a number of symptoms from the symptom index and items from the performance index of Peters et al. study (1977) mirrored the depression scale used in this study. Items from the sociability-satisfaction index could be correlated with items from the interpersonal sensitivity scale used in this study. Peters et al. (1977) found a statistically significant improvement on each of the four indices of well-being for the group practicing the relaxation technique as compared to the group that received no relaxation instruction.

Significant findings did not occur for the obsessive-compulsive or hostility symptom dimensions as had been expected for the study sampling. Other researchers also report this dimension unchanged by selected stress-management intervention strategies. Grimm (1971) reported that muscle tension and relaxation effected changes in the anxiety scale but not in the hostility scale of the Multiple Affect Adjective Checklist. Baker and Lynn (1979) found significantly lower anxiety and depression but no change in hostility levels in nurses who received interventions designed to assist them in dealing with stress.

The finding that the symptom dimensions of obsessive-compulsive and hostility were not relieved by relaxation training raises the question of whether these dimensions reflect symptomatology impervious to change or whether specific psychologic interventions other than relaxation training might be necessary to alleviate these symptoms. A study on the effect of hospitalization in supporting the coping mechanisms of cancer patients that showed a reduction in the obsessive-compulsive and hostility dimensions of the SCL-90-R merely as a result of hospitalization (Craig and Abeloff, 1974) would tend to make this first interpretation less likely. In support of the second interpretation, Novaco (1976) found a combination of cognitive self-control procedures and relaxation to be an effective tech-

• *Table 5* **Pretest, Posttest, and Adjusted Posttest Means for SCL-90-R Symptom Scores**

Scale		Pretest	Posttest	Adjusted posttest
Somatization	Experimental	5.67	2.67	2.46
	Control	4.84	4.52	4.72
Depression	Experimental	6.72	3.61	3.41
	Control	5.89	5.26	5.45
Anxiety	Experimental	4.33	1.78	1.42
	Control	2.95	2.74	3.08
Interpersonal sensitivity	Experimental	4.11	1.94	1.89
	Control	3.95	3.74	3.79
Obsessive-compulsive	Experimental	8.06	6.06	5.55
	Control	6.58	5.47	5.95
Hostility	Experiment	3.11	2.44	2.21
	Control	2.53	1.89	2.12

• *Table 6* **Summary of ANCOVAS for SCL-90-R Symptom Measures**

Scale	Adjusted means between	Adjusted means within	$F(1, 34)$
Somatization	46.73	3.93	11.88**
Depression	38.25	5.69	6.72*
Anxiety	24.15	3.04	7.94*
Interpersonal sensitivity	33.36	3.12	10.68**
Obsessive-compulsive	1.39	5.73	0.24
Hostility	0.08	2.09	0.04

$*p < .05$
$**p < .01$

nique in the treatment of chronic anger problems. The cognitive procedures involved cognitive restructuring of experiences to provoke anger and the use of self-statements to manage anger. Friedman and Roseman (1974) advocated behavior modification techniques as a strategy for reducing hostility and obsessive-compulsive behavior.

Conclusions

The investigation demonstrated that it is feasible to incorporate relaxation training into a cardiac exercise program; and that, compared to a control group, cardiac patients trained in relaxation techniques demonstrate significant improvement in psychologic distress measures. The findings of this study indicate that multiple dependent variables are required to sufficiciently evaluate the effects of a relaxation training program. Other researchers point out that "the relaxation response appears to influence many different aspects of physical and psychic health, but not necessarily the same aspects in different individuals" (Peters et al., 1977, p. 952). Therefore, measures of a number of parameters are necessary for satisfactorily evaluating the effectiveness of relaxation training.

The significant findings of this study show a need for more extensive research regarding the use of relaxation training as a stress management technique for cardiac patients. In this study, relaxation training was introduced as a technique that must be regularly practiced for positive effects of treatment to be accrued and maintained. However, it was acknowledged

that once learned, some subjects would practice the technique only during periods of increased stress. Follow-up studies are indicated to determine patterns in the use of the technique. Studies that investigate alternate indices of changes with relaxation training would be helpful. Finally, studies that include not only pretreatment and posttreatment data but also a series of follow-up long term assessments are needed to investigate the duration of the effect of relaxation training.

Progressive relaxation training is a stress-reducing technique advocated for use in clinical nursing practice (Garbin, 1979). Identifying methods for validating the effectiveness of this investigation is important. The positive findings of this study suggest that relaxation may be an effective nursing intervention in promoting rehabilitation of cardiac patients.

• References

Baker, B.S., and Lynn, M.R. (1979). Psychiatric nursing consultation: the use of an inservice model to assist nurses in the grief process, *Journal of Psychiatric Nursing and Mental Health Services,* **17**:15-19.

Bengtsson, C., Hallstrom, R., and Tibblin, G. (1973). Social factors, stress experience and personality traits in women with ischemic heart disease, compared to a population sample of women, *Acta Medica Scandinavica,* **54**:82-92.

Borovec, T.D., Grayson, J.B., and Cooper, K.M. (1978). Treatment of general tension: subjective and physiologic effects of progressive relaxation, *Journal of Consulting and Clinical Psychology,* **46**:518-528.

Bauhn, J.G., Paredes, A., Adsett, C.A., and Wolf, S. (1974). Psychological predictors of sudden death in myocardial infarction, *Journal of Psychosomatic Research* **18**:187-191.

Craig, T.J., and Abeloff, M.D. (1974). Psychiatric symptomatology among hospitalized cancer patients, *American Journal of Psychiatry,* **131**:1323-1327.

Derogatis, L.R. (1977). SCL-90-R (Revised) version, *Manual I.* Baltimore, Johns Hopkins University.

Derogatis, L.R., Lipman, R.S., Rickels, K., Uhlenhulth, E.H., and Covi, L. (1974). The

Hopkins symptom checklist (HSCL): a self-report symptom inventory, *Behavioral Science,* **19**:1-15.

Eastwood, M.R., and Trevelyan, H. (1971). Stress and coronary heart disease, *Journal of Psychosomatic Research,* **15**:289-292.

Edelman, R. (1970). Effects of progressive relaxation on automatic processes, *Journal of Clinical Psychology,* **26**:421-425.

Edwards, D.W., Yarvis, R.M., Mueller, D.P., Zingale, H.C., and Wagman, W.J. (1978). Test-taking and the stability of adjustment scales, *Evaluation Quarterly,* **2**:275-291.

Friedman, G., Ury, H.K., Klatsky, A.L., and Siegelaub, A.B. (1974). A psychological questionnaire predictive of myocardial infarction: results from the Kaiser permanenta epidemiologic study of myocardial infarction, *Psychosomatic Medicine,* **36**:327-349.

Friedman, M., and Rosenman, R.H. (1974). *Type A behavior and your heart,* New York, Alfred A. Knopf, Inc.

Garbin, M. (1979). Stress research in clinical settings, *Topics in Clinical Nursing,* **1**:87-95.

Goldfried, M.R., and Davison, G.C. (1976). *Clinical behavior therapy,* New York, Holt, Rinehart, and Winston, Inc.

Grimm, P.F. (1971). Anxiety change produced by

self-induced muscle tension and by relaxation with respiration feedback, *Behavior Therapy,* **2:**11-17.

Hellerstein, H.K., and Horsten, T. (1966). Assessing and preparing the patient for return to a meaningful and productive life, *Journal of Rehabilitation,* **22:**46-52.

Medalie, J.H., Synder, M., Groen, J.J., Neufeld, H.N., Goldbourt, V., and Riss, E. (1973). Angina pectoris among 10,000 men: 5 year incidence and univariate analysis, *American Journal of Medicine,* **55:**583-594.

Novaco, R.W. (1979). Treatment of chronic anger through cognitive and relaxation controls, *Journal of Consulting and Clinical Psychology,* **44:**681.

Parloff, M.B., Kelman, H.C., and Frank, J.D. (1954). Comfort, effectiveness and self-awareness as criteria of improvement in psychotherapy, *American Journal of Psychiatry,* **111:**343-351.

Paul, G.L. (1969). Physiological effects of relaxation training hypnotic suggestion, *Journal of Abnormal Psychology,* **74:**425-437.

Peters, R.K., Benson, H., and Porter, D. (1977). Daily relaxation response breaks in a working population: Part I. Effects on self-reported measures of health performance and well-being, *American Journal of Public Health,* **67:**946-952.

Rime, B., and Bonami, M. (1973). Specificite psychosomatique et affections cardiaques coronariennes: Essai de verification de la theorie de Dunbar au moyen du MMPI, *Journal of Psychosomatic Research,* **17:**345-352.

Spielberger, C.D., Gorsuch, R.L., and Lushene, R.E. (1970). *STAI manual for the state-trait-anxiety inventory,* Palo Alto, Calif., Consulting Psychologists Press.

Stoudenmire, J. (1975). A comparison of muscle relaxation training and music in the reduction of state and trait anxiety, *Journal of Clinical Psychology,* **31:**490-492.

Thiel, H.G., Parker, D, and Bruce, T.A. (1973). Stress factors and the risk of myocardial infarction, *Journal of Psychosomatic Research,* **17:**43-57.

Wardwell, W.I., and Bahnson, C.B. (1973). Behavior variables and myocardial infarction in the Southeastern Connecticut heart study, *Journal of Chronic Disease,* **26:**447-461.

Williams, B., and White, P.D. (1961). Rehabilitation of the cardiac patient, *American Journal of Cardiology,* **7:**317-319.

• Introduction to Critique

The introduction of the study immediately informs the reader about the topical nature of this study's focus. The focus is specific, that is, modes of intervention that decrease psychological distress in cardiac patients. The delineation of the focus is immediately followed by supporting statements that provide a rationale for the direction of the study. This includes a reference to previous work in the area. The points that substantiate the evaluation are the following:

- Investigators report that patients who have suffered myocardial infarctions tend to be more depressed and anxious than the general population.
- Following participation in an exercise training program, three patients showed less depression and anxiety.
- Another technique that shows promise as a useful treatment for psychiatric distress is progressive relaxation training.
- Since cardiac patients are apt to experience psychological distress, it is important to provide various modes for managing this distress to ensure full rehabilitative efforts.

The problem statement is not identified in a separate section, nor is it clearly embedded in the context of the introductory section. The reader is able to infer that the independent variable is a relaxation training program of some kind. However, it remains unclear at this point as to what the dependent variable will be. It would be helpful to the reader if a firm sense of which of the many psychological variables the investigator intended to study were provided.

The literature review is very well done. The author cites selected studies pertinent to the investigation that have specific significance to supporting the premise of the study. A logical continuity between previous work and this project is evident throughout the two subsections of the literature review.

A theoretical framework is not clearly evident. It seems as if the author might have been using a stress and adaptation theory. The use of multiple psychological variables such as anxiety, depression, somatization, and obsessive-compulsive symptoms suggests that there might be a logical unifying theoretical framework. However, none is specified in the article.

Conceptual definitions are presented in Table 1 and operationalized by the Anxiety State Scale of the STAI as well as the Symptom Checklist-90-Revised (SCL-90-R). The conceptual definition of state anxiety is also included in the section titled *Psychological Distress Measures*. The completeness of the aforementioned section provides a clear picture of the nature of the variables.

There is one hypothesis in this study. It is declarative, directional, clear, testable, and concise. The hypothesis indicates the use of an experimental group and a control group. However, it does not precisely specify the sample under consideration.

• Methodology

The methodology section informs the reader of how the researcher conducted the study. Enough detail should be provided that would permit the study to be replicated if so desired. In addition, enough description should be evident so that the reader is able to evaluate the appropriateness of the methodology.

Two problems regarding the nature of the sample and its selection are evident. First, the precise nature of the subjects in the sample is not adequately presented. The common subject criteria presented besides the sample size (n = 37) were that all subjects were participants in a cardiac exercise program and that subjects did not differ significantly in pretest psychological variables. However, this does not indicate important demographic variables, such as age, sex, mental status, type and duration of cardiac problem, length of time in exercise program, and any medication regimen. These variables are important considerations to control for in the data analysis, because they have implications for the external validity or generalizability of the study. Indeed, these variables may have been considered and controlled for by the researcher, but the lack of data presented leaves the critiquer in a quandary about the equivalence of the subjects in this area.

Second, it is unclear whether probability or nonprobability sampling procedures were utilized. For example, the author states that an experimental group and a control group were employed. However, it is not evident whether random selection was used to assign subjects to the experimental and control groups, or if a quota form of a convenience sample was used instead. The type of sampling method that was used has implications for internal validity. For example, if random selection was used, the integrity of the experimental design is maintained. On the other hand, if a convenience sample was used, selection bias may have been introduced to the study.

The instruments selected as the tools for this study are both psychometrically well developed. The author logically presents the reliability and validity data related to the instruments as well as their conceptual basis. For example, the internal consistency reliability for the STAI's Anxiety State Scale and the SCL-90-R Symptom Dimensions are reported and discussed by the author. She also discusses the appropriateness of the tools in light of the variables being measured in *this* study. This point is being stressed because research studies may sometimes employ tools that are *not* theoretically consistent with the variables being studied. Authors then go on to make generalizations regarding the data based on tool results that are not comparable with the variables being explored.

A summary of the steps of the procedure, of what and how the researcher operationalized the investigation, is evident. Although the author does not present a step-by-step format of how the relaxation training program was conducted, she does give a basic description and goal of the technique. The reader is then referred to Goldstein and Davison's technique of progressive relaxation training (1976) for further details. This type of presentation enables the reviewer to have a brief, but clear picture of what the procedure was and how it was accomplished. There is also adequate description of the pretest and posttest procedure for assessing the psychological variable that is consistent with the standards of a quasi-experimental design.

Ethical procedures designed to protect the human rights of the subjects are addressed. The researcher notes that confidentiality was assured. This assurance meets ethical standards for the conduct of a research project.

• Results

In this study, the collected data and its statistical treatment are appropriately summarized. The statistical tests applied to the pretest and posttest data are named; how the statistical tests were applied in the testing periods was explained. Tabular presentation of the data facilitates the reporting of the results. It is evident which of the psychological variables were statistically significant and which were not. The succinct presentation of the results allows the critiquer to move into the discussion section where decisions regarding the evaluation and interpretation of the research results are made.

• Discussion

An important aspect of the discussion is how the researcher finally weaves together the findings with every other element of the research process. This investigator makes excellent use of the discussion section. Each aspect of the measurement tools and findings was reexamined in light of theoretical underpinnings of the study. For example, the author indicates that the decrease in state anxiety was significantly lower than that of a comparable group of untrained patients and goes on to state that this finding is consistent with other investigators who also report a reliable drop on the State Anxiety Scale of the STAI in response to relaxation procedures and cites the appropriate reference.

The author's unbiased approach to the discussion is apparent in that she also examines the results in terms of questions raised by the nonsignificant findings. She attempts to draw inferences based on both supportive and nonsupportive results. For example, the author cites that:

> Significant findings did not occur for the obsessive-compulsive or hostility symptom dimensions. . . .

She used the lack of support regarding this finding to raise the question:

> . . . of whether these dimensions reflect symptomatology impervious to change or whether specific psychologic interventions other than relaxation training might be necessary to alleviate the symptoms (p.286-287).

A question raised for the reviewer in the discussion section is whether the Hawthorne effect was operative in this study. The reader is told that the experimental subjects may have been more careful in recalling or reporting their symptoms in anticipation of an intervention strategy. Indeed, if the intervention group knew that they were the experimental subjects, their response to the relaxation program and in the recall or reporting of symptoms may have been biased. That is, the subjects may have felt that they were part of a "special" group and might have tended to respond to the testing and relaxation program in a way that spuriously enhanced the seeming effect of the treatment program. A critiquer must raise a question about whether or not this contaminating factor could have influenced the differential findings between the experimental and control groups.

The author does not specifically indicate the limitations of the study, especially with regard to generalizability. However, she does explicitly propose the need for further research in this area. For example, she indicates the need for a follow-up study to determine the patterns in the use of the relaxation technique, alternate indices of changes with relaxation training, and longitudinal follow-up to determine the duration or effect of relaxation training. The critiquer should also be aware of the value of replicating a study such as this so that the knowledge base about this phenomenon can be refined and extended.

The findings and recommendations of the study have implications for nursing. Theoretically, in this study it builds on the concept of anxiety in relation to cardiac patients. However, anxiety is a concept integral with the delivery of care to a broad scope of patients as well. As such, this research impinges on related aspects of nursing theory, education, and practice.

• Other Aspects of the Study

The type of design is not explicitly stated. However, the author's presentation implies to the critiquer that a quasi-experimental design was employed. This design appears appropriate to the problem being studied. If the investigator had used random assignment of subjects to experimental and control groups, a true experimental design would also have been appropriate.

The title of the study clearly reflects the investigator's intent and reflects the focus of the study. The abstract was presented at the beginning of the study and briefly summarizes the content and purpose of the study. The review can quickly survey the content of the abstract to gain an idea of the nature of the study.

• • •

In summary, this study represents a quasi-experimental investigation that has many merits. The researcher's effort to adhere to the scientific approach is evident. The weaknesses of the study that were noted in the critique may, in fact, have been a function of the many realistic pragmatic constraints that a researcher inevitably encounters. This research project is an excellent example of how a nurse has utilized the research process to add to the body of nursing knowledge. The critiquer can now evaluate the strengths and weaknesses of the study to determine its potential applicability to clinical practice.

• References

Bohachick, P. (1984). Progressive relaxation training in cardiac rehabilitation: effect on psychological variables, *Nursing Research,* Sept./Oct., **33**:(5)283-287.

Downs, F.S., and Newman, M.A. (1977). *A source book of nursing rsearch,* Philadelphia, F.A. Davis Co.

Jaecox, A. and Prescott, P. (1978). Determining a study's relevance for clinical practice, *American Journal of Nursing,* **78**:1822-1889.

Kerlinger, F.N. (1973). *Foundations of behavioral research,* (2nd ed.) New York, Holt, Rinehart, & Winston, Inc.

Publication Manual of the American Psychological Association (1983). Washington, D.C.

Stetler, C.B., and Marram, G. (1976). Evaluating research for applicability in practice, *Nursing Outlook,* **24**:559-563.

20

Utilizing Nursing Research

Rona F. Levin

•

LEARNING OBJECTIVES

After reading this chapter, the student should be able to do the following:
- Identify the factors that contribute to the gap between the dissemination and the use of nursing research findings.
- Describe the mechanisms that facilitate the utilization of research findings in nursing practice.
- Apply the criteria for research utilization to the evaluation of findings for implementation in practice.
- Compare and contrast nursing research and the evaluation of practice innovations.

KEY TERMS

construct replication
replication
research base
scientific merit

Previous chapters have explored the significance of research to the practice of nursing, described the research process, and provided guidelines for the critical evaluation of research reports. Throughout this book the emphasis has been placed on your role as a consumer of nursing research. The reason for this emphasis is that the goal of research and theory development in nursing is to develop knowledge that will guide professional practice (Donaldson and Crowley, 1978). As a profession, nursing is ultimately responsible for the provision of safe and effective health care to society. Thus the ultimate purpose of research and theory development in nursing is to provide a "validated body of knowledge on which to base [this] practice" (Fawcett, 1984, p. 62).

This chapter will focus on the implementation of the role of the nursing research consumer. It begins by highlighting the present gap between research and practice, the factors that contribute to that gap, and suggestions for bridging, if not closing, the gap. The section on *utilization criteria* explores how to go about integrating research findings into practice. In other words, now that you have acquired some knowledge of the research process, what do you do with it? Unless professional practitioners of nursing use research in their practice, the goal of research and theory development in nursing will not be reached.

• The Gap Between Research and Practice

Unfortunately, a tremendous gap exists between the dissemination and the use of research findings in nursing practice. Studies conducted by Ketefian (1975a) and Kirchoff (1982) highlight this problem.

For example, Ketefian wanted to find out if nurses were using research findings in client care settings. She identified oral temperature determination as a common, frequent practice that had been studied and replicated. *Replication* is the repetition of a study in different settings with different samples, taken from the same or different populations. The findings of these studies had been widely disseminated for at least 5 years before her investigation.

The *research base* or group of studies on oral temperature determination indicated that the usual practice of placing a thermometer sublingually for 2 to 4 minutes did not reflect an accurate body temperature. More specifically, Nichols and Verhonick found that the optimum placement time was 9 minutes (cited in Ketefian, 1975a).

Ketefian (1975a) surveyed 87 registered nurses in New York and Massachusetts from a variety of employment settings regarding their practices of temperature determination. She found that only one nurse gave the correct placement time for an oral thermometer. Furthermore, although the majority of respondents indicated that they thought the rectal mode was more accurate, they continued to use the oral mode in practice.

Another example of the gap that exists between the reporting of research findings and their use in practice is the results of Kirchoff's study (1982). She surveyed a nation-wide sample of critical care nurses to "assess the impact of the published studies on the practices of restricting ice water and the measurement of rectal temperature" in cardiac patients (p. 196). Although reported research findings did not validate that these coronary precautions were necessary, they were still widely practiced. In addition, nurses' awareness of the published research was not related to changes in their practice.

Thus, as Horsley, Crane, and Bingle (1978) have pointed out, little evidence exists to indicate that research findings are being incorporated into practice. Nursing must come to terms with this issue to be accepted as a professional discipline that bases its practice on a valid body of knowledge.

CONTRIBUTING FACTORS

What are the reasons for the gap between research and practice? They can be broadly classified under the categories of educational preparation, communication, organizational resources, and resistance to change.

Educational Preparation

In nursing, the professional practitioner is prepared at the baccalaureate level. Therefore the inclusion of research-related content in undergraduate nursing curricula is usually reserved for baccalaureate programs. However, it is well known that the majority of practicing nurses are graduates of diploma or associate degree programs. Thus the majority of nurses who are expected to implement research findings in their practice do not have the educational preparation required to do this. Moreover, the focus of many research courses at the baccalaureate level is on the process of conducting research and the critical evaluation of research reports. Rarely has the area of utilization been dealt with in an adequate fashion (Kirchhoff, 1983). Thus neither the professional nor the technical nurse have had the knowledge and skill needed for using research findings in practice.

Communication

Another factor that contributes to the gap between the dissemination and the use of research findings is the way that studies are communicated to the profession. For the most part, research reports appear in research journals, publications that the majority of practicing nurses do not read. Even if practitioners do read the published reports, they do not fully understand them. The presentation, which includes the use of research jargon, is aimed at an audience with an advanced knowledge of research design and statistics, namely, other researchers.

Furthermore, nurses who are involved in either direct client care or in the management of that care do not usually attend conferences where research findings are disseminated. They either do not know of their existence, have not been encouraged to attend, or do not see the relevance of these conferences to their practice. As a consequence, those nurses who are in the best position to use the research findings disseminated at these conferences do not know of their existence.

Organizational Resources

The organizational factors that can either facilitate or hinder research utilization in a service setting include the research climate, the availability of consultation, and the financial support.

The Research Climate   To be able to question current practices within our profession, an atmosphere of intellectual curiosity and freedom of thought must prevail in the workplace as well as in our educational institutions. Unfortunately, as Ketefian (1957b) has stated, "there is a deeply ingrained adherence to tradition, authoritative sources, the 'procedure manual,' 'the way we were taught,' that makes it difficult to make room for the new" (p.26). Coupled with the nonresearch attitudes that may exist within nursing services are the attitudes of physicians and administrators regarding nursing's place within the organization. For the most part, the latter group still believes nursing's primary role is to carry out the physician's orders. The majority of physicians and hospital administrators are not even aware that nursing has its own body of knowledge that is different from medical knowledge. Even fewer are cognizant of the fact that some nurses are prepared educationally at the doctoral level to conduct their own research related to nursing phenomena, or that nurses are capable of collaborating on interdisciplinary research projects as peers.

The Availability of Consultation   Traditionally, doctorally prepared nurses who possess the skills needed to carry out research related activities have been employed in academic settings. Concurrently, the nurses who are involved in the delivery of care and who are most familiar with the kinds of clinical problems that need to be addressed are employed in service settings. Unfortunately, there has been little communication between these two groups. Ketefian (1975b) suggested that the functions of developing and applying knowledge "cannot be adequately performed either by the practitioner or the researcher-scholar as that role is presently conceived, and that we probably need to conceive of new researcher roles or, in any case, a breed that has one foot in the world of research and the other in the world of practice" (p. 14).

However, many nurses, concerned about the lack of communication between researchers and practitioners have begun to reach out to each other and realize each other's worth. A few schools of nursing and clinical agencies have begun to work together in both formal and informal relationships. The establishment of joint appointments in research between education and service is an example of a formal mechanism that provides an available research consultant to both groups. An example of an informal mechanism is the establishment of a consultative relationship between a staff nurse and her former teacher for the purpose of engaging in a research study or utilization project.

Financial Support   In today's health care system with the advent of Diagnostic Related Groupings (DRGs) and the push toward cost containment, financial resources are limited. Thus even if the research climate in a given organization is favorable and consultation is readily available, the researcher still has to contend with the limited amount of funds available for both the conduct and utilization of nursing research.

Financial resources consist of the time that the nurse is released from the usual nursing responsibilities as well as the direct outlay of funds. In a recent survey conducted by Levin et al. (1983) to assess the research climate in a large suburban medical center, the great majority of nurses responded that lack of time was the greatest barrier to their involvement in research activities.

Resistance to Change

Most people are comfortable with the status quo. They are used to established routines and traditional ways of approaching problems. Every individual or group has a system of internalized values, beliefs, or attitudes that guide behavior. A proposed change that is perceived as threatening to this system is likely to result in resistance. Other factors that contribute to resistance to change include the following (Mauksch and Miller, 1981):

1. Lack of a felt need.
2. Lack of knowledge about the change program.
3. Threat to security.
4. Behavior of the change agent.

For example, when the introduction of a practice innovation is the change that is planned, the nursing staff may perceive it as a threat to their security because of a real inadequacy. That is, they are not familiar with the new practice and may question their ability to implement it. When the sources of resistance are known, they can be dealt with in a constructive manner.

However, not all opposition to change is defined as resistance. When change is opposed for logical reasons based on valid data it is considered rational behavior (Mauksch and Miller, 1981). For example, a policy established at hospital X requires nurses to discard intravenous bags that have been removed from their outer wrappings and not used within 24 hours. Nurse Y has become attuned to cost-effective practices, sees this policy as very expensive, and wonders if it is supported by research findings. She reviews the literature and calls the company that manufactures the intravenous bags to obtain information related to the growth of organisms in unwrapped bags. Her search indicates that the outer wrap is not sterile to begin with, and studies have shown that bacterial growth does not occur any more often in unwrapped bags than it does in wrapped bags. Thus she opposes the new policy on logical grounds and is supported by facts.

It is also important to distinguish between resistance and interference. *Interference* is defined as those forces that hamper progress toward the change objective without being directly concerned with it (Lippett, Watson, and Westley, 1958, Chapter 4). It usually stems from a lack of resources needed to implement the change.

These resources consist of time, energy, money, and qualified personnel. Let us imagine that you and your colleagues have read several studies that you believe to have relevance to your practice. You have obtained an informal consultation with a former teacher to evaluate these studies and validate your thinking. You wish to develop a proposal for implementation and evaluation of the research findings in your client care area. Because the members of your group have not attempted such a project before, you are not sure how to proceed and need additional consultation. Your former teacher, although interested in helping you, does not consider it possible to devote the necessary time and energy to the project without receiving financial reimbursement from your agency. Your group approaches the director of nursing, who has shown enthusiasm for your ideas, to ask for the necessary funds. She informs you that the nursing budget has already been submitted and approved for this year, and it did not include the services of a nursing research consultant. She goes on to say that she will try to include such an item in next year's budget, and so the project will have to be postponed. This is an example of an interfering force.

CLOSING THE GAP

Although the factors that contribute to the gap between the production and the use of knowledge may appear to be overwhelming, several mechanisms for narrowing the gap can be suggested. Some of these have been attempted on a limited basis. These mechanisms will be discussed in relation to the contributing factors outlined earlier.

Educational Preparation

Professional nursing practitioners should be prepared to be intelligent research consumers. This includes the ability to critically evaluate reported studies and to determine which findings may be applicable to practice. One course in research methods taught in isolation from the rest of the curriculum fails to do this. As Levin (1983) has pointed out previously, "students do not come to perceive research as real or as related to their role as clinical practitioners" (p. 258).

One approach that may foster critical thinking about practice is to integrate research concepts throughout the curriculum. Instead of teaching fundamental nursing skills from the perspective of tradition and authority, research findings that support the demonstrated technique can be cited (Levin, 1983). For example, placing a client in a prone position with femurs internally rotated for the administration of a dorsogluteal injection has been taught for years as a valid practice to reduce discomfort. In theory, this position was supposed to result in a relaxed muscle that would reduce the discomfort of an injection. However, only recently was this hypothesis supported by research findings (Kruszewski, Lang, and Johnson, 1979).

Granted that the educator has the responsibility of integrating such concepts into a curriculum, it behooves you, as a nursing student or practitioner, to question and challenge the principles and procedures that you are taught either in school or on the job. As a professional nurse, you are responsible and accountable for seeking validation for your practice and for guiding the practice of those nurses who are not prepared at the professional level and who may not have been exposed to the perspective and methods of scientific inquiry.

Consider the following example, based on an actual incident. A staff nurse working on a surgical unit had taken a course on the uses of acupuncture and acupressure. She decided to try using an acupressure technique with some clients for the alleviation of postoperative pain. Her experience suggested that the technique might be an effective pain reduction innovation. It so happened that a nurse researcher employed by the hospital and an undergraduate student interested in participating in a research project as part of her clinical practicum were assigned to this unit. Because of the staff nurse's interest in acupressure, it was decided that the student would conduct a literature review to determine what prior research had been done in this area. The search revealed that no studies on the effectiveness of acupressure for pain relief had been published. Furthermore, the only literature found on the topic consisted of "how to" manuals. In reading these manuals, it was discovered that the administration of a great deal of pressure on various body areas was advocated for pain relief. However, this treatment was not suggested for postoperative pain. It became obvious that the administration of unusual pressure to a client postoperatively could result in deleterious effects. The staff nurse was, therefore, requested to discontinue her "experimentation." The point of this anecdote is to share with you the potential danger of using a treatment or technique that has not been validated through research and to encourage you to think critically about nursing practice.

Communication

The issue of communicating research findings to nurses who are involved in direct client care has begun to be addressed by some members of our profession. One direction that needs to be taken is to publish research-based articles in journals that are read by the majority of practicing nurses. In such a spirit, the *American Journal of Nursing (AJN)* recently added a regular column, "For the Research Record," that publishes summaries of completed and ongoing studies. Although some researchers are attempting to publish the results of their studies in a form that the practicing nurse would find easier to read and understand, a review of *AJN* for the period June, 1983 through June, 1984 revealed only one research-based, full-length article (Taylor, West, Simon, Skelton, and Rowlingson, 1983).

The content and format of articles that appear in journals are based on what the publisher believes will appeal to the readers. If professional nurses began writing to the journals that they read and requesting more research-based content, the appearance of such articles would increase. By the same token, more nurses at all levels of practice could encourage our profession's research journals, for example, *Nursing Research* and *Research In Nursing and Health,* to publish articles that are written in terms more understandable to the practicing nurse.

Another approach to closing the communication gap might be for you to request staff development programs on the research process, the evaluation of research studies, and research utilization. Many in-service education departments in clinical agencies survey the nursing staff to plan their educational activities. If a nurse who is able to teach this content is not available within the agency, it may be possible to contact a nearby school of nursing to arrange continuing education courses, or to request a faculty member to present classes for the nursing staff at the agency.

Finally, many nursing research conferences in the past few years have focused on the presentation of studies that are of a clinical nature and have direct applicability to practice. Some examples are the following: the comparison of different techniques for treating decubitus ulcers, the use of various relaxation techniques for decreasing pain, and the development and validation of nursing diagnoses. Attendance at these conferences would enhance a practitioner's awareness of potential practice innovations and increase her ability to understand and evaluate research findings. It is the responsibility of every professional nurse to keep up to date with the expanding body of knowledge of the discipline.

Because participation at these conferences can be costly, many nursing service departments have an educational fund that can be used to defray the cost of attending such programs. However, to receive reimbursement for expenses, for example, registration fees, transportation, and lodging, a formal request must be submitted. Ask your head nurse, supervisor, or in-service educator how to go about this. You may be asked to justify the relevance of these programs to your position at the agency. It is hoped that the information contained in this chapter will assist you in emphasizing the importance of your role as a research consumer.

Organizational Resources

The Research Climate   Clearly, the key to making the conduct and utilization of research an integral part of nursing practice is the administrator of a nursing service (Fawcett, 1980). Without this individual's support, any attempt at establishing a research utilization program cannot succeed. Therefore, it is essential that a nurse ask relevant questions about the nursing service administrator's attitude toward nursing research in general, and utilization in particular, when interviewing for a position within an organization. Ascertaining the level of education of the head of a nursing department as well as that of the nurses in middle management can be a helpful place to start. If you know that the Director of Nursing has a doctorate, you are almost assured that she or he is at least aware of the significance of nursing research to practice. On the other hand, if she or he has a bachelor's degree in another field, such as in health education or business, such an awareness may be lacking. It is also important to find out whether or not these nurses have been involved in research activities, either in their educational programs or in the practice setting, and their attitudes toward innovation and positive change.

Obtaining this kind of information may be a difficult task for you, especially if you are applying for your first job. The answers to these questions, however, will tell you something about the general attitude toward nursing within the institution as well as the specific attitude toward nursing research and its application in practice.

The following are some nonthreatening questions that can elicit these answers:
1. Can you share a copy of the job description for a staff nurse with me? Are there any additional expectations?
2. Do staff nurses get involved with research? How?
3. What are the criteria for promotion?
4. What kinds of committees does the nursing department have? Is there a research committee? How could I participate?

The manner in which these kinds of questions are answered as well as the answers themselves indicate the prevailing attitude toward nursing research within the department. If you perceive a negative attitude, you have the option of withdrawing your application for employment.

Given the existence of a positive attitude toward research within the nursing department, an ideal mechanism for facilitating the utilization of research in practice is the employment of a nurse researcher by the service agency. Such a position can take several forms, such as the following: (1) a full-time position, (2) a part-time position, (3) a consultant position, or (4) a joint appointment with a school of nursing. However, the employment of a doctorally prepared nurse who can guide research efforts within a service setting is expensive. Few agencies have been able to develop such a position within the nursing department, although there is an increasing trend in this direction.

However, there are several ways you can assist your nursing colleagues to become aware of and integrate research into their practice. A relatively simple way to begin is to form a journal club. Such a group can meet periodically to review research articles that have potential applicability to practice. Members can rotate the responsibility for finding and critiquing these studies and presenting them to the group. The discovery of a new technique or practice approach in one article may generate enough interest in the group to pursue a more thorough literature search on that topic, which can form the research base for a potential utilization project.

A more formal approach is the establishment of a nursing research committee within a department of nursing service. Among the purposes of such committees are the following: (1) creating an awareness of the need for using research findings in practice; (2) identifying clinical practice problems that require investigations (3) providing educational programs related to research utilization to nursing staff; and (4) planning, implementing, and evaluating utilization projects. Of course, to carry out these purposes, committee members must possess some knowledge of research and be able to obtain the resources they do not already possess.

The Availability of Consultation   If nurses who have the necessary educational preparation and research skill are not available within the organization, faculty members from nearby schools of nursing can be asked to join the committee. Such an arrangement not only provides needed expertise for the research committee, but can provide faculty members with a clinical setting and ideas for the conduct of their own research. It can also foster collaborative research efforts between service and education.

Intradisciplinary (within nursing) collaboration is one way of facilitating the use of research in practice. *Interdisciplinary* (between professions) collaboration is another alternative. Many innovations may be interdependent in nature and therefore would require the joint efforts of medicine and nursing. The use of a clean, as opposed to a sterile, technique for tracheostomy suctioning is one example. Another is the early discharge of a specified group of clients from the acute care setting.

Interdisciplinary collaboration begins with a colleagial relationship between different health care providers. It means having respect for the perspective and knowledge that each one brings to the client care or research situation. Because other health care providers, such as physicians, may not be aware of nursing's increasing knowledge and capabilities relative to research or its unique contribution to client care, it may be necessary to convey this in informal conversation about specific client problems or situations before broaching the idea for a collaborative research project. For example, I was part of an interdisciplinary hospital Professional Standards Review Committee a number of years ago. The committee's task was to review the records of surgical clients to determine the adequacy of postoperative pain management. The focus of the physicians and pharmacists was on the proper use of analgesics. However, as a nurse, I was able to present the potential benefits of other techniques of pain management that had previously not be considered by this group and to gain the committee's support for including items regarding these interventions (for example, positioning, touching, and relaxing) as part of the audit. When a subsequent nursing research project on the use of relaxation techniques for postoperative pain was initiated, full cooperation of these health professionals was apparent.

Implicit in interdisciplinary collaboration is the notion of equal status. That means that nurses function as coinvestigators on a study or utilization project, not just as research assistants or data collectors. To be a coinvestigator means being involved in determining the purpose and method of a research project as well as coauthoring any publications that result from it.

As nurses become more articulate about the uniqueness of their profession and more knowledgeable about the research process and implementation of research in practice, and as physicians and other members of the health care team begin to realize the unique and valuable contribution that nurses make in health care, interdisciplinary collaboration in research utilization will increase.

Financial Support   Collaborative approaches to research utilization not only provide the skill and expertise needed for the development, implementation, and evaluation of such projects, but may also decrease the investment of time and energy required by any one individual. Furthermore, expenses such as consultation fees and the purchase of computer time for data analysis can be defrayed. Faculty from a nearby school of nursing may be willing to forgo a consultation fee in exchange for authorship on a publication about the project. In addition, faculty may be able to draw on other resources that are more available in an academic setting than in a service setting. The use of computer services for statistical analysis of data, for example, may be available to faculty members for a minimal charge or at no cost.

Resistance to Change

When evaluating the potential for change, the first step is to assess the existence of interfering forces and try to eliminate them. As you will recall, these forces have to do with an absence of needed resources, such as time, energy, money, and skill. Measures that can decrease interfering forces have been described earlier.

The next step is to assess the actual or potential sources of resistance to change, described previously (see p. 298). When the sources of resistance are known, they can usually be dealt with in a constructive manner. For example, if nurses do not know what to expect from the introduction of a practice innovation, their fear of the unknown may become a resistive force. One way of preventing this is to explicitly communicate what the utilization project entails, why it is being carried out, how they will or will not be involved, and when it will take place. Such information should be provided before the project is a fait accompli so that there is time to deal with the concerns of those nurses whose support is essential to a successful project outcome.

So far we have looked at forces that can hinder the process of change. There are also forces that can facilitate the process of change, called *driving* forces. Driving forces can be both initial and emergent facilitators of the change process. Initial facilitators include the following: (1) a dissatisfaction with the present situation; (2) a realization that the situation can be improved; and (3) feelings of external pressure, such as role expectations or competitiveness. Emergent facilitators include the following: (1) the need to complete a task or project that has begun; (2) the need to meet expectations, both external and internal, and (3)an increase in insight or a developed need on the part of the individual or group involved in the change (Lippett et al., 1958, Chapter 4).

Horsley, Crane, Crabtree, and Wood (1983) have emphasized the importance of fostering an awareness of the need for change among those who will be involved in the process. They state, "Both administrative and practicing nurses must perceive some need for the change if it is to succeed" (p.4). Participation in decision making by all persons whom the change will affect can enhance interest and motivation. The use of a suggestion box, regularly scheduled meetings where new ideas are encouraged between staff nurses and those in middle management, and participation by representatives from all levels of practice in decision-making groups are all ways to increase an awareness of the need for change.

After the development of a need for a practice change is realized and relationships among involved individuals are established, planning for the change can occur. Change takes time; a great deal of frustration can result from expecting it to occur too rapidly. However, in the long run a careful, deliberative approach to the change process will increase the chances of a successful outcome.

• Utilization Criteria

Given a climate that encourages and supports the conduct and use of nursing research, how do you decide which areas of clinical research are ready for incorporation into practice? Before 1979, little assistance in this area was available in the nursing literature. As a result of a federally funded project in the mid-1970s, *Conduct and Utilization of Research in Nursing,* criteria to guide utilization efforts were established. They fall into the following three major categories (Haller, Reynolds, and Horsley, 1979):

1. Evaluating the knowledge base
2. Assessing relevance to practice
3. Determining the potential for clinical evaluation

Despite the existence of these criteria as a guide, it is not realistic to expect that you will be able to accomplish the task of research utilization on your own. However, it is essential that you understand the process and that you participate actively in it as a knowledgeable consumer. Consultation and collaboration are a necessary component of the process.

EVALUATING THE KNOWLEDGE BASE

The identification of studies that can provide a valid research base for application to practice involve the following three criteria (Haller et al., 1979; Fawcett, 1982):

1. Replication
2. Scientific merit
3. Risk

Replication

As you may recall, *replication* is the repetition of a study in different settings with different samples, taken from the same or different populations. The replication study may be conducted by the same or different investigators. The purpose of replication is to increase the generalizability of findings (Fawcett, 1982) and to decrease the chances of committing a type I error (Haller et al., 1979). This error occurs when a researcher concludes falsely that a treatment or intervention has a significant effect, but in reality, this effect has occurred by chance alone.

It has been noted that replication is not commonplace in nursing research (Fawcett, 1982). When direct replication of a study has not been attempted, it is important to find instances of *construct replication*. "Construct replication is achieved when a second investigator begins with a similar problem statement but formulates original methods of measurement and design to verify the first author's findings" (Haller et al., 1979, p.47).

The following two studies demonstrate construct replication. In the first study, Flaherty and Fitzpatrick (1978) tested the effects of a relaxation exercise on postoperative clients' comfort level when they were getting out of bed for the first time. A sample of 42 male and female clients who underwent elective surgery, such as cholecystectomy, herniorraphy, or hemorrhoidectomy, were divided into experimental and control groups. The experimental group was taught a relaxation exercise the night before surgery and was reminded to use it when getting out of bed 6 to 8 hours following surgery. Comfort level was measured by a scale on which clients indicated both the degree of sensation they were experiencing and how much distress this sensation was causing them. In addition, the investigators collected data on the amount of analgesics each group required during the first 24 postoperative hours. The results of this study showed that the experimental group experienced significantly less discomfort and required fewer analgesics than the control group.

Wells (1982), building on the work of Flaherty and Fitzpatrick, used a sample of 12 clients undergoing cholecystectomy to study a similar problem: however, she looked at clients' comfort levels during the first 3 postoperative days, not during their first ambulation. A relaxation technique that differed somewhat from the one used by Flaherty and Fitzpatrick was taught to the experimental group on the night before surgery. Wells used the same scale to measure postoperative discomfort, but her method of determining analgesic usage differed. The results did not support a difference between experimental and control groups in their use of analgesics or in sensation scores. However, in agreement with the former study, Wells found self-reported distress to be significantly different between the groups. Taken together, these studies indicate that the use of a relaxation technique has potential for the reduction of postoperative discomfort.

Ideally, a research base should consist of a synthesis of the knowledge gained from several studies whose findings are consistent. In reality, this is not always possible. It is suggested that at least two valid investigations of a similar problem be identified before an innovation is considered for application to practice (Horsley et al., 1983).

Scientific Merit

Once a research base has been identified, the scientific merit of each study that constitutes this base must be considered. Chapter 19 provides the criteria for critiquing research reports. The findings and conclusions of a study must always be evaluated in terms of the theoretical framework and design. When the goal is utilization, the population from which study samples were drawn is particularly important. Are they appropriate for the clinical problem? Has at least one study used a clinical population for hypothesis testing (Haller et al., 1979)? The results of laboratory experiments using a "normal" population cannot be generalized to a clinical setting. For example, a recent study by Geden, Beck, Hauge, and Pohlman (1984) investigated the effects of five different pain-coping strategies on the self-reported sensation of labor contractions. The sample for this research consisted of 100 nulliparous female college undergraduates. The subjects were exposed to a laboratory stimulus that simulated labor contractions. Although one of the strategies (sensory transformation) was found to have a significant effect on self-reported pain, these results cannot be generalized to a population of women who are experiencing the actual process of labor. Replication of this study using a clinical population would be necessary before these findings could be considered for use in practice.

During the process of evaluating the scientific merit of the research base, you may come across studies that have contradictory findings. As Haller et al. (1979) pointed out, "attempts are made to resolve contradictory findings either through identification of methodological weakness or through a theoretical explanation for the discrepancy. It is also recognized that in a series of replications of the same study, a nonsignificant difference may be expected to occur a certain number of times on the basis of chance alone" (p.48).

Risk

The third criterion that should be applied when evaluating research for its applicability to practice is the degree of risk involved in the new intervention. Teaching clients how to use a relaxation technique to decrease postoperative discomfort or leaving an oral thermometer in place a few more minutes are innovations that entail very little if any risk. On the other hand, the elimination of coronary precautions, such as avoiding the rectal mode of temperature determination, does involve a certain degree of risk. When an innovation has risks associated with it, a "stronger, more established" knowledge base is required than when no risk is evident (Fawcett, 1982, p.57). That is, if there is any risk to a client, it is imperative that several studies with a high degree of scientific merit that have been replicated with clinical populations form the knowledge base and support the benefits of the practice. You must always question whether the potential benefits of a new practice outweigh the risks.

ASSESSING RELEVANCE TO PRACTICE

Given a sound research base that supports the efficacy of a clinical innovation, an assessment of its relevance to practice follows. The following are questions to be addressed in such an assessment (Fawcett, 1982, p. 58):

> Does the study focus on a significant clinical practice problem?
> Do nurses have clinical control of the study variables?
> Is it feasible to implement the nursing action (if any such action was part of the study)?
> What is the cost of implementing the nursing action?

The first question involves a determination of the clinical merit of the research base. Simply put, you want to know if a problem of practical significance to nurses will be solved by instituting a new intervention. Fawcett (1982) cautions us to guard against the premature application of study findings. Even if findings appear to be ready for clinical use, they may lack a clear theoretical structure. When knowledge consists of a collection of atheoretical facts, it usually cannot be generalized to situations or settings outside of those where it was obtained. Therefore, the clinical merit and the scientific merit of a research base must be balanced.

The second question addresses the degree of clinical control nurses have over the implementation and the evaluation of the new practice. Implementation involves the degree of independence nursing has in manipulating the independent variable. For instance, the introduction of a relaxation exercise to clients preoperatively for their use after surgery is clearly within the purview of nursing. However, the innovation sometimes requires an interdependent activity that can only achieve clinical control through collaborative efforts with other disciplines. Haller et al. (1979) provide the example of nonsterile intermittent urinary catheterization as an innovation that requires medical cooperation.

Clinical control in the measurement of outcomes, the dependent variable(s), is also of concern. What kind of instruments have been used in the research base to measure the dependent variables? Are these readily available and applicable in practice? What new skills might be needed to use the research tools (Haller et al., 1979)? If you are introducing a new protocol based on research findings for oral hygiene with clients who are receiving chemotherapy, you would want to evaluate its effectiveness. One client outcome that may be indicative of the protocol's effectiveness is a decrease in the growth of organisms in the mouth at specific intervals. To measure this you would need to gain the cooperation of physicians in ordering periodic cultures.

Sometimes it is not possible to use the same tools that have been used in studies. In such cases a clinical approximation needs to be made. As an example, instead of using spirometry to measure respiratory status as an indication of the efficacy of a preoperative teaching protocol, one hospital "chose to substitute tape measurement of chest expansion and auscultation" (Haller et al., 1979, p. 49).

The third factor needed to be considered when assessing the relevance of an innovation to practice is *feasibility*. Are the resources, such as time, personnel, equipment, and skill, available in your practice setting (Haller et al., 1979)? Recall the research cited earlier that studied the effectiveness of relaxation techniques for postoperative discomfort. Although the implementation of a simple relaxation exercise during preoperative teaching sessions would not involve a great deal of time or additional personnel it would require other resources. If an audio recording of the technique was used as a teaching tool there would be a need for equipment, such as tape recorders and earphones. In addition, skill in using and teaching the relaxation technique would be needed by the involved nurses. Learning this skill can be accomplished in a relatively short period of time, but an organized program of instruction conducted by a knowledgeable individual would be required. To attend the classes, nurses would most likely need to be given released time from their client care responsibilities.

Finally, the *cost-effectiveness* of a new practice needs to be estimated. This includes the costs of both implementation and evaluation. The research base may include variables that are related directly to cost, such as days in hospital or prevention of complications. However, it is more likely for the research base to contain variables that possess an indirect relationship to cost, such as client or staff satisfaction. In the latter case, it may be necessary for you to "make a case for" the potential of an innovation to decrease actual costs before administrators are willing to invest the financial resources needed for research utilization.

CLINICAL EVALUATION

Once a research base for a practice innovation has been identified and its relevance to clinical practice has been established, the next step is to determine the potential for clinical evaluation of the new innovation. It is important to realize that the research variables, measurement techniques, and experimental procedures may not always be amenable to direct translation into practice. Thus you need to consider how these will be transformed for purposes of implementation and evaluation.

Because utilization of research findings usually involves a transformation of the independent variable in some way, it is essential that its effects in practice or outcomes be evaluated. For example, tight controls over the administration of an experimental treatment are needed to increase the internal validity of a research design. Such controls would probably include limiting the number of nurse research assistants who perform the treatment; using data collectors who are blind to the subjects' experimental condition, such as a treatment group versus a control group; and attempting to keep the setting or situation where the treatment is administered the same for all subjects. It cannot be assumed that the translation of experimental procedures into practice will achieve the same outcomes as demonstrated in controlled studies. Thus careful planning of how the experimental treatment will be incorporated into practice is essential. At the very least, those nurses who will be involved in using a practice innovation need to be taught a standardized approach for implementation.

How will client or staff outcomes be measured? Are the measurement tools used in the research studies appropriate for clinical use? Have all the variables of interest to nursing been assessed in the studies? Have variables that nursing does not have control over been included as outcome measures? Haller et al. (1979) explicate these problems with the following example:

> The original work on nonsterile intermittent catherization was done by physicians. Some of the dependent variables, such as cystoscopy results, were not felt to be appropriate as nursing outcomes. On the other hand, some of the variables of keen interest to nursing were not accounted for in the research base; these included patient satisfaction, patient mobility, and degree of interaction. Therefore, an evaluation procedure was devised that included variables from the research base and also drew on introspection about clinical practice (p.50).

Sometimes the dependent variable or outcome measure is appropriate for clinical evaluation, but the research instrument is not easily incorporated into a practice situation. Many studies have used lengthy questionnaires to assess such variables as self-concept, client satisfaction, locus of control, and anxiety. The State-Trait Anxiety Inventory (STAI) (Spielberger, Gorsuch, and Lushene, 1970), for instance, has been shown to be a valid and reliable instrument and has been used in many recent studies to measure situational or characteristic anxiety. It is a 40-item questionnaire that takes approximately 15 minutes to complete. If anxiety was an outcome measure that you were interested in assessing, you might have to find a more convenient way of measuring it in your setting.

Recently, I was faced with just such a situation. Staff nurses in a general hospital were looking for a simple tool to assess clients' anxiety levels. Graphic rating scales were developed (see Fig. 20-1) and compared with the STAI. Both instruments were administered to a sample of 30 nurses who were enrolled in graduate research courses at a nearby university. Using the Pearson product moment coefficient of correla-

HOW DO YOU USUALLY FEEL?

0	1	2	3	4
Calm	Slightly anxious	Moderately anxious	Very anxious	Extremely anxious

HOW DO YOU FEEL RIGHT NOW?

0	1	2	3	4
Calm	Slightly anxious	Moderately anxious	Very anxious	Extremely anxious

Fig. 20-1   Graphic anxiety scale.

tion *(r)*, the following results were obtained: (1) scores of state anxiety correlated 0.80 and (2) scores of trait anxiety correlated 0.70. Given the relatively high positive relationship between the scores, the graphic rating scales were deemed to be useful for measuring anxiety in clinical practice (Levin and Crosley, in press).

The process of evaluating a new innovation can be costly. Therefore, it is imperative that a budget be drafted and approved before any efforts at implementation begin. Items such as released time for nurses to learn the new technique as well as for nurse educators or clinical specialists to teach it, the development of an evaluation protocol, purchase or development of measurement tools, direction of the project, and data collection and analysis must all be considered. As mentioned earlier, because the cost of introducing and evaluating a nursing practice innovation can be high, justification of these expenditures must be documented in the form of potential savings for the institution and the consumer.

If the service agency cannot afford to support a utilization project on its own, alternatives are available. Outside funding may be one way of obtaining the needed financial resources. As an example, the U.S. Department of Health and Human Services (DHHS), through the Division of Nursing of the Public Health Service (PHS), offers a competitive grants program for nursing research utilization projects. However, to compete for these grants, the principal investigator must possess the appropriate credentials, for example, doctoral preparation, previous research, and publications. Few service agencies employ such an individual; most doctorally prepared nurses with research expertise are affiliated with academic institutions. Therefore, collaborative efforts between service and education, as discussed previously, may facilitate the implementation and evaluation of research findings in practice.

• Research Versus Clinical Evaluation

There are differences between conducting a research study and evaluating the use of research findings in practice. Although clinical evaluation requires a systematic process that involves standardization of treatments (independent variable), measurement of outcomes (dependent variables), and analysis of data, it does not usually require the tight methodological controls of research studies (Haller et al., 1979). In addition, the purposes of the projects differ. The New York State Nurses Association Council on Nursing Research, in an effort to clarify the differences between evaluation and research, identified the following criteria to use when judging whether a project is a nursing research study (NYSNA Council on Nursing Research, 1983, p.43):

1. Rigorous scientific method is employed throughout the process from the statement of hypotheses or research question through the conclusion.
2. The purpose of the study is the discovery of new knowledge.
3. The knowledge sought falls within the body of knowledge needed for nursing.

The purpose of a clinical evaluation project is to assess the worth or effectiveness of an innovation in a specific setting. The selection of clients does not usually include probability sampling techniques. Hypothesis testing using inferential statistics is not employed. The design of an evaluation is usually preexperimental, such as a comparison of preimplementation and postimplementation data using frequencies, percentages, ranges, rates, and means (Haller et al., 1979). Thus the results of a clinical evaluation can guide the decision about whether or not to incorporate a nursing practice innovation in a specific setting with a particular group of clients, but cannot be generalized to the entire client population or to other settings.

For too long a gap has existed between research and practice. Nursing has been so engrossed in elevating its status in the health care arena that at times it has perhaps lost sight of its primary goal: the development of knowledge to guide professional practice, not the development of knowledge for its own sake. Nurse researchers and practitioners have sometimes forgotten the need to communicate with one another if this goal is to be achieved. It is up to the new generation of professional nurses, both researchers and practitioners, to work together to improve the care we provide to society. This can only be accomplished by using valid research findings in practice. In your role as a knowledgeable consumer of nursing research, you have an important part to play in this effort.

• Summary

The members of a professional discipline use research findings as a basis for practice. In this chapter, factors related to the gap between the dissemination and the use of nursing research findings in practice were discussed. These included the educational preparation of nurses, the way that research is communicated to the profession, the lack of organizational resources, and the resistance to change. Suggestions for closing the gap were provided. Criteria that can be used to evaluate research findings and assess their applicability to clinical practice were presented. The factors involved in determining the potential for clinical evaluation of a practice innovation were outlined. Finally, the differences between a research study and a clinical evaluation were highlighted.

• References

Donaldson, S., and Crowley, D. (1978). The discipline of nursing, *Nursing Outlook,* **26**:113.

Fawcett, J. (1980). A declaration of nursing independence: the relation of theory and research to nursing practice, *Journal of Nursing Administration,* **10**:36.

Fawcett, J. (1984). Another look at utilization of nursing research, *Image,* **16**:59.

Fawcett, J. (1982). Utilization of nursing research findings, *Image,* **14**:57.

Flaherty, G., and Fitzpatrick, J. (1978). Relaxation technique to increase comfort level of postoperative patients: a preliminary study, *Nursing Research,* **27**:352.

Geden, E., Beck, N., Hauge, G., and Pohlman, S. (1984). Self-report and psycho physiological effects of five pain-coping strategies, *Nursing Research,* **33**:260.

Haller, K., Reynolds, M., and Horsley, J. (1979). Developing research-based innovation protocols: process, criteria, and issues, *Research in Nursing and Health,* **2**:45.

Horsley, J., Crane, J., and Bingle, J. (1978). Research utilization as an organizational process, *Journal of Nursing Administration,* **8**:4.

Horsley, J., Crane, J., Crabtree, M., and Wood, D. (1983). *Using research to improve nursing practice: a guide,* New York, Grune & Stratton, Inc.

Ketefian, S. (1975a). Application of selected nursing research findings into nursing practice, *Nursing Research,* **24**:89.

Ketefian, S. (1975b). Problems in the dissemination and utilization of scientific knowledge: how can the gap be bridged? *Translation of Theory into Nursing Practice and Education,* New York, New York University Press.

Kirchhoff, K. (1982). A diffusion survey of coronary precautions, *Nursing Research,* **31**:196.

Kirchhoff, K. (1983). Using research in practice: should staff nurses be expected to use research? *Western Journal of Nursing Research,* **5**:245.

Kruszewski, A., Lang, S., and Johnson, J. (1979). Effect of positioning on discomfort from intramuscular injections in the dorsogluteal site, *Nursing Research,* **28**:103.

Levin, R. (1983). Research for the undergraduate: too much, too soon? *Nursing Outlook,* **31**:258.

Levin, R., and Crosley, J. (in press). Evaluation of focused data collection for the generation of nursing diagnoses, *Journal of Nursing Staff Development.*

Levin, R., Fitzgibbon, A., Belevich, R., and McDonald, A. (1983). *Assessment of nursing research climate,* Unpublished manuscript.

Lippett, R., Watson, J., and Westley, B. (1958). *The dynamics of planned change,* New York, Harcourt, Brace, Jovanovich, Inc.

Mauksch, I., and Miller, M. (1981). *Implementing change in nursing,* St. Louis, The C.V. Mosby Co.

NYSNA Council on Nursing Research (1983). What constitutes nursing research? *Journal of New York State Nurses' Association,* **14**:42.

Spielberger, C., Gorsuch, R., and Lushene, R. (1970). *STAI manual,* Palo Alto, Calif., Consulting Psychologists Press.

Taylor, A., West, B., Simon, B., Skelton, J. and Rowlingson, J. (1983). How effective is tens for acute pain? *American Journal of Nursing,* **83**:1171.

Wells, N. (1982). The effect of relaxation on postoperative muscle tension and pain, *Nursing Research,* **31**:236.

Glossary

accidental sampling   A nonprobability sampling strategy that utilizes the most readily accessible persons or objects as subjects in a study.

alternate form reliability   Two or more alternate forms of a measure are administered to the same subjects at different times. The scores of the two tests determine the degree of relationship between the measures.

antecedent variable   A variable that affects the dependent variable, but occurs before the introduction of the independent variable.

anonymity   A research participant's protection in a study, so that no one, not even the researcher, can link the subject with the information given.

applied research   Tests the practical limits of descriptive theories, but does not examine the efficacy of actions taken by practitioners.

assumptions   Basic principles assumed to be true without the need for scientific proof.

basic research   Theoretical or pure research that generates, tests, and expands theories that explain or predict a phenomenon.

bias   A distortion in the data analysis results.

case study   An in-depth study of an individual, group, or institution.

chance errors   Attributable to fluctuations in subject characteristics that occur at a specific point in time and are often beyond the awareness and control of the examiner.

clinical research   Examines the effects of nursing processes on health status.

close-ended items   Questions that the respondent may answer with only one of a fixed number of choices.

cluster sampling   A probability sampling strategy that involves a successive random sampling of units. The units sampled progress from large to small.

concept   An image or symbolic representation of an abstract idea.

conceptual definition   Conveys the general meaning of the concept. It reflects the theory used in the study of that concept.

conceptual literature   Published material that deals with theory and propositions about phenomena.

confidentiality   Assurance that a research participant's identity cannot be linked to the information that was provided to the researcher.

constancy   Methods and procedures of data collection are the same for all subjects.

construct   An abstraction that is adapted for a scientific purpose.

313

construct replication   The use of original methods, such as sampling techniques, instruments, or research design, to study a problem that has been investigated previously.

construct validity   The extent to which an instrument is said to measure a theoretical construct or trait.

consumer   One who actively uses and applies research findings in nursing practice.

content analysis   A technique for the objective, systematic, and quantitative description of communications and documentary evidence.

content validity   The degree to which the content of the measure represents the universe of content, or the domain of a given behavior.

control   Measures used to hold uniform or constant the conditions under which an investigation occurs.

control group   The group in an experimental investigation that does not receive an intervention or treatment; the comparison group.

correlation   The degree of association between two variables.

correlational studies   A type of nonexperimental research design that examines the relationship between two or more variables.

criterion-related validity   Indicates the degree of relationship between performance on the measure and actual behavior either in the present (concurrent) or in the future (predictive).

critique   The process of objectively and critically evaluating a research report's content for scientific merit and application to practice, theory, or education.

cross-sectional studies   A nonexperimental research design that looks at data at one point in time, that is, in the immediate present.

data   Information systematically collected in the course of a study; the plural of datum.

data base   A compilation of information about a topic organized in a systematic way.

data-based literature   Published material that reports results of research studies.

deductive reasoning   A logical thought process in which hypotheses are derived from theory; reasoning moves from the general to the particular.

degrees of freedom   The number of quantities that are unknown minus the number of independent equations linking these unknown; a function of the number in the sample.

delimitations   Those characteristics that restrict the population to a homogeneous group of subjects.

dependent variable   In experimental studies, the presumed effect of the independent or experimental variable on the outcome.

descriptive statistics   Statistical methods used to describe and summarize sample data.

developmental studies   A type of nonexperimental research design that is concerned with not only the existing status and interrelationship of phenomena, but also with changes that take place as a function of time.

direct observation   A method for measuring psychological and physiological behaviors for purposes of evaluating change and facilitating recovery.

directional hypothesis   One that specifies the expected direction of the relationship between the independent and dependent variable.

ecological validity   Generalization of results to other settings or environmental conditions.

element   The most basic unit about which information is collected.

error variance   The extent to which the variance in test scores is attributable to error rather than a true measure of the behaviors.

ethics   The use of a moral code in research.

evaluative research   The utilization of scientific research methods and procedures for the purpose of making an evaluation.

ex post facto studies   A type of nonexperimental research design that examines the relationships among the variables after the variations have occurred.

experiment   A scientific investigation where observations are made and data are collected utilizing the characteristics of control, randomization, and manipulation.

experimental group   The group in an experimental investigation that receives an intervention or treatment.

external criticism   Establishment of genuineness, validity, and credibility of a document.

external validity   The degree to which findings of a study can be generalized to other populations or environments.

extraneous variable   Variables that interfere with the operations of the phenomena being studied.

findings   Statistical results of a study.

frequency distribution   Descriptive statistical method for summarizing occurrences of events being studied.

generalizability   The inferences that the data are representative of similar phenomena beyond the studied sample to a population.

hardware   The electronic equipment that makes a computer. Usually includes an input device, an output device, a central processing unit, and a memory.

historical research   Studies designed to systematically compile data, and critically present, evaluate, and interpret facts regarding former people, events, or occurrences.

history   The internal validity threat that refers to events outside of the experimental setting that may affect the dependent variable.

homogeneity   Similarity of conditions.

hypothesis   An assumptive statement about the relationship between two or more variables.

independent variable   The antecedent or the variable that has the presumed effect on the dependent variable.

inductive reasoning   A logical thought process in which generalizations are developed from specific observations; reasoning moves from the particular to the general.

inferential statistics   Procedures that combine mathematical processes and logic to test hypotheses about a population using sample data.

informed consent   An ethical principle that requires a researcher to obtain the voluntary participation of subjects after informing them of potential benefits and risks.

Institutional Review Board   A board established in agencies to review biomedical and behavioral research involving human subjects within the agency or in programs sponsored by that agency.

instrumentation   Changes in the measurement of the variables that may account for changes in the obtained measurement.

internal criticism   Establishment of the reliability or consistency of information within a document.

internal validity   The degree to which it can be inferred that the experimental treatment, rather than an uncontrolled condition, resulted in the observed effects.

interrater reliability   An index of the constituency between observers or scorers. This is usually used with the direct observation method.

interrelationship studies   The classification of a nonexperimental research design that attempts to trace relationships among variables. The four types are correlational, ex post facto, prediction, and developmental.

interval   The level of measurement that provides different levels or gradations in response, and the differences or intervals between responses are assumed to be approximately equal.

interval measurement scales   Scales used to show rankings of events or objects on a scale with equal intervals between numbers, but with an arbitrary zero, for example, centigrade temperature.

intervening variable   A variable that occurs during an experimental or quasi-experimental study that affects the dependent variable.

kurtosis   The relative peakness or flatness of a distribution.

level of significance (alpha level)   The risk of making a type I error, set by the researcher before the study begins.

levels of measurement   Categorization of the precision that an event can be measured with, such as nominal, ordinal, interval, and ratio.

limitations   Weaknesses of a study.

longitudinal studies   A nonexperimental research design where a researcher collects data from the same group at different points in time.

manipulation   The provision of some experimental treatment, in one or varying degrees, to some of the subjects in the study.

maturation   Developmental, biological, or psychological processes that operate within an individual as a function of time and are external to the events of the investigation.

mean   A measure of central tendency; the arithmetic average of all scores.

measurement   The assignment of numbers to objects or events according to rules.

measures of central tendency   Descriptive statistical procedures that describe the average member of a sample, such as mean, median, and mode.

measures of variability   Descriptive statistical procedures that describe how much dispersion there is in sample data.

median   A measure of central tendency; the middle score.

memory   The amount of working space that the computer has; an IBM PC is usually sold with 64K bytes of RAM (random access memory). Different amounts of memory are required for specific uses.

methodological research   The controlled investigation and measurement of the means of gathering and analyzing data.

modal percentage   A measure of variability; percent of cases in the mode.

modality   The number of peaks in a frequency distribution.

mode   A measure of central tendency; most frequent score or result.

modem   The device needed to communicate from a terminal to a mainframe computer.

mortality   The loss of subjects from time one data collection to time two data collection.

nominal   The level of measurement that simply assigns data into categories that are mutually exclusive.

nominal measurement scales   Scales used to classify objects or events into categories without any relative ranking, such as sex or hair color.

nondirectional hypothesis   One that indicates the existence of a relationship between the variables but does not specify the anticipated direction of the relationship.

nonexperimental research   Research where an investigator observes a phenomenon without manipulating the independent variable or variables.

nonparametric statistics   Statistics that are usually utilized when variables are measured at the nominal or ordinal level because they do not estimate population parameters and involve less restrictive assumptions about the underlying distribution.

nonprobability sampling   A procedure where elements are chosen by nonrandom methods.

normal curve   A curve that is symmetrical about the mean and unimodal.

null hypothesis   A statement that there is no relationship between the variables and that any relationship observed is a function of chance or fluctuations in sampling.

objectivity   The use of facts without distortion by personal feelings or bias.

open-ended items   Questions that the respondent may answer in his or her own words.

operational definition   The measurements utilized to observe or measure a variable; delineates the procedures or operations required to measure a concept.

operationalization   The process of translating concepts into observable, measurable phenomena.

ordinal   The level of measurement that systematically categorizes data in an ordered or ranked manner. Ordinal measures do not permit a high level of differentation among subjects.

ordinal measuremment scales   Scales used to show rankings of events or objects; numbers are not equidistant and zero is arbitrary (class ranking).

parameter   A characteristic of a population.

parametric statistics   Inferential statistics that involve the estimation of at least one parameter, require measurement at the interval level or above, and involve assumptions about the variables being studied. These assumptions usually include the fact that the variable is normally distributed.

percentile   A measure of variability; percent of cases a given score exceeds.

phenomenological research   Based on the investigation of the description of experience as it is lived.

philosophical research   Based on the investigation of the truths and principles of existence, knowledge, and conduct.

population   A well-defined set that has certain specified properties.

population validity   Generalization of results to other populations.

prediction studies   A type of nonexperimental research design that attempts to make a forecast or prediction derived from particular phenomena.

primary sources   First-hand accounts of events, such as reports of research studies written by the investigator.

probability   The probability of an event is the event's long-run relative frequency in repeated trials under similar conditions.

probability sampling   A procedure that utilizes some form of random selection when choosing the sample units.

problem statement   An interrogative sentence or statement about the relationship between two or more variables.

programs   A list of instructions in machine-readable language written so that a computer's hardware can carry out an operation; software.

propositions   The linkage of concepts that lays a foundation for the development of methods that test relationships.

prospective studies   Nonexperimental studies that begin with an exploration of assumed causes and then move forward in time to the presumed effect.

psychometrics   The theory and development of measurement instruments.

purposive sampling   A nonprobability sampling strategy where the researcher selects subjects who are considered to be typical of the population.

qualitative measurement   The items or observed behaviors are assigned to mutually exclusive categories that are representative of the kinds of behavior exhibited by the subjects.

quantitative measurement   The assignment of items or behaviors to categories that represent the amount of a possessed characteristic.

quasi-experimental   A study design where random asignment is not utilized, but the independent variable is manipulated and certain mechanisms of control are utilized.

questionnaire   A self-administered, highly structured instrument that is a direct method for studying relationships and testing hypotheses.

quota-sampling   A nonprobability sampling strategy that indentifies the strata of the population and proportionately represents the strata in the sample.

random access memory (RAM)   A computer's memory that the user can read or change.

random selection   A selection process in which each element of the population has an equal and independent chance of being included in the sample.

randomization   A sampling selection procedure in which each person or element in a population has an equal chance of being selected to either the experimental group or the control group.

range   A measure of variability; difference between the highest and lowest scores of sample data.

ratio   The highest level of measurement that possesses the characteristics of categorizing, ordering, and ranking and also has an absolute or natural zero that has empirical meaning.

ratio measurement scales   Scales used to rank the order of events or objects on scales with equal intervals and an absolute zero, such as height or weight.

reactivity   The distortion created when those who are being observed change their behavior because they know that they are being observed.

read only memory (ROM)   A computer's memory that can be read but not changed.

recommendations   Applications of a study to practice, theory, and future research.

reliability   The consistency or constancy of a measuring instrument.

replication   The repetition of a study, using different samples and conducted in different settings.

representative sample   A sample whose key characteristics closely approximate those of the population.

research   The systematic, logical, and empirical inquiry into the possible relationships among particular phenomena to produce verifiable knowledge.

research base   The accumulated knowledge, gained from several studies that investigate a similar problem.

research hypothesis   A statement about the expected relationship between the variables; also known as a scientific hypothesis.

retrospective data   Data that have been manifested, such as scores on a standard examination.

retrospective studies   A nonexperimental research design that begins with the phenomena of interest (dependent variable) in the present and examines its relationship to another variable (independent variable) in the past.

review of the literature   An extensive, exhaustive, systematic, and critical examination of publications relevant to a research endeavor.

sample   A subset of sampling units from a population.

sampling   A process in which representative units of a population are selected for study in a research investigation.

sampling error   The tendency for statistics to fluctuate from one sample to another.

sampling interval   The standard distance between the elements chosen for the sample.

sampling unit   The element or set of elements used for selecting the sample.

scale   A self-report inventory that provides a set of response symbols for each item. A rating or score is assigned to each response.

scientific approach   A logical, orderly, and objective means of generating and testing ideas.

scientific hypothesis   The researcher's expectation about the outcome of a study.

scientific merit   The degree of validity of a study or group of studies.

secondary sources   Accounts of events written by someone other than the person involved; may include summaries of research, textbooks, or biographies.

selection bias   The internal validity threat that arises when pretreatment differences between the experimental group and the control group are present.

semiquartile range   A measure of variability; range of the middle 50% of the scores.

simple random sampling   A probability sampling strategy where the population is defined, a sampling frame is listed, and a subset from which the sample will be chosen is selected; members randomly selected.

skew   Measure of asymmetry of a set of scores.

software   Computer programs, or lists of instructions in machine language, that allow the computer to perform specified operations such as statistics or word processing.

split-half reliability   An index of the comparison between the scores on one half of a test with the other half to determine the consistency in response to items that reflect specific content.

standard deviation   A measure of variability; measure of average deviation of scores from the mean; dispersion of a distribution.

standard error of the mean   The standard deviation of a theoretical distribution of sample means; it indicates the average error in the estimation of the population mean.

statistical hypothesis   States that there is no relationship between the independent and dependent variable. If a statistically significant relationship emerges between the variables at a specified level of significance, the statistical, or null, hypothesis is rejected.

statistical reliability   An index of the interval consistency of responses to all items of a single form of a measure that is administered at one time.

stratified random sampling   A probability sampling strategy where the population is divided into strata or subgroups. An appropriate number of elements from each subgroup are randomly selected based on their proportion in the population.

survey research   A type of nonexperimental research design that collects descriptions of existing phenomena for the purpose of using the data to justify or assess current conditions, or to make plans for improvement of conditions.

systematic errors   Attributable to lasting characteristics of the subject that do not tend to fluctuate from one time to another.

systematic sampling   A probability sampling strategy that involves the selection of subjects randomly drawn from a population list at fixed intervals.

terminals   An input device for a mainframe consisting of a keyboard and a monitor.

test   A self-report inventory that provides for one response to each item that the examiner assigns a rating or score. Inferences are made from the total score about the degree to which a subject posess whatever trait, emotion, attitude, or behavior the test is supposed to measure.

testability   Variables of a proposed study that lend themselves to observation, measurement, and analysis.

testing   The effects of taking a pretest on the scores of a posttest.

test-retest reliability   Administration of the same instrument twice to the same subjects under the same conditions within a prescribed time interval with a comparison of the paired scores to determine the stability of the measure.

theoretical framework   A context in which to examine a problem; the theoretical rationale for the development of hypotheses.

theory   A set of interrelated constructs or concepts, definitions, and propositions that present a systematic view of phenomena by specifying relations among variables, with the purpose of explaining and predicting phenomena.

time-sharing   Several users working on one mainframe via terminals at the same time.

type I error   The rejection of a null hypothesis that is actually true.

type II error   The acceptance of a null hypothesis that is actually false.

validation sample   The sample that provides the initial data for determining the reliability and validity of a measurement tool.

validity   Determination of whether a measurement instrument actually measures what it is purported to measure.

A

Pediatric Surgical Patients' and Parents' Stress Responses and Adjustment

As a Function of Psychologic Preparation and Stress-Point Nursing Care

John A. Wolfer
Madelon A. Visintainer

The purpose of this study was to test the hypotheses that children who receive systematic psychologic preparation and continued supportive care, in contast to those who do not, would show less upset behavior and more cooperation in the hospital and fewer post-hospital adjustment problems and that their parents would be less anxious and more satisfied with information and care received. Eighty children scheduled for minor surgery and their parents were randomly assigned to experimental and control conditions. The experimental intervention consisted of accurate information about sequences of events, sensory experiences, role expectations and appropriate responses, previews of procedures through play techniques, and supportive care given at critical points pre- and postoperatively. Significant differences between experimental and control children and parents on ratings of upset behavior, painful procedures, resistance to induction, time to first voiding, posthospital adjustment, and parental anxiety and satisfaction with information and care consistently supported the hypotheses. Results were also analyzed in relation to the age and sex of the children and whether parents roomed with the children.

☐ This study was supported in part by U.S. Public Health Service Research Development Grant NU 00314.

Many children show adverse reactions to the stressful experience of hospitalization and surgery, both immediate reactions while in the hospital and once they have returned home (Blom, 1958; Chapman *et al.*, 1956; Deutsch, 1942; Fagin, 1964; Gellert, 1958; Jackson *et al.*, 1953; Jessner and Kaplan, 1949; Levey, 1945; Prugh *et al.*, 1953). The term, "psychologic upset," has been used to refer to a variety of these immediate and longer lasting behavioral problems (Chapman *et al.*, 1956; Gellert, 1958).

• Background

MITIGATION OF HOSPITAL STRESS

That the stress of hospitalization and surgery can be mitigated by appropriate psychologic preparation and supportive care has been an assumption underlying many clinical practices for several decades (Beverly, 1936; Francis and Cutler, 1957; Godfrey, 1955; Jackson, 1951; Oremland and Oremland, 1973; Plank and Ritchie, 1971) and partially documented by descriptive and experimental studies (Cassell, 1963; Coleman, 1952; Jackson, 1951; Jessner *et al.*, 1952; Mahaffy, 1965; Prugh *et al.*, 1953; Scahill, 1969; Skipper *et al.*, 1968; Vaughan, 1957; Weinick, 1958).

The popularity of the idea is reflected in the wide use of preparatory booklets. Clinical research in medicine and nursing in this area over the past 20 years has helped to delineate relevant variables, develop methods of measuring adverse reactions, demonstrate the apparent beneficial effects of various types of special preparation and continued care, and, in a few instances, articulate the theoretic basis for these special practices. Although much has been learned and many changes have been made in pediatric care, few of the practices have been tested systematically for their effectiveness, and much of the underlying theory is obscure or superficial. The published work in this area contains little sustained research where critical variables regarding psychologic preparation, special care, and outcome are taken into account from one study to the next under similar conditions. Moreover, there has been virtually no replication. In addition, although some of the studies are highly suggestive of what should be done to improve the preparation and care of pediatric patients, the clinical circumstances under which the investigations were conducted may not be appropriate or feasible for normal operations where practice must be congruent with the availability of scarce human and material resources. For example, in a number of studies the caregiver who provided the special preparation and care was a highly trained person whose only responsibility on a floor was to give the time-limited special care.

As far as possible, clinical experiments designed to test the stress-reducing effects of special procedures should be conducted in such a way that effective procedures have a chance of being implemented. Finally, although there has been a proliferation of techniques and subspecialties for giving hospitalized children special preparation and supportive care in the last two decades, there have been no published attempts to implement and evaluate systematically coordinated programs for psychologic preparation and supportive care since a study by Prugh *et al.* in 1953.

In 1965, under the title, *The Psychological Responses of Children to Hospitalization and Illness: A Review of the Literature,* Vernon *et al.* provided an excellent comprehensive review of over 200 articles and books dealing with theories and data concerning why hospitalization is psychologically upsetting for children and what has been done to mitigate the problem. Only six of the studies reviewed were some form of clinical experiment where preparation was given to children of their parents along with an attempt to determine if the preparatory communication had a positive outcome (Cassell, 1963; Jackson *et al.,* 1953; Jessner *et al.,* 1952; Prugh *et al.,* 1953; Vaughan, 1957; Weinick, 1958. Outcome variables were either immediate responses, meaning indications of psychologic upset while the children were in the hospital, or posthospital responses, referring to indications of psychologic upset occurring after the children returned home. Discussions of psychologic preparation focused on three major themes: the factual information given to the child or parent, encouraging emotional expression, and establishing trust and confidence with hospital staff. The beneficial effects of information were assumed to result because vague, undefined threats are more upsetting than threats which are known and understood, and unexpected stress is more upsetting than expected stress.

Methodologic limitations in these studies, combined with the fact that they were not comparable in terms of design, type of preparation, measurement techniques, and outcome variables, allow only tentative conclusions about the positive effects of psychologic preparation and other supposedly beneficial procedures. As Vernon *et al.* (1965) noted, there is some support for the hypothesis that unfamiliarity with the hospital setting is a determinant of the level of psychologic upset experienced following hospitalization. Four of the six studies provided some findings to the effect that psychologic preparation either reduced the incidence of posthospital upset or increased the incidence of posthospital benefit.

With regard to measures of psychologic upset during hospitalization, of the three studies that provided data on psychologic preparation and immediate upset, two showed no positive findings and one had mixed findings. Again, methodologic limitations prevented definitive conclusions. In addition, these studies combined different aspects of the process of preparation, such as the provision of factual information, the establishment of a trusting relationship with a staff member, and the provision of other supportive care measures following surgery and other threatening procedures. Consequently, it is impossible to determine the relative contribution of these different sets of treatment variables.

EFFECT OF PSYCHOLOGIC PREPARATION

A review of the medical, nursing, psychiatric, and psychologic literature from 1965 to the present revealed only three further experimental investigations of the effect of psychologic preparation and special supportive care procedures on hospitalized children's stress reactions and adjustment. In a related series of experiments, Mahaffy (1965) and Skipper *et al.* (1968) took a different approach from the previous investigations by concentrating the preparatory and supportive efforts on the mothers rather than the children who were having minor surgery.

The basis for the preparatory and supportive intervention was social interaction theory, the emotional contagion hypothesis (Campbell, 1957; VanderVeer, 1949), which holds that a parent's emotional state may be transmitted to a young child, and the clinical observation that uninformed or emotionally upset parents are often unable to assist their children in coping with stress. The research nurse saw mothers randomly assigned to the experimental group at admission in order to determine their emotional states, concerns, and need for information. The nurse then provided the necessary information, emotional support, and assisted them in participating meaningfully in the care of their children. Further nurse-mother contacts occurred at several points during the hospitalization: twice during the evening before surgery, when the child returned from the recovery room, twice during the first evening after surgery, and at discharge. Hence, the treatment variable consisted of a combination of advanced preparatory information and continued supportive care at potential stress points throughout the hospitalization. Mothers randomly assigned to the control group did not receive these preparatory communications and supportive attention.

It was predicted that mothers in the experimental group would experience less emotional distress, would be more satisfied with the information and medical and nursing care they received and would feel more helpful to their child than control mothers. In turn, it was predicted that experimental group children would experience less emotional distress and evidence better adaptation and recovery in the hospital and upon returning home than control children. Outcome measures were staff nurses' observations of mothers' anxiety and adaptation, mothers' questionnaire responses regarding their level of anxiety at key points, their need for information, their trust and confidence in the staff, and their general satisfaction with the hospital experience. The children's temperature, blood pressure, and pulse were recorded at four potential stress points during the hospitalization as indicators of emotional arousal. Time to first voiding and incidence of emesis in the recovery room and amount of fluid intake were also recorded. Posthospital adjustment was determined from a questionnaire mothers completed eight days later. Results based on 80 patients in the three studies significantly and consistently supported the hypotheses on all outcome variables. A subgroup of the experimental group mothers and their children who were seen only at admission showed almost as much stress reduction and improved adaptation as those who were seen by the research nurse at six other critical points throughout the hospitalization. This finding suggested that admission is the crucial time and place to initiate stress-reducing interaction. However, the distinction between admission-only and admission-plus-follow-up interventions may have been confounded by the fact that the admission-only intervention was done by a female nurse, while the admission-plus subsequent interaction was made by a male nurse.

In these studies, consistent with the hypotheses being tested, the major focus of the preparation and supportive care was the parent. It is not clear how or to what extent children were included in the nurse-mother transactions, particularly at admission. Consequently, it cannot be determined if some of the positive effects for the children may have resulted from the preparation and support they received directly from the experimental nurse rather than, or in addition to, the indirect effects of mothers' lowered distress and improved coping.

From a theoretical point of view, it would be valuable to determine the possible independent and relative effects of parent preparation and support as distinct from child preparation and support. On the other hand, in the light of the suspected and known undesirable effects of separating young children from their parents, particularly during stressful events (Vernon *et al.,* 1967), it would be questionable procedure. In addition, it is awkward and impractical to separate a child from his parents shortly after admission up until the evening meal because separate rooms and additional personnel would be necessary in most pediatric units.

If the patient and his immediate family are taken as a dynamic unit in the planning of care, rather than the individual patient, it is illogical to separate them in order to give them different types of interventions. Further, when the nurse works with both parent and child, they learn from each other during the three-way transaction. This is particularly true of the parent who may see, for the first time, what his child knows and doesn't know about what is going to happen as the nurse interacts with the child. Therefore, it did not seem desirable to attempt to differentiate the parent and child components of the preparation and support procedures.

Another consideration in this line of search is who should provide the special preparation and supportive care. In the Mahaffy (1965) and Skipper *et al.* (1968) studies, the research nurses who gave the special care were essentially visitors on the unit with highly specialized and limited functions. They were not responsible for or involved in other nursing care activities over and above what they did for the purpose of their studies. This raises the question of whether the special psychologic preparation and continued supportive care can be given with the same beneficial effects when the "research" nurse is actively involved in general nursing care on the unit and functions more as a regular member of the staff.

Finally, except for Prugh *et al.* (1953), none of the experimental investigations reviewed above systematically examined the effect of psychologic preparation and supportive care as a function of age or sex of the children or in relation to whether the parent roomed in. Are the apparent benefits of reduced emotional distress and a lower incidence of behavioral upset the same for younger and older and male and female patients? Verson *et al.* (1967) did not find a relationship between age or sex and children's degree of upset behavior at admission or at the time of induction. However, the admission procedure in the study was not found to be very distressing and the age range was restricted to two to five years. Because of the major differences in children's behavior associated with developmental level, it is especially important to take age (as an approximate indication of developmental level) into account. Whether the parent remains with the child overnight, i.e., rooms in, especially for younger children, may make an important difference in how the child responds.

• Purpose

The purpose of this investigation as the first of a planned series of studies was to: provide a partial replication of the Mahaffy (1965) and Skipper *et al.* (1965) studies; operationalize the independent variable, psychologic preparation and supportive care for parent and child, in the form of a more complete nursing role on a pediatric unit; consider and explicate the transactional process of communicating with both the mother and the child; and examine the effects of the experimental preparatory and supportive transactions in relation to the age and sex of the child and whether the mother roomed in.

• Hypothesis

It was hypothesized that children and parents who receive special psychologic preparation and continued supportive care, in contrast to control children and mothers, would show less upset behavior and better coping and adjustment as indicated on the following ten dependent variables: blind observer ratings of the children's upset behavior and cooperation with procedures at five potential stress points; pulse rates at admission and before and after the blood test and preoperative injections; resistance to induction; recovery room medications; ease of fluid intake; time to first voiding; posthospital adjustment; mother's self-ratings of anxiety at potential stress points throughout the hospitalization; mother's rated satisfaction with various aspects of the nursing and medical care they received; and mother's ratings of the adequacy of information they received.

These dependent variables were operationalized in a similar fashion to the dependent variables in the Mahaffy (1965) and Skipper *et al.* (1968) studies. It was also expected that older children (seven to 14) would generally show less upset behavior and better coping and adjustment than younger children (three to six variables.

There was no strong basis for making a hypothesis regarding sex.

• Method

DESIGN

A two-group experimental design was used with random assignment of children and parents to either a control or an experimental group. The control group received regular nursing care. The experimental group received special preparation and supportive care which was provided by the same nurse at six different times during the hospitalization. Children's pulse rates, which were taken at admission and before and after the blood test and the preoperative injections, were treated as repeated measures. The upset behavior and cooperation ratings were analyzed separately for each of the four events when they were made (admission examination, blood test, preoperative injection, and transport to the operating room).

SETTING

The clinical setting for the study was the 30-bed pediatric unit in a 400-bed Catholic, general hospital located in a metropolitan area of 60,000. The pediatric unit admits children from infancy to 16 years of age. Over 90 percent of the elective surgical procedures in pediatrics are private cases admitted by the surgeon in the particular specialty. Children who have minor elective surgery are admitted from Sunday through Thursday, are scheduled for the operating room on the day following admission, and are discharged the day after surgery.

The nursing staff on the unit consists of ten registered nurses (RNs), four licensed practical nurses (LPNs) and ten nurses' aides (NAs), full- and part-time, divided over three eight-hour shifts. In a foster grandmother program, 17 grand-mothers rotate through the day shift to escort children and their parents to their rooms and to provide comfort and support, especially for children hospitalized for extended periods of time. LPN students rotate through the pediatric service for six-week periods and are responsible for the care of one to three patients a day during the six hours they are on the ward. They were not assigned to study patients. A play therapist supervises the playroom on the ward and organizes school activities and arts and crafts for the children. She did not engage in special preparation or supportive activities of play therapy during this study.

ROUTINE (CONTROL) PROCEDURES

On admission to the ward the parents and child saw the admission nurse (a part-time LPN who does admission procedure for all patients throughout the hospital). The child was weighed and measured and his vital signs recorded. The child then waited with his parents until the hospital pediatrician examined him, after which he was assigned to a room. In the afternoon a laboratory technician, accompanied by a pediatric nurses' aide, took a blood sample via vena puncture.

During the afternoon, an anesthesiologist reviewed the child's chart and wrote orders for medication. He did not routinely see the parents or child unless the child had a physical or developmental problem that might complicate surgery. No specific nursing contact, except during change of shift, was made with the child or parent unless a problem arose. No preoperative instruction was given. Vital signs were taken twice during the evening, and one parent was allowed to stay overnight on a cot beside the child's bed.

In the morning all children scheduled for surgery had their temperature taken, were dressed in hospital pajamas, and received the preoperative medication (intra-muscular Demerol® and Vistaril® or Seconal® and Atropine® given 45-60 minutes prior to induction).

The child was taken to the operating room on a stretcher by a surgical technician and was accompanied as far as the operating suite by a pediatric aide or nurse. Parents were not allowed to go with the children.

Until the operating room was ready, the child, often awake, waited with the technician in the hall of the surgical suite. Induction for children under 12 was usually by inhalation of halothane or Fluothane®. Older children frequently received intra-venous Pentothol®. After the recovery period, the child was returned to the ward by the recovery room aide.

Contact between the parents and the surgeon occurred late in the afternoon after surgery. Overall, the nursing contact, except for answering call lights and special requests by parents, was limited for the control patient. In general, the nurses were friendly, courteous, and concerned in their interactions with parents and children. However, there was no formal preparation nor systematic attempt to determine parents' and children's information or emotional needs.

SAMPLE

During the data collection period, 80 children met the following criteria and were included in the study. They: 1) were between the ages of three and 14, 2) had had no previous hospitalization within the past year, 3) were English-speaking, 4) were free from chronic diseases, 5) had no medical or psychologic condition that required consultation or special care, and 6) were admitted for elective tonsillectomy, adenoidectomy, myringotomy, polyethylene tubes (and any combination of these), or inguinal or umbilical herniorraphy. Informed consent was obtained from all parents. There were no refusals to participate in the study.

GROUP ASSIGNMENTS

With random assignment of individual children to the experimental or control conditions, some children and their parents who received different nursing interventions could have been placed in adjacent beds. Consequently, there might have been the possibility of some interaction between control and experimental subjects. Furthermore, some children or parents might have been concerned or disturbed by experiencing a type of nursing care different from that given a child in the next bed. To reduce this possibility, all children and parents admitted to the study on a given day who were assigned to the same room received the same treatment, either the control or the experimental nursing regimen. Treatment given each of the six rooms on the ward each day was determined randomly. Room assignment was made in advance by the admission office roughly on the basis of the age and sex of the child without knowledge of the experimental conditions. Forty-five children were assigned to the experimental group and 35 to the control.

EXPERIMENTAL PREPARATION AND STRESS-POINT SUPPORTIVE CARE

Hospitalization and surgery create a series of real, imagined, or potential threats for the child. The exact nature of the threats depends on many factors, such as the age and developmental level of the child, his previous experience with similar threats, amount and type of relevant information he possesses, and amount and type of support from parents and others. The threats can be classified into five general categories, each of which assumes a need or a cluster of needs: 1) physical harm or bodily injury in the form of discomfort, pain, mutilation, death; 2) separation from parents and the absence of trusted adults (especially for preschool children); 3) the strange, the unknown, the possibility of surprise; 4) uncertainty about limits and expected "acceptable" behavior; and 5) relative loss of control, autonomy, and competence. To the extent these threats are not removed, minimized, or coped with more or less effectively, the child is under varying degrees of stress. The purpose of the experimental preparation and stress-point supportive care was to remove or minimize stress and assist the child in coping through the provision of information, instruction, and support from a single nurse who was present at critical times. The exact content of the information and the manner in which it was given depended on the child's intellectual and cognitive development following Piaget's (1958) formulations. Generally, there was a greater use of play techniques for preschool children (three to six) and more direct verbal interactions for the older children (seven to 14), depending on the individual child's ability and willingness to interact and communicate in a given way. Throughout the preparatory communications, a distinction was made between external events and sensations the children would experience in order to maximize their understanding of what would happen, when, how long it would last, and how it would feel (Johnson, 1972).

The experimental condition was a combination of psychologic preparation and supportive care provided at six points: admission, shortly before the blood test, late in the afternoon the day before the operation, shortly before the preoperative medications, before transport to the operating room (OR), and upon return from the recovery room (RR). Admission, the blood test, preoperative medication, transport to the OR, and return from the RR are stressful events for many children. The provision of information about what to expect and how to respond shortly before these events, along with support and reassurance during the events, constitutes stress-point nursing care. The preparation and support was integrated for the parent and child, and the parental component followed the rationale and procedure used by Mahaffy (1965) and Skipper *et al.* (1968) and the theory and process of deliberative nursing (Orlando, 1961; Wiedenbach, 1964). During all interactions the preparation attempted to provide individualized attention to the mothers, to explore and clarify their feelings and thoughts, to provide accurate information and appropriate reassurance, and to explain how the mother could help care for her child. The preparation stressed the parent's importance to the child, her continued control over him during hospitalization, and the importance of her approval of his being in the hospital and reassuring him that she would return if she left.

The child component of the preparation included information, sensory expectations, role identification, rehearsals, and support. The initial contact with the child at admission was used to establish a relationship through an expression of interest in home or school activities and likes and dislikes. During all interactions the child's fears and concerns were explored and his understanding of and past experience with the procedures assessed. The child was asked to present his impressions of what was happening and how it involved him. Any misconceptions were clarified by using his own terms whenever possible or by asking his parents to express what the nurse had said in more familiar words. Information included the time of the procedure, who would do it and how, why it was done, how it would begin and end, and what could be expected after it was completed. The sensations and emotions he would or might experience were described and demonstrated whenever possible; for example, the cold sensation and smell of the alcohol, the pressure and smell of the alcohol, the pressure and smell of the anesthesia mask, and a dizzy feeling after the medication was given. For the younger child the information and sensations were presented in story form using a doll and the hospital equipment. The child was encouraged, through play, to exchange roles with the nurse and to conduct the procedure on the doll, himself, while the story was repeated. For the older child the equipment and the doll were also used; the child's curiosity about the mechanics of the procedure was recognized and more detail was given, but not in story form.

The identification of the child's role and the expected behaviors was considered essential to increasing his feelings of control and involvement in the procedure. After the information was given, the child was encouraged to express his feeling about the event. The child was then helped to identify goals and to recognize those which were obtainable. It was believed that this would direct his effort away from activities that would only lead to frustration and failure. For example, he was helped to recognize that avoiding the blood test was impossible, but shortening the length of time it would take to do it was something he could control.

After identifying the goal, the child was shown the behavior he would need to attain it. For example, for a short blood test, he would need to hold his arm still; for a fast induction, he would have to blow up the "balloon" (anesthesia bag) using the mask. The specific behaviors were then rehearsed and the child was assured of help if he needed it.

Because children have different expectations of themselves, either because of age or experience, after the prescribed behavior was determined, other actions were decided upon by the child himself. For example, holding still for the preoperative medication was essential; however, the verbal response during the test could vary within certain limits. The child was told that crying was permissible and something that even adults do during the same procedure. If the child rejected crying as unacceptable behavior, or if crying did not seem appropriate for a particular age level, alternatives were offered, such as counting or giving verbal command to the nurse, i.e., repeating the words, "hurry up." Older children did not have to focus on verbal response, but could concentrate on muscle relaxation instead. In each case, the child's choice of behavior was supported, and the behaviors practiced during the preparation period. This preparation format was followed during the interactions prior to the blood test, preoperative medication, and transport to surgery.

During the interaction on the afternoon of admission, the nurse explained in detail what would happen the next day. This contact was considered important because of the short period of time available the morning of surgery. Doll play was used for the younger children to demonstrate equipment, sequence of events, and perceptions. A simple explanation of the surgical procedure was given, including the point that no incision would be made and no other part of the body would be touched. The sequence of events from transport to the operating room to return to the room was described in detail in terms of what the child would experience through this period.

During the interaction after surgery, the nurse reassured the child the operation was over, that he was doing fine, and that he should take fluids. She also discussed with the mother her role after surgery, what she could expect for the remainder of the recovery period, and from whom to seek help.

A brief predischarge visit was made for the purpose of explaining that the child was ready to go home, he had done very well, he would feel the same as usual in a few days, and what the mother could expect for the next few days.

ROLE OF THE RESEARCH NURSE

Before the study began the research nurse spent approximately a month on the unit, participating in all aspects of direct patient care. Throughout the study she was present on the unit from 7:00 A.M. to 4:00 P.M., six days a week, and provided direct care and supervision of care for many nonstudy patients. Typically, she played a key role in conjunction with the head nurse and team leader in the management of care for the more seriously ill cases. Essentially, she functioned as a clinical specialist in such a way that the special preparation and supportive care she provided the experimental group patients was an integral part of her overall role.

OUTCOME VARIABLES

Behavioral Ratings   Two ratings of the child's emotional state and cooperation were made. 1) The manifest upset scale is a five-point scale designed to reflect the emotional state of a child at a given point in time, primarily in terms of verbal and nonverbal expressions of fear, anxiety, or anger. A rating of one indicates little or no fear or anxiety (calm appearance, no crying, no verbal protest). A rating of three, a moderate amount (some temporary whimpering and/or mild verbal protest), and a rating of five indicates extreme emotional distress (agitated, hard crying or screaming and/or strong verbal protest). 2) The cooperation scale is a five-point scale for indicating the degree to which a child cooperates with a procedure. A rating of one indicates complete cooperation including active participation in and assistance with the procedure. A rating of three indicates mild or initial resistance or passive participation without assistance. A rating of five indicates extreme resistance, strong avoidance, and the necessity to retrain the child.

The children's manifest upset and cooperating rating scales were completed by a nurse observer for five different events: admission examination, blood test, preoperative medication, transport to the operating suite, and while waiting in the hall in the operating suite. The observer also noted whether there was resistance to induction in the form of attempts to get off the operating table, verbal protest, refusing to hold the mask, fighting the mask, squirming and restlessness once the mask was applied. This observation was coded simply "yes" or "no."

All rating scales were repeatedly field tested by the investigators and the nurse observer until there was essential agreement on what types of observable behaviors were to correspond to the scale points. After the final revisions, the second author and the nurse observer made independent simultaneous ratings of a small sample of children at each of the observation points. The mean percentage of agreement between the two raters over 123 separate ratings for seven children and their parents was 90 percent. On only three individual scales was the agreement less than 80 percent—60 percent in each case. Interrater reliability was considered adequate. The nurse observer was unaware of whether parents and children were in the experimental or control groups.

Ease of Fluid Intake   When the child first took fluids following the operation, a rating of ease of fluid intake was made by the observer on a four-point scale; one, great ease; two, ease; three, difficulty; four, great difficulty.

Pulse Rates   An indication of physiologic arousal accompanying fear, anxiety, or general emotional distress, pulse rates were recorded by the nurse observer at admission before any contact with the research nurse, before and after the blood test, and before and after the preoperative injections. The admission pulse (along with the admission upset and cooperation ratings) permitted a before-treatment comparison of subjects.

Recovery Room Medication   A further measure of upset was indicated by the way the child recovered from anesthesia in the recovery room. The first reaction to sensations of pain and fears about the surgery may vary from a quiet awakening to thrashing, uncontrolled movements, and crying. Because there was routinely an order for medication to relieve pain and reduce the restlessness, if needed, the administration of pro re nata medication in the recovery room indicated the presence of upset behavior. Although it depended upon the nurses' subjective evaluation of the child's upset, the recovery room staff were completely blind to the groups to which the children were assigned.

Time to First Voiding   A final outcome measure in the hospital was time to first voiding following surgery. This has been considered a recovery measure which reflects a patient's emotional state; the more emotionally upset a patient is, the longer before he voids (Elman, 1951, p.42; Hollender, 1958). In the Mahaffy (1965) and Skipper *et al.* (1968) studies, children whose parents received the special preparation and supportive care had a significantly shorter time to first voiding than did control children.

Posthospital Adjustment   This variable was measured with the Vernon *et al.* (1966) Posthospital Behavior questionnaire, a list of 27 behavioral times most frequently cited in the literature as occurring in children following hospitalization. For each item the parent compares the child's typical behavior before hospitalization with his behavior during the first week after hospitalization. Five response alternatives are provided: "much less than before"—scored one; "less than before"—two; "same as before"—three; "more than before"—four, and "much more than before"—five. Vernon *et al.* performed a factor analysis of the questionnaires of 387 hospitalized children which revealed six orthogonal factors: 1) general anxiety and regression; 2) separation anxiety; 3) anxiety about sleep; 4) eating disturbance; 5) aggression toward authority; and 6) apathy–withdrawal. Comparison of the mean factor and total scores for the full sample with the levels indicative of no overall change indicated that the combination of illness and hospitalization is a psychologically upsetting experience for children in general, resulting in increased separation anxiety, increased sleep anxiety, and increased aggression toward authority. Vernon *et al.* (1966) also reported a test-retest reliability coefficient of .65 for 37 children, along with a significant correlation between questionnaire responses and a psychiatric interview intended to get at the same information. Further evidence of the predictive validity of the questionnaire came from its detection of changes as predicted in studies by Vernon *et al.* (1966, 1967).

The Posthospital Behavior questionnaire was given to parents along with detailed instructions on how and when to complete it at the time of discharge. On the eighth day postdischarge they were contacted by phone and reminded to complete the questionnaire and return it by mail. This procedure resulted in an 87 percent return rate.

Parental Measures   Five aspects of parental experience during the hospitalization were assessed. During the admission examination, an independent observer, blind to conditions, rated each parent on two separate scales: 1) manifest upset, a five-point scale designed to indicate the degree of anxiety, apprehension, nervousness, or general emotional distress as expressed in the mother's verbal and nonverbal behavior (a rating of one indicates no signs of emotional distress; of three, a moderate degree of anxiety; of five, a high degree of emotional distress); and 2) coping and cooperation, a five-point scale designed to reflect the degree to which the mother was dealing effectively with the immediate situation as expressed in her verbal and nonverbal behavior while she interacted with the admissions nurse and her child (a rating of one indicates that the mother was in complete control in appropriately assisting with the examination, answering the nurse's questions, as well as asking questions, and appropriately supporting her child, while a rating of five indicates a complete loss of control, inappropriate and/or ineffective interaction with the nurse and her child).

Three other measures for parents were obtained from a questionnaire which was administered shortly before discharge. One assessment was the parent's self-rating of anxiety experienced at eight different points: at admission, immediately after the admission examination, during the blood test, bedtime the night before surgery, any other time during that night, before the child was taken to the operating room, during the operation, and when the child first took fluids. Each was a five-point scale with one indicating no anxiety and five an extreme degree of anxiety. The nine scales were summed to give an overall mean rating of anxiety.

A final rating obtained from the questionnaire was a satisfaction with care score which was based on 20 items that covered nursing and medical procedures and the quality and effectiveness of nurse-child transactions. Each item has a four-point scale: needs much improvement—one; needs improvement—two; satisfactory—three; very good—four, and a "did not observe" box. A mean overall satisfaction score was obtained from these items.

Another score from the questionnaire was an indivation of the adequacy of the information received. This consisted of items regarding whether mothers considered they were adequately informed about 18 points such as the type of operation, expected length of stay, general hospital routines, reasons for various procedures, what they could do to help. The items were coded "yes" or "no" to indicate whether mothers were adequately informed. A score of 18 indicated adequate information on all 18 items. Each item also asked from whom the information was received, including the project nurse. This not only provided a check on whether mothers received more information from the research nurse than from other sources but also indicated the number of items of information (of a possible total of 18) the mother received from only the research nurse.

• Results

Table 1 shows sample characteristics for experimental and control groups. As the chi-square analysis revealed, the two groups did not differ significantly in terms of sex, age, birth order, whether the parent stayed overnight, or type of surgery. Thus, the groups appeared to be comparable on these variables. For the remaining analyses, the total number of subjects in each of the groups fluctuated somewhat from variable to variable because of missing observations.

During the admission examination, before they were seen by the research nurse, all children were rated on manifest upset behavior and cooperation; all parents were also rated on manifest upset behavior and coping-cooperation. The means for these ratings were: upset behavior—children (experimental) 1.73, (control) 1.82, parents (experimental) 1.57, (control) 1.71; cooperation—children (experimental) 1.28, (control) 1.48; parents (experimental) 1.42, (control) 1.46. Comparison of the group means with t-tests showed no significant difference between experimental and control children and parents on these variables before the experimental nursing intervention began.

The results on each child's outcome measures were subjected to a three-way analysis of variance (treatment condition by age by sex) (Table 2). Upset behavior and cooperation ratings were analyzed separately for each of the four events (blood test, preoperative injections, transport to the operating suite, and waiting in the hall in the operating suite). There were no significant main effects for sex on any of these variables. Therefore, there were no consistent differences between girls and boys on these measures.

As predicted, children in the experimental group were significantly less upset and more cooperative than control children for all four events. They also had signif-

• *Table 1*   **Sample Characteristics of Experimental and Control Subjects (N = 80)**

Characteristics	Experimental (N = 45)	Control (N = 35)	χ^2
Female	16	14	.16
Male	29	21	
Age			
3-6	22	20	
7-14	23	15	.26
Mean age	7.1 years	7.1 years	
Birth order			
Only child	7	6	
First child	22	10	3.64
Later born	16	19	
Parent stayed			
Yes	17	17	.94
No	28	18	
Type of surgery			
Tonsillectomy	35	25	
Ear	6	5	.63
Hernia	4	5	

icantly lower ease of fluid intake ratings, fewer minutes to first voiding, and lower posthospital adjustment scores than the control group, again as predicted. A significant *F* was also obtained for age on all the behavioral ratings except upset and cooperation while waiting in the operating room and ease of fluid intake. This reflected the general tendency for older children to exhibit less upset and more cooperation than younger children as expected.

The results of the analysis of variance indicated there were no significant treatment by age interactions on any of the children's outcome variables. There were, however, three significant age by sex interactions for the transport cooperation rating, the upset rating, and the cooperation rating while waiting in the operating suite. For each of these three ratings, three- to six-year-old males had relatively lower ratings than the same age females independent of the treatment condition. This difference was reversed for the seven- to 14-year-old males versus females. This age by sex pattern did not appear on other outcome measures.

The results for the resistance to induction indicated that five of 43 children (two observations were missed) in the experimental group showed resistance, compared to 11 of the 35 control children. A chi square of 4.64 indicated that significantly fewer children in the experimental group resisted induction ($p < .05$).

Table 3 shows the mean pulse rates for experimental and control children classified by sex and age, and time of measurement: at admission, before, and after the

Table 2 Mean Scores and Significance Levels for Children's Dependent Variables

Variable	Children's age	N E	N C	Mean scores Experimental	Control	Total	Effect	ANOVA df	F	p
Blood test										
Upset	3-6	22	20	2.01	3.10	2.55	Treatment:	1	8.88	.005
	7-14	20	11	1.33	1.93	1.63	Age:	1	10.46	.002
Total				1.67	2.52					
Cooperation	3-6	22	20	1.60	2.88	2.24	Treatment:	1	6.36	.001
	7-14	20	11	1.04	1.27	1.15	Age:	1	13.25	.01
Total				1.32	2.07					
Preoperative medication										
Upset	3-6	22	20	2.07	3.62	2.85	Treatment:	1	25.55	.001
	7-14	20	11	1.16	2.48	2.06	Age:	1	11.08	.002
Total				1.86	3.05					
Cooperation	3-6	22	20	1.41	3.49	2.45	Treatment:	1	24.07	.001
	7-14	20	11	1.15	2.12	1.63	Age:	1	6.95	.01
Total				1.28	2.81					
Transport										
Upset	3-6	22	20	1.61	2.14	1.88	Treatment:	1	4.89	.03
	7-14	20	11	0.81	1.65	1.23	Age:	1	4.36	.04
Total				1.21	1.70					
Cooperation	3-6	22	20	1.48	2.14	1.81	Treatment:	1	4.58	.04
	7-14	20	11	0.81	1.40		Age:	1	5.87	.02
Total				1.15	1.77					
Waiting in operating suite										
Upset	3-6	22	20	1.64	1.87	1.76	Treatment:	1	6.05	.02
	7-14	20	11	.95	2.22	1.59	Age:	1	0.31	—
Total				1.30	2.04					
Cooperation	3-6	22	20	1.38	1.65	1.52	Treatment:	1	7.06	0.01
	7-14	20	11	0.85	1.97	1.41	Age:	1	0.17	—
Total				1.12	1.81					
Ease of fluid intake	3-6	22	20	1.69	2.07		Treatment:	1	3.34	.07
	7-14	20	11	1.52	1.97		Age:	1	0.37	—
Total				1.61	2.02					
Minutes to first voiding	3-6	20	17	226.3	343.6		Treatment:	1	10.91	.001
	7-14	19	8	248.1	366.0		Age:	1	0.38	—
Total				237.2	354.8					
Posthospital adjustment score	3-6	19	18	79.6	85.5		Treatment:	1	12.31	.001
	7-14	15	9	80.8	87.7		Age:	1	1.22	—
Total				79.8	84.9					

338   Appendix

Table 3   Mean Pulse Rates for Experimental and Control Groups at Admission and Before and After the Blood Test (N = 70)

| | | | Mean pulse rates | | | | | | |
| | | Experimental | | | | Control | | | |
Sex	Age	N	Admission	Before	After	N	Admission	Before	After
Male	3-6	17	91.3	111.2	104.1	11	91.7	112.9	106.1
	7-14	13	85.4	103.3	84.7	5	90.8	117.6	107.2
Female	3-6	4	102.0	133.0	112.0	7	88.0	134.3	129.4
	7-14	7	86.0	106.3	94.6	5	96.0	100.0	94.4
TOTAL		41	91.2	113.4	98.8	28	91.6	116.2	109.3

blood test. A two (treatments) by two (age groups) by two (sex) analysis of variance was performed on the pulse rates across the three measurement times (repeated measures). An unweighted-means analysis for unequal cell entries was used (Winer, 1962). The summary of the analysis of variance in Table 4 contains only significant ($p \leq .05$) or near significant ($p < .10$) effects. There was no overall significant effect for the treatment condition. The significant effects for age and sex indicated a reliable tendency for younger children to have higher pulse rates than older children and for girls to have higher pulse rates than boys, independent of the treatment condition. The significant age by sex interaction resulted largely from the younger girls' having substantially higher pulse rates at, before, and after the blood test than the other groups. The significant effect for measurement times indicated a significant ($p < .001$)

Table 4   Summary of Analysis of Variance for Blood Test Pulse Rates (Significant or Near-Significant Fs Only)

Source	df	F	p
Age	1	14.81	.001
Sex	1	3.19	.079
Age × sex	1	5.73	.020
Time	2	56.56	.001
Time × treatment	2	2.82	.064
Time × age	2	6.04	.004
Time × age × sex	2	5.18	.007
Treatment × age × sex × time	2	5.49	.006

overall change in mean pulse rates from the time of admission to immediately before and after the blood test. These three means (91.4, 114.8, and 104.7) were significantly ($p < .001$) different from each other, indicating that independent of age, sex, and the treatment condition, there was a significant increase in pulse from admission to before the blood test ($t = 12.0$), and a significant decrease from admission to after ($t = 6.8$) and from before to after the blood test ($t = 5.2$) as would be expected if changes in heart rate reflect changes in physiologic arousal accompanying threatening events. In addition, there was no significant difference between the experimental and control means at admission before the experimental intervention began (91.2 versus 91.6). Before the blood test the experimental group had a lower pulse than the control, but not significantly so (113.4 versus 116.2), but had a highly significantly lower pulse after the blood test (98.8 versus 109.3; $t = 5.38$, $p < .001$).

The remaining significant interactions in Table 4 for combinations of repeated measures for pulse in relation to age, sex, and treatment indicated there were complicated differential heart rate changes across measurement times which were related to the age, sex, and type of experience or preparation of the child. However, these interactions did not occur with the preoperative medication heart rates.

Table 5 contains the mean pulse rates at admission and before and after the preoperative medication injections. Table 6 presents the results of the analysis of variance of these data which was the same type as for the blood test pulses. In this case there was a near significant ($p = .057$) tendency for experimental group children to have an overall lower mean pulse rate than controls. Again, the main effects for age and sex indicated that overall the younger children and girls tended to have higher pulse rates independent of the treatment condition. The significant treatment-by-sex interaction resulted largely from much lower means before and after the injections for the experimental males compared to the other three groups. There was a significant

• *Table 5*   **Mean Pulse Rates for Experimental and Control Groups at Admission and Before and After Preoperative Medication (N = 70)**

			Mean pulse rates						
			Experimental				Control		
Sex	Age	N	Admission	Before	After	N	Admission	Before	After
Male	3-6	17	91.3	113.1	107.5	13	91.7	125.8	119.5
	7-14	11	85.4	95.6	88.9	5	90.8	114.8	108.4
Female	3-6	4	102.0	122.5	119.0	6	90.0	129.3	121.3
	7-14	8	89.2	115.0	104.0	6	94.7	110.0	100.7
TOTAL		40	92.0	111.5	104.9	30	91.8	120.0	112.5

($p < .001$) F for pulse rates across the three measurement times, and the individual t-tests indicated, as with the blood test pulse rates, a significant mean pulse rate increase from admission (91.9) to before the injection (115.8), followed by a significant decrease after the injection was completed (108.7). Admission versus before mean rate showed $t = 13.0$, admission to after, $t = 9.2$; before and after, $t = 3.9$. The experimental children had a significantly lower pulse before (111.5 versus 120.0; $t = 4.84$, $p < .001$) and after (104.9 versus 112.5; $t = 4.42$, $p < .001$) the preoperative medications. The nearly significant treatment by pulse interaction indicated that the changes in mean pulse rate across the three measurement times tended to be different for the two groups, which resulted largely from the much smaller increase from admission to before the injection for the experimental children (92.0 to 111.5 = 19.5) compared to the controls (91.8 to 120.0 = 28.2). The decreases in pulse from before to after the injections was of about the same magnitude for both groups (111.5 to 104.9 = 6.6 versus 120.0 to 112.5 = 7.5). The significant age by pulse interaction resulted from the younger children's exhibiting a relatively greater increase in mean pulse rate from admission to before the injections and a relatively smaller decrease from before to after the injections than the older children.

Results of parents' rating of anxiety, adequacy of information received, and satisfaction with care—analyzed in separate two (treatments) by two (age) by two (sex) analyses of variance—indicated no significant effects for sex of the child (Table 7). Experimental group parents had significantly lower self-ratings of anxiety, rated information received significantly higher in adequacy, and were significantly more satisfied with their care. Except for the anxiety rating where parents of younger children had significantly higher anxiety ratings, there were no significant interactions between the treatment and the age of the child. The mean number of information items (out of a possible 18) parents in experimental and control groups indicated they received from only the research nurse were 11.1 and 1.3, respectively. A t of 11.7 indicated that parents in the experimental group received significantly more information from the research nurse only than control group parents ($p < .001$).

• Discussion

The results of the study supported the hypothesis that children and parents who received systematic psychologic preparation and continued supportive care, in contrast to those who did not, would show less upset behavior and more cooperation in the hospital and fewer posthospital adjustment problems. The experimental group had significantly lower mean upset ratings and higher mean cooperation ratings at each of the stress points than the control group. Children in the experimental condition demonstrated nearly significantly greater ease of fluid intake, significantly less time to first voiding, had significantly lower heart rates after the blood test and before and after the preoperative medication, had a significantly lower incidence of resistance to induction, and obtained significantly lower posthospital adjustment scores. Children

• *Table 6* **Summary of Analysis of Variance for Preoperative Medication Pulses (Significant or Near-Significant *F*s Only)**

Source	df	F	p
Treatment	1	3.77	.057
Age	1	17.20	.001
Sex	1	3.93	.052
Treatment × age	1	5.26	.026
Time	2	71.77	.001
Treatment × time	2	2.72	.070
Age × time	2	5.35	.006

between the ages of three and six, compared with those between seven and 14, consistently demonstrated greater upset and less cooperation, but did not differ significantly in terms of ease of fluid intake, minutes to first voiding, or posthospital adjustment scores. Except for heart rate where girls tended to have higher pulses than boys before and after the blood test and preoperative medication, there were no significant sex differences on the outcome measures.

Parents in the experimental group had significantly lower self-ratings of anxiety, higher ratings of the adequacy of the information received, and greater satisfaction with care than parents in the control group.

Taken at face value and in conjunction with the positive findings of other preparation studies, these results seemed to provide strong support for the beneficial effect of systematic preparation and support for hospitalized children and parents. Apparently, the treatment condition which consists of preparatory communications designed to impart accurate information about events, procedures, sensations, and role expectations, combined with supportive care in the form of encouragement, reassurance, and reinforcement from a single care-giver who attends to the child and parent throughout the hospitalization, and especially at critical points, enables children to cope more effectively with and adjust to the various stresses encountered. The treatment condition seems also to result in less anxiety and greater satisfaction for parents. The exact causal sequence of this involved process is complex and unknown. Presumably the preparatory instruction and rehearsal produce accurate expectations about the nature and sequence of events which in turn create an enhanced sense of control and capability for both children and parents (Miller *et al.*, 1960). Part of this preparation, especially for the young child, is the emotional support which comes from having a sustained relationship with a consistent danger control figure who communicates in a manner appropriate for the child's developmental level. The net effect of the preparation and supportive care can be described as stress reducing. However, the precise nature of this dynamic cognitive and affective process remains to be determined.

• *Table 7* **Mean Ratings and Significant *F*s for the Three Parents' Dependent Variables**

Variable	Children's age	Group						ANOVA			
		Experimental		Control		Total					
		N	$\bar{X}$	N	$\bar{X}$	N	$\bar{X}$	Effect	df	F	p
Self-rating anxiety	3-6	22	2.51	19	3.27	41	2.89	Treatment:	1	9.03	.004
	7-14	20	2.27	11	2.62	31	2.44	Age:	1	5.78	.02
TOTAL			2.39		2.94						
Adequacy of information received	3-6	22	16.20	19	6.00	41	11.72	Treatment:	1	84.82	.001
	7-14	20	17.00	11	7.50	31	11.63				
TOTAL			15.84		7.40						
Satisfaction with care	3-6	22	3.74	17	2.65	39	3.19	Treatment:	1	17.99	.001
	7-14	20	3.68	8	2.95	28	3.32				
TOTAL			3.71		2.80						

LIMITATIONS AND SUGGESTIONS FOR FURTHER STUDY

Before the present results can be taken as conclusive, a number of questions need further investigation. First, there is the question of the possibility of observer bias. Although every attempt was made to keep the nurse observer blind to conditions while she made her behavioral ratings, possibly, part of the time, at least, there may have been cues regarding which group a particular child and parent were in. The observer was free to move about the unit and had no other responsibilities during the observation periods. When she was to make an observation, she entered the room immediately before the rating was to be made and left immediately after. Since the experimental nurse was present at each of these times for both experimental and control patients, her presence or absence was not a sign of which group a child was in. Throughout the study the observation nurse was aware of the possibility of bias and made a deliberate attempt to keep herself blind to group assignment. Nevertheless, at times it was unavoidable for her to witness some interactions between the experimental nurse and the patients which would indicate their group assignment. She reported this happened only in a few cases and for some of the ratings. Most of the time she reported she was either clearly unaware or uncertain of which group the patients were in. To the extent there was observer bias in the direction of the hypothesized effects, this was a limitation of the methodology. In future studies, it would be better if, at the very least, observers were uninformed of the purpose of the study and the nature of the experimental conditions.

There is also a possibility of bias on the part of the parents in the experimental group. Although the control parents clearly knew they were participating in a study, were given the same instructions in the use of the questionnaires at the time of discharge, and saw the experimental nurse throughout their hospital stay, the research nurse was much more involved with the experimental parents. Consequently, there is the possibility that in order to please the nurse for her extra effort, they may have been inclined to rate themselves as being less anxious and more satisfied with the information and care they received. It seems much less likely that this type of bias would be present ten days later when they rated their children's behavior at home. In a future study this possible source of bias might be controlled by having an additional condition where a single nurse spent approximately as much time with the child and parent as under the experimental condition but without providing the systematic preparation. Whether participation in a study along with special attention would produce a positive effect on parents' ratings could then be ascertained.

Another question which can be raised is whether the positive effects of the experimental condition resulted from the process and content of the preparation and supportive care as such, or from the personality and interpersonal style of the experimental nurse, or both. That is, something about the characteristics of the particular nurse might have been responsible or largely responsible for the positive effects. The answer to this requires a replication of the experimental treatment with one or more different nurses following the same principles and using the same process and content. The replication should further determine if the principles and techniques of preparation and supportive care for stressful events can be implemented effectively by other nurses.

Closely associated is the possibility that the obtained effects resulted from the establishment of a warm, trusting relationship with a single nurse who was present at critical times throughout the hospitalization, independent of the special preparation and communication techniques. Again, to test this possibility the experimental treatment needs to be compared to a condition where a single nurse establishes a warm relationship with the child and is present at the same points throughout the hospitalization, but does not provide the systematic preparation.

Finally, assuming the positive effects on the outcome measures are primarily the result of psychologic preparation and supportive care, there is the question of whether this type of preparation and care can be given as a regular part of the nursing care in a pediatric service. The attempt in the current study was to incorporate the treatment condition into a full nursing role. Nevertheless, the research nurse functioned more in the capacity of a clinical specialist with special responsibilities for difficult cases and for preparation and support rather than as a staff nurse. Ideally, following a primary nursing organizational plan, it would seem that each staff nurse with primary assignments to individual patients should include stress-point preparation and support for child and parent as an integral part of the care. Further research is necessary in order to determine if this is clinically and administratively feasible.

John A. Wolfer (Ph.D., University of Utah, Salt Lake City) is chairman of the Nursing Research Program and associate professor at Yale University School of Nursing, New Haven, Connecticut.

Madelon Visintainer (University of Maryland School of Nursing, Baltimore; M.S.N., Yale University, New Haven, Connecticut) is an instructor in pediatric nursing at Yale University School of Nursing, New Haven, Connecticut.

The assistance of Eileen Korman; Kathleen Tauer, head nurse; Mrs. Diana Brown, director of nursing service; William Lattanzi, M.D., chairman of pediatrics; and the medical nursing staff and administration at St. Raphael Hospital, New Haven, Connecticut, is acknowledged.

*Credentials at time of article's publication.

• References

Beverly, B.I. The effects of illness upon emotional development. *J Pediatrics* 8:533-543, 1936.

Blom, G.E. The reactions of hospitalized children to illness. *Pediatrics* 22:590-600, Sept. 1958.

Campbell, E.H. *Effects of Mothers' Anxiety on Infants' Behavior.* New Haven, Conn., Yale University, 1957. (Unpublished doctoral dissertation)

Cassell, S.E. *The Effect of Brief Puppet Therapy upon the Emotional Responses of Children undergoing Cardiac Catheterization.* Evanston, Ill., Northwestern University, 1963. (Unpublished doctoral dissertation)

Chapman, A.H., and others. Psychiatric aspects of hospitalizing children. *Arch Pediatrics* 73:77-88, Mar. 1956.

Coleman, L.L. Children need preparation for tonsillectomy. *Child Study J* 29:18-19ff, 1952.

Deutsch, H. Some psychoanalytic observations in surgery. *Psychosom Med* 4:105-115, 1942.

Elman, Robert. *Surgical Care: A Practical Physiologic Guide.* New York, Appleton-Century-Crofts, 1951.

Fagin, Claire. The case for rooming in when young children are hospitalized. *Nurs Sci* 2:324-333, Aug. 1964.

Francis, L., and Cutler, R. Psychological preparation and premedication for pediatric anesthesia. *Anesthesiology* 18:106-109, Jan-Feb. 1957.

Gellert, E.: Reducing the emotional stresses of hospitalization for children. *Am J Occup Ther* 12:125-129ff, May-June 1958.

Godfrey, A.E. Study of nursing care designed to assist hospitalized children and their parents in their separation. *Nurs Res* 4:42-70, Oct. 1955.

Hollender, Marc. *Psychology of Medical Practice.* Philadelphia, W.B. Saunders Co., 1958.

Jackson, K. Psychologic preparation as a method of reducing the emotional trauma of anesthesia in children. *Anesthesiology* 12:293-300, May 1951.

Jackson, K., and others. Behavior changes indicating emotional trauma in tonsillectomized children. *Pediatrics* 12:23-27, July 1953.

Jessner, Lucie, and Kaplan, Samuel. Observations of the emotional reactions of children to tonsillectomy and adenoidectomy. In *Problems of Infancy and Childhood: Transactions of the Third Conference,* ed. by M.J.E. Senn., New York, Josiah Macy, Jr. Foundation, 1949.

Jessner, Lucie, and others. Emotional implications of tonsilectomy and adenoidectomy on children. In *The Psychoanalytic Study of the Child,* ed. by R.S. Eissler and others. New York, International Universities Press, 1952, pp. 126-169.

Johnson, J.E. Effects of structuring patients expectations on their reactions to threatening events. *Nurs Res* 21:499-504, Nov.-Dec. 1972.

Levy, D.M. Psychic trauma of operations in children. *Am J Dis Child* 69:7-25, Jan. 1945.

Mahaffy, P.R., Jr. Effects of hospitalization on children admitted for tonsillectomy and adenoidectomy. *Nurs Res* 14:12-19, Winter 1965.

Miller, G.A., and others. *Plans and the Structure of Behavior.* New York, Holt, Rinehart & Winston, 1960.

Oremland, E., and Oremland, J.D., eds. *The Effects of Hospitalization on Children: Models for Their Care.* Springfield, Ill., Charles C Thomas, Publisher, 1973.

Orlando, I.J. *The Dynamic Nurse-Patient Relationships.* New York, Putnam, 1961.

Piaget, Jean. *The Growth of Logical Thinking from Childhood to Adolescence,* translated by A. Parsons and S. Seagren. New York, Basic Books, 1958.

Plank, E.N., and Ritchie, M.A. *Working with Children in Hospitals.* 2d ed. Cleveland, Press of Case Western Reserve University, 1971.

Prugh, D.G., and others. A study of the emotional reactions of children and families to hospitalization and illness. *Am J Orthopsychiatry* 23:70-106, Jan. 1953.

Scahill, Mary. Preparing children for procedures and operations. *Nurs Outlook* 17:35-38, June 1968.

Skipper, J.K., and others. Child hospitalization and social interaction: An experimental study of mothers' feelings of stress, adaptation and satisfaction. *Med Care* 6:496-306, Nov.-Dec. 1968.

Vander Veer, A.H. The psychopathology of physical illness and hospital residence. *Q J Child Behav* 1:55-71, 1949.

Vaughan, G.F. Children in hospital. *Lancet* 272:1117-1120, June 1, 1957.

Vernon, D.T.A., and others. *The Psychological Responses of Children to Hospitalization and Illness.* Springfield, Ill., Charles C Thomas, Publisher, 1965.

Vernon, D.T.A., and others. Changes in children's behavior after hospitalization. *Am J Dis Child* 111:581-593, June 1966.

Vernon, D.T.A., and others. Effect of mother-child separation and birth order on young children's responses to two potentially stressful experiences. *J Pers Soc Psychol* 5:462-474, 1967.

Weinick, H.M. *Psychological Study of Emotional Reactions of Children to Tonsillectomy*. New York, New York University, 1958. (Unpublished doctoral dissertation)

Wiedenbach, E. *Clinical Nursing: A Helping Art*. New York, Springer Publishing Co., 1964.

Winer, B.J. *Statistical Principles in Experimental Design*. New York, McGraw-Hill Book Co., 1962.

B

The Effect of Oxygen Inhalation on Oral Temperature

Fidelita Lim-Levy

variables:-

A study was conducted to determine the effect of oxygen inhalation by nasal cannula on oral temperatures. One hundred healthy adult subjects were randomly assigned to a control and to three experimental groups that received 2, 4, and 6 liters per minute of oxygen for 30 minutes. Oral temperatures were measured 30 minutes after oxygen treatment. The data analysis did not show any significant effect of the treatment. This study encourages review of the common empirical practice of changing temperature sites from the preferred oral to the less acceptable rectal or axillary sites in patients receiving oxygen inhalation treatments.

Oxygen inhalation by nasal cannula is believed to affect oral temperature. It has been thought that the increased air current directed to the nasal cavity lowers the oral temperature. Consequently, in the presence of oxygen inhalation, body temperature monitoring is changed from the usual oral site to either rectal or axillary.

Many persons find that having rectal temperature taken is emotionally uncomfortable. Nursing personnel consider taking rectal and axillary temperatures more time-consuming than oral temperatures.

Patients who receive oxygen on a continual basis are repeatedly embarrassed by having their rectal temperatures taken. This could result in anxiety and subsequent increase in the metabolic rate, a need for more oxygen, and possibly changes in body temperature (Renbourn, 1960). Patients who receive intermittent oxygen inhalation have temperatures taken orally when they are off the oxygen inhalation and rectally

---

☐ Accepted for publication July 17, 1981.

when they are on oxygen inhalation. This results in two baselines from which to consider the patient's temperature pattern.

This study sought to determine how oxygen inhalation by nasal cannula affects oral temperature. If oral monitoring is not adversely affected, there is no need for the rectal or axillary procedures.

Few studies have been done on the effect of oxygen inhalation on oral temperatures. Beland and Passos (1975) and Wolff, Weitzel, and Fuerst (1979) recommend examining the practice of changing temperature monitoring from oral to other sites during oxygen inhalation. Du Gas (1977) and Levine (1973) stated that it is customary for a rectal temperature to be taken when a person is receiving oxygen therapy. Twenty other textbooks in nursing fundamentals, medical-surgical nursing, and intensive care nursing reviewed for this study did not discuss the relationship between oxygen inhalation and oral temperatures.

Grass (1974) studied the effects of 15 minute oxygen inhalation by nasal cannula at a rate of three liters per minute (LPM) on nine subjects. Kintzel (1967) used 40 subjects (320 paired oral-rectal readings) using mask and nasopharyngeal catheter as the methods of oxygen inhalation. Both studies showed no significant effect of oxygen inhalation on oral temperatures.

This study used a large sample, three different treatments, and the nasal cannula, which is the most common method of giving oxygen inhalation (Sweetwood, 1979).

The hypothesis tested was: Oxygen inhalation by nasal cannula of up to 6 LPM does not affect oral temperature measurement taken with an electronic thermometer.

[handwritten margin note: — answers research question — Clearly stated]

• Methods

The study sample consisted of 100 healthy adults (59 females, 41 males) ranging in age from 18 to 56 years. It included employees of a general hospital and students of its school of nursing. Informed consent was obtained from all subjects. Most of them were familiar with oxygen administration, but only a few had previously received oxygen inhalation. Each subject was randomly assigned to one of three treatment levels of oxygen flow (2, 4, or 6 LPM), or to control. Oral temperature was taken before and 30 minutes after oxygen inhalation.

One electronic thermometer[1] was used for the entire study to eliminate variations between measuring instruments (Beck and Campbell, 1975). The thermometer was a solid-state instrument capable of registering temperatures of 94°F to 108°F, ±2°F. An audible tone and a red light signal when the subject's maximum temperature has been reached. Compressed oxygen in tanks was used with a flowmeter indicating LPM. A humidifier[2] was used following the usual procedure of oxygen inhalation by nasal cannula. A nasal cannula[3] was used for each subject.

The study controlled for several local factors known to affect oral temperature:

[1]IVAC model 811®, donated by IVAC Corporation, San Diego, California.
[2]Ohio Medical Company, Madison, Wisconsin.
[3]Donated by Hudson Oxygen Therapy Sales Company, Wadsworth, Ohio.

recent ingestion of food and beverages, smoking, gum chewing, and local inflammatory process. Subjects were requested verbally and in writing to refrain from vigorous activity, eating, drinking, and smoking for one hour before the procedure.

Subjects who were mouth breathing or hyperventilating were excluded, even though an open mouth does not affect temperature monitoring done electronically at the sublingual pocket area (IVAC). This restriction increased uniformity in the testing condition. All subjects automatically closed their lips on the probe. Conversation was discouraged during the actual temperature monitoring (approximately 30 seconds).

Activity has long been known to raise body temperature and is an important mechanism for heat production. Subjects were requested to sit quietly for at least 15 minutes before starting the experiment. A change in body position from standing to supine and vice versa causes a fall in temperature (Cranston et al., 1954). This was controlled by having the subjects remain lying down throughout the procedure. Subjects changed their position from supine to lying on their sides at will. Conversations were not controlled, except during the actual temperature monitoring. Many subjects carried on conversations with other subjects or with the investigator.

Possible short-term effects of anxiety were controlled by providing a comfortable position, a calm approach by the investigator, and a chance to observe and question other subjects undergoing the procedure. Subjects had ample opportunity to touch and inspect the cannula and the thermometer while their informed consent was being obtained. Both the nasal cannula and the electronic thermometer were foreign to the subjects. However, no one refused to participate in the study because of a negative perception of the cannula or the electronic thermometer.

Data was collected using at least 15-minute intervals so that one subject was started while another was in the middle of the procedure. A predetermined randomized classification from a table of random numbers was consulted to assign the subjects to the treatments groups. Group One received no oxygen (control); Group Two received 2 LPM; Group Three, 4 LPM; and Group Four, 6 LPM. The subject lay on the examining table with one pillow. Oral temperature was taken using the slow-slide technique suggested by the manufacturer (IVAC) and Beck and Campbell (1975). The probe was held loosely during insertion, placed under the front of the tongue, and slid back along the gumline to the right sublingual pocket area at the base of the tongue. The right sublingual pocket area was used consistently in this study, since different sublingual areas are known to register different temperatures (Beck and Campbell, 1975; and Erickson, 1980). The investigator held the thermometer in place at all times. After the body's maximum temperature was reached, the reading was manually recorded on the data sheet.

Groups Two, Three, and Four received oxygen by the nasal cannula for 30 minutes. Oxygen flow was regulated before the nasal cannula was adjusted in place. At the end of 30 minutes, the oral temperature was adjusted in place. At the end of 30 minutes, the oral temperature was taken again, as described above, while the subject continued to receive the oxygen. After recording the temperature, the oxygen was discontinued, the subject dismissed from the study, and the cannula discarded.

• *Table 1*   Mean Temperatures and Differences

Group	N	Sex[a]	Oral temperatures (°F)		Difference
			Initial	After 30 min.	
	11	M	98.85	98.67	−.18
1. (Control)	14	F	98.81	98.99	+.18
	25	C	98.83	98.85	+.02
	12	M	98.93	98.71	−.22
2. (2 LPM)	12	F	99.0	98.82	−.18
	24	C	98.96	98.76	−.20
	9	M	98.97	98.92	−.05
3. (4 LPM)	17	F	98.16	98.85	+.69
	26	C	98.44	98.87	+.43
	9	M	98.87	98.89	+.02
4. (6 LPM)	16	F	98.89	98.68	−.21
	25	C	98.88	98.76	−.12

[a]M = Male; F = Female; C = Combined.

• **Results and Discussion**

Pre-oxygen administration temperatures were compared with temperature taken 30 minutes after the start of oxygen. Table 1 shows the temperature differences in Groups One, Two, and Four to be small (−22°F to +18°F). Group Three who received oxygen at 4 LPM showed an increase of .43°F. The Group Three females had the lowest initial temperature, 98.16°F, and the increased temperature observed after oxygen administration might reflect, in part, a return to a higher normative temperature. The inter-subject variability was greater than the differences observed following experimental treatment, suggesting that the temperatures were all within the limits of expected temperature variation.

An analysis of the data using mixed type analysis of variance showed no statistically significant change in the temperatures, regardless of sex and oxygen treatment. This finding is similar to Grass (1974) in its lack of statistical significance but different in one sense: Grass's study showed a general increase in oral temperature after 15 minutes of oxygen inhalation while this study showed a decrease after 30 minutes of oxygen treatment. This difference could be attributed to the longer oxygen treatment in this study or the different type of thermometer used (Erickson, 1980).

In clinical practice, there are many factors that contribute to inaccuracies of the actual temperature monitoring as well as the interpretation of its pattern. When temperatures are taken orally at times and rectally or axillary at another, the procedure calls for using different thermometers. Even when using an electronic thermometer, a different probe is used for orals and axillary and a different one for rectals. In some facilities that use electronic thermometers for the oral site, the procedure may call for the use of a glass thermometer when rectal temperature is taken.

• *Table 2*   **Analysis of Variance for Oxygen Treatment, Sex and Duration of Treatment**

Source	SS	df	Mean square	F	p
O_2	.43708	3	.14569	.51	.679
sex	.18768	1	.18768	.65	.422
$O_2 \times$ sex	.39768	3	.13256	.46	.711
error	26.49	92	.28796		
time	.51759	1	.51759	2.97	.088
time $\times O_2$	.25992	3	.9664	.50	.685
time $\times$ sex	.03315	1	.03315	.19	.664
time $\times$ sex $\times O_2$	.90471	3	.30157	1.73	.166
error	16.021	92	.17415		

Erickson reported variations associated with different types of instruments (1980). When temperatures are recorded, some nursing personnel subtract 1°F from a rectal reading to translate it into an oral reading. Other nursing personnel do not practice this procedure. They record the actual reading but identify the rectal temperature. Since most temperature records are in the form of a linear graph, the pattern becomes obscure when some of the points represent oral and some represent rectal or axillary readings. This situation can occur when a patient is receiving oxygen intermittently.

This study did not show a significant effect of oxygen inhalation on oral temperature. Embarrassment and anxiety may result from the rectal procedure and should be considered, especially in patients whose oxygenation status are already compromised. Other factors to be considered are the increased expenditure of time and energy by nursing personnel in taking rectal or axillary temperatures and the inaccurarcy in determining the individual's temperature pattern, when different instruments are used and temperatures from different sites are recorded.

Further research using higher oxygen flow, longer treatment, and including febrile patients are recommended.

Fidelita Lim-Levy, M.S.N., R.N., C.S., is a clinical specialist, Medical-Surgical Nursing, Wm. Middleton Memorial Veterans' Hospital, Madison, Wisconsin.

The author wishes to thank the Bohol Provincial Hospital Staff. Tagbilaran, Philippines, Dr. Jesus Ceballos, Guidette Borja, M.S.N., R.N.; Pilar Bucia, B.S.N., R.N.; Neil S. Levy, PH.D.; Signe Cooper, PH.D., R.N.; Audrey Chang, PH.D.; Jerry Homzie, PH.D., and Cindi Birch.

*Credentials at time of article's publication.

• References

Beck, W.C., and Campbell, Robert. Clinical thermometry. *Guthrie Bull* 44:175-194, Spring 1975.

Beland, L., and Passos, Joyce. *Clinical Nursing, Pathophysiological and Psychological Approach.* 3rd ed. New York, Macmillan Co., 1975, pp. 826-827.

Cranston, W.I., and others. Oral, rectal and oesophagial temperatures and some factors affecting them in man. *J Physiol* 126:347-358, Nov. 29, 1954.

Du Gas, B.W. *Introduction to Patient Care.* 3rd ed. Philadelphia, W.B. Saunders Co., 1977, p. 160.

Erickson, Roberta. Oral temperature differences in relation to thermometer and technique. *Nurs Res* 29:157-164, May-June 1980.

Grass, Suzanne. Thermometer sites and oxygen. *Am J Nurs* 74:1862-1863, Oct. 1974.

IVAC Electronic Thermometer User Information. IVAC Corp. n.d. (P.O. Box 2385, La Jolla, Calif. 92038).

Kintzel, K.C. Recognition of clinical problems requiring investigation: A comparative study of oral and rectal temperatures in patients receiving two forms of oxygen therapy. *ANA Clin Sess* 99-103, 1966.

Levine, M.E. *Introduction to Clinical Nursing.* 2nd ed. Philadelphia, F.A. Davis Co., 1973.

Renbaum, E.T. Body temperature and pulse rate in boys and young men prior to sporting contests. A study of emotional hypothermia: with a review of literature. *J Psychosom Res* 4:149-175, Mar. 1960.

Sweetwood, H.M. *Nursing in the Intensive Respiratory Care.* 2nd ed. New York, Springer Publishing Co., 1979, p. 225.

Wolff, Luverne, and others. *Fundamentals of Nursing.* 6th ed. Philadelphia, J.B. Lippincott Co., 1979, p. 295.

Index